Reasoning, Inference, and Judgment in Clinical Psychology

Reasoning, Inference, and Judgment in Clinical Psychology

Dennis C. Turk and
Peter Salovey, Editors

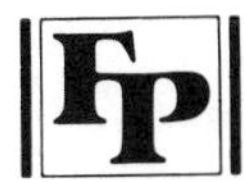

THE FREE PRESS
A Division of Macmillan, Inc.
NEW YORK

Collier Macmillan Publishers
LONDON

The Free Press
A Division of Macmillan, Inc.
866 Third Avenue, New York, N.Y. 10022

Collier Macmillan Canada, Inc.

Printed in the United States of America

printing number
1 2 3 4 5 6 7 8 9 10

Library of Congress Cataloging-in-Publication Data

Reasoning, inference, and judgment in clinical psychology.

Includes bibliographies and index.
1. Psychology, Clinical—Decision making.
I. Turk, Dennis C. II. Salovey, Peter. [DNLM:
1. Decision Making. 2. Judgment. 3. Psychology, Clinical—methods. WM 105 R2884]
RC467.R38 1987 150 87-17812
ISBN 0-02-933190-0

We dedicate this volume to:

Lorraine, Kenneth Matthew, and Katharine Elizabeth—three decisions that turned out exceptionally well even though made under conditions of uncertainty (D.C.T.)

Marta Elisa Moret, who inspires all my inferences (P.S.)

and especially to the memory of Hillel J. Einhorn, whose untimely death cut all too short a brilliant career.

When I was at last obliged to recognize that the scenes of seduction had never taken place, and that they were only fantasies which my patients had made up or which I myself had perhaps forced on them . . . . *My confidence alike in my technique and its results suffered a severe blow; it could not be disputed that I had arrived at these scenes by a technical method which I considered correct.*

Sigmund Freud quoted by Janet Malcolm
in *The New Yorker,* December 3, 1983

Contents

Preface

THE practice of clinical psychology can be defined operationally in terms of the decisions required. Clinicians spend the greatest amount of their time performing assessment and providing counseling and psychotherapy. To accomplish these tasks, they must (a) determine what information is needed to make a diagnosis or to plan appropriate treatment, (b) decide what assessment procedures to employ (e.g., interviews, behavioral observations, projective techniques) that will inform subsequent decisions about treatment (e.g., individual versus group, inpatient versus outpatient, insight-oriented versus problem-focused), and (c) integrate the diversity of information acquired.

Clinicians' activities are subject to two sources of influence: as human information processors, their inferences and decisions are shaped by universal human characteristics; as individuals, their judgments are affected by their own personal histories. The reliance on clinical judgment to predict behavioral outcomes holds many of the pitfalls first described in Meehl's (1954) classic monograph on clinical versus statistical prediction. The controversy raised by Meehl remains unresolved. As long as clinicians must make decisions about outcomes on the basis of limited data and quickly formulated hypotheses, no statistical or technical assistance is likely to eliminate completely human biases and cognitive limitations.

Many judgments are made before the clinician and client have met for the first time. A clinician's preconceptions and prior expectations influence the initial encounter with a client. For example, one of the most basic professional expectations is that clinicians will observe pathology. This process may reduce judgmental accuracy, or at least introduce systematic biases in the direction of overestimating psychopathology. Think of the attributes that come to mind when a client is referred to as a "castrating female" or a "passive–aggressive personality." Both of these labels instigate a host of associated attributes and expectancies. These expectancies are likely to influence the questions clinicians ask; the information that is encoded, stored, and retrieved in memory; as well as the behavioral consistencies observed. Likewise, the clinician's theoretical orientation provides preconceptions that will determine the nature of the information regarded as relevant.

The therapist, despite training in statistics and experimental methodology, is an "intuitive psychologist" and thus is prey to foibles in data gathering, memory processes, and judgment that have been documented in the literature on social cognition (e.g., Nisbett & Ross, 1980). The clinician is theory-driven in data gathering and interview techniques. Thus, a psychoanalytically oriented therapist enters a clinical interview with a very different set of preconceptions than does a behavior therapist (Langer & Abelson, 1974). Psychoanalysts focus on psychosexual stages, are interested in information about childhood experiences, and elicit information from the client about dreams and fantasies. Behavior therapists, on the other hand, enter the interaction with a set of beliefs about specific behavioral problems, are concerned with the current environments in which clients are operating, and ask questions about current situational stresses and goals. The course of these clinical interactions is shaped, at least to some degree, by clinicians' particular beliefs and expectancies and by their tendency to focus on, ask about, and differentially recall certain aspects of clients' current and past lives. Moreover, the clinical hour is a social interaction subject to the same problems of cognitive and behavioral confirmation that are present in any other interpersonal encounter. In order to "get into the client's head," clinicians must strive to overcome the many biases that characterize social information processing in general—and these are not unique to clinical practice (Cantor & Kihlstrom, 1982).

The intention of this volume is to identify sources of these biases; illustrate how these biases might affect assessment, diagnosis, treatment, and clinical research; and explore alternative strategies for reducing the negative consequences stemming from these sources of bias. To accomplish this goal, we have brought together a collection of experts from diverse areas of psychology whose work is relevant to the field of mental health but is largely unknown to mental health practitioners.

In the first chapter, Turk, Salovey, and Prentice introduce mental health workers to a range of concepts from the research literature in social cognition that bear directly on clinical practice. This chapter sets the tone and delineates the vocabulary used throughout the volume. The following two chapters, by Elstein and Einhorn, respectively, provide a theoretical framework for understanding the cognitive processes involved in all inferential and decision-making tasks and the importance of those processes for all aspects of clinical practice. In the next section, four chapters describe specific sources of bias in clinical practice. Smith identifies the very basic way in which our cognitive system organizes information about people. Jordan, Harvey, and Weary describe biases emanating from attempts to explain the causes of another person's behavior. Salovey and Turk reflect on how clinicians' moods influence the kinds of clinical information that is attended to and that is stored in and retrieved from memory. Snyder and Thomsen discuss the biases inherent in any social interactions in which one individual must form a hypothesis about another person. Then, Mahoney describes the importance of two competing information-processing orientations and their implications for clinical reasoning. Singer addresses a basic tenet of psychoanalytic theory, the importance of the transference in clinical practice, but reinterprets it within the framework offered by researchers of social cognition. In the final two chapters, Arnoult and Anderson provide suggestions on how clinicians can engage in reasoning, inference, and judgment while minimizing some of the difficulties described in previous chapters, and Robert Holt reflects on the importance of these issues for day-to-day clinical practice.

References

Cantor, N., & Kihlstrom, J. F. (1982). Cognitive and social processes in personality: Implications for behavior therapy. In C. M. Franks & G. T. Wilson (Eds.), *Handbook of behavior therapy.* New York: Guilford Press.

Langer, E. J., & Abelson, R. P. (1974). A patient by any other name . . . : Clinical group differences in labeling bias. *Journal of Consulting & Clinical Psychology, 42,* 4–9.

Meehl, P. E. (1954). *Clinical versus statistical prediction: A theoretical analysis and review of the evidence.* Minneapolis, MN: University of Minnesota Press.

Nisbett, R. E., & Ross, L. (1980). *Human inference: Strategies and shortcomings of social judgment.* Englewood Cliffs, NJ: Prentice-Hall.

Acknowledgments

We could not have completed this volume without the help of others. We both offered seminars in clinical decision making in the Department of Psychology at Yale University, and the lively discussions with graduate students in those classes convinced us of the importance of the material presented here. In addition, several individuals offered helpful advice along the way, including John D. (Jack) Mayer, Mahzarin Banaji, and Jefferson A. Singer. We both profited from being in environments at Yale University and the University of Pittsburgh in which others cared about the issues raised in this volume. And the financial support of the National Institutes of Health in the form of Biomedical Research Support Grant S07 RR07015 to Peter Salovey is gratefully acknowledged. Finally, the staff at The Free Press patiently guided this book to completion with considerable thoughtfulness and care. We are particularly appreciative of the efforts of our editor, Laura Wolff, who, over the course of nearly two years, stimulated, encouraged, advised, and sometimes prodded us into organizing a truly integrated set of chapters. Ms. Wolff is one of the best in the business! To all, we extend our thanks and appreciation.

About the Contributors

Craig A. Anderson received his Ph.D. in social psychology from Stanford University and is an associate professor of psychology at Rice University. His research interests include social judgment, attribution theory, aggression, and the application of social psychological theories to clinical problems.

Lynn H. Arnoult has clinical experience both within agencies and in private practice. She holds master's degrees in social work and psychology and is currently a doctoral student in psychology at Rice University, where she has researched causal reasoning problems.

Hillel J. Einhorn was a professor at the Center for Decision Research of the University of Chicago, Graduate School of Business. An expert in judgment and decision making, Dr. Einhorn died while this volume was in production.

Arthur S. Elstein received his Ph.D. in human development from the University of Chicago. His research has concentrated on clinical judgment and decision making, especially on analyzing strategies in clinical diagnosis and on identifying differences between the intuitive decision making of experienced clinicians and the choices implied by normative approaches. He is currently on the faculty of the Center for Educational Development, University of Illinois at Chicago.

John H. Harvey is professor and chair at the department of psychology, University of Iowa. He is co-editor, with William Ickes and Robert Kidd, of the three-volume *New Directions in Attribution Research;* co-author, with Gifford Weary, of *Perspectives on Attributional Processes;* and co-editor, with Weary, of *Attribution: Basic Issues and Applications.*

Robert R. Holt is a professor of psychology and the director of the Program on Peace and Global Policy Studies at New York University. He has been an active psychotherapy researcher for many years and has been particularly interested in clinical versus statistical prediction in clinical psychology.

John S. Jordan is assistant professor of medical psychology at Duke University Medical Center, where he coordinates research and psychological services for the Combined Medical Specialties ("stress disorders") Program. He received his A.B. from Dartmouth College and his Ph.D. from Ohio State University.

Michael J. Mahoney is director of the Personal Development Laboratory at the University of California, Santa Barbara. His numerous books and publications have focused primarily on basic principles and processes in human change, the psychological aspects of science, and sports psychology.

Deborah A. Prentice is a doctoral candidate in psychology at Yale University. Her research interests include the functional approach to attitudes, the attitude–memory relationship, persuasion by fiction, and self–other differences in information processing.

Peter Salovey received his Ph.D. in clinical psychology from Yale University, where he is now an assistant professor. His research interests concern mood and emotion, especially their cognitive and behavioral consequences; complex affective states, such as envy and jealousy; beliefs and behaviors concerning health; and the application of social psychological theories and research to clinical problems. He and V. J. D'Andrea wrote *Peer Counseling: Skills and Perspectives.*

Jerome L. Singer received his Ph.D. in clinical psychology from the University of Pennsylvania in 1950 and his certificate in psychoanalysis from the William Alanson White Institute in 1958. He is currently professor of psychology and director of the Graduate Program in Clinical/Community Psychology, Yale University.

Albert F. Smith is a member of the faculty of the department of psychology at the State University of New York, Binghamton. His research interests include selective attention, judgment and decision making, memory functions, and the interface of cognitive psychology with social and personality psychology.

Mark Snyder is professor of psychology at the University of Minnesota. He is the author of *Public Appearances/Private Realities: The Psychology of Self-Monitoring.* He obtained his Ph.D. at Stanford University.

Annette D. Telgarsky is a doctoral candidate in clinical psychology at Yale University. Her research is in the areas of health psychology and client expectations in psychotherapy.

Cynthia J. Thomsen is a doctoral student in social psychology at the University of Minnesota. Her research interests include stereotyping and prejudice, and the self-fulfilling nature of social perception.

Dennis C. Turk is the director of the Center for Pain Evaluation and Treatment at the University of Pittsburgh School of Medicine, where he is also professor of psychiatry and anesthesiology. His research interests are primarily in health psychology and behavioral medicine, and concern assessing and treating chronic pain, coping with chronic illness, and clinical decision making. Among his many books and articles is the widely acclaimed *Pain and Behavioral Medicine: A Cognitive–Behavioral Perspective.*

Gifford Weary is associate professor of psychology at Ohio State University, where she is on the faculty of both the Social and Clinical Psychology Graduate Training Programs. Her research interests include attribution and self-presentation processes, particularly as they relate to depression.

1 Psychotherapy: An Information-Processing Perspective

Dennis C. Turk
Peter Salovey
Deborah A. Prentice

THROUGHOUT clinical practice, therapists decide what questions to ask, what topics to pursue, what interpretations or advice to offer, and when to offer it. Clinicians must rely largely upon their judgment, based on experience, their intuition, and their ability to make accurate inferences. These concepts have often been discussed by experimental psychologists within a paradigm called "information processing."

The Information-Processing Perspective

The information-processing approach to psychology emphasizes mental activities including learning, memory (and memorial structures), language, thinking, and understanding. Investigators are concerned with how people collect, store, modify, interpret, understand, and use both internally generated information and environmental stimuli (e.g., Merluzzi, Rudy, & Glass, 1981). Within the information-processing perspective, humans are viewed as active seekers, creators, and users of information. This approach may be contrasted with behavioral (and associationist) perspectives that emphasize the historical and environmental control of behavior. Information-processing psychologists and social learning theorists (e.g., Bandura, 1978; Mischel, 1973) view the individual's behavior as reciprocally determined: Behavior is both a product and an initiator of mental acts and environmental changes.

Currently, clinical psychologists are seeking to integrate the behavioral and cognitive perspectives (Mahoney, 1974, 1977; Meichenbaum, 1977). Certainly, social learning theory (Bandura, 1977, 1986) and cognitive–behavioral interventions (e.g., problem-solving training) employ principles from learning theory within an information-processing paradigm (Bower, 1978). From this perspective, clients' maladaptive behavior patterns are viewed as rooted in cognitive processes. Likewise, the errors to which clinicians are prone are seen as based on the same limited cognitive processes. This chapter will take an information-processing perspective on the interactions of clients and therapists in an attempt to understand better the process of psychotherapy.

Clinicians have often experienced considerable difficulty in changing their clients' self-conceptions, even after months and months of intensive therapy (e.g., Wylie, 1979). However, the very difficulty we observe in bringing about changes in our clients is endemic in our own beliefs, expectancies, and a priori preconceptualizations, which influence all aspects of clinical practice. There are numerous cognitive processes that contribute to the recalcitrant maintenance of our theories (see Snyder & Thomsen, this volume). Little formal attention has been given to the importance of these processes in the therapeutic context. In this chapter and, indeed, in this entire book, consideration will be given to some of the influences on clinicians' inferences and judgments that are rooted in the processing of information in general and not solely dependent on clinical orientation. It is our intention to inform clinicians of the relevance of these concepts to their clinical practice.

Limitations of Human Information-Processing Capabilities

From intake to termination of treatment, practitioners collect information, formulate hypotheses, and make judgments and decisions. The data in clinical practice do not "speak for themselves"; they must be interpreted. Clinicians are constantly confronted by an enormous amount of information, and they can only process a subset of it at a given time. Cognitive psychologists have labeled this phenomenon "selective attention" (e.g., Broadbent, 1958; Garner, 1974; Smith, 1986 and this volume), and it is necessary to consider what mechanisms guide clinicians' attentional processes.

Experimental psychologists have identified a variety of guiding knowledge structures that help the information processor focus attention on relevant data, ignore irrelevant data, fill in missing data, and decide how to act on this information. These higher order knowledge structures go by many names (see the appendix at the end of this volume for a comparison of these terms) and serve different functions; most trace their origins to the work of Bartlett (1932) and Neisser (1967). In the following sections, we will focus on the cognitive structures and cognitive processes that help the clinician make decisions about the course of therapy.

Traits

Historically, one of the first structures proposed to organize information about people was the *trait.* A trait is a label describing personality that is based on a collection of consistent behaviors exhibited by an individual. The label is used to summarize this information about the individual's usual behavior and to guide others (including clinicians) in their perception of that individual. The construct is discussed in depth by Smith in this volume. We introduce it here because traits represent expectations about how an individual is likely to behave. Individuals construct images of other people in ways that serve to stabilize their view of the social world (Heider, 1958; Kelly, 1955) and make it predictable and manageable. To the extent that we attribute stable traits and enduring dispositions to other people, we may feel better able to understand their actions and to predict their future behavior. Moreover, we may use these beliefs to guide our interactions with others.

For example, if a client is labeled "passive-aggressive," the therapist is likely to perceive any behavior on the part of this client as indicative of this trait and caused by it. Such reasoning is circular in that behavior is used as evidence for the existence of a trait while the trait is simultaneously proposed as motivating the behavior. Even a single trait can serve as a powerful influence on perceptions of an individual. Berman, Read, and Kenny (1983) found that people formed expectations about a stimulus-person on the basis of just one trait; when confronted with information that contradicted this initial trait, they discounted the new information.

Clinicians may hold theories about how traits are associated with each other. These constitute "implicit personality theories" (Asch, 1946) and are based on the expectations of the perceiver rather than on the properties of the stimulus-person. For example, the "passive-aggressive" client may be judged likely to be hostile, even in the absence of any indications of hostility. These implicit personality theories can become quite complex and resistant to change. When the clinician uses implicit personality theories as labels (e.g., "paranoid schizophrenic"), no amount of contradictory evidence generated by the client is likely to alter them (Rosenhan, 1973).

Schemas

Schemas, or *schemata,* are collections of expectations about a stimulus domain (see Taylor & Crocker, 1981, and the appendix at the end of this volume for more detailed definitions). To illustrate the schema concept from the clinician's viewpoint, consider the stimulus domain "major affective disorders." The cognitive schema for this stimulus domain includes three key components. One component consists of the characteristics requisite for category membership (as outlined in the *Diagnostic and Statistical Manual of Mental Disorders, Third Edition* [DSM-III], Research Diagnostic Criteria [RDC] etc.). A second component is a list of probable features of major affective disorders (e.g., more likely in women than in men) and of exemplars (e.g., particular clients who have been evaluated or treated). The final component is an affective valence about the domain (e.g., type of client with whom I do or do not like to work). When confronted with a client who exhibits many of the necessary attributes, the major affective disorder schema is activated.

Once this framework is adopted, inconsistent or novel attributes of the depressed client may, under some circumstances, lead to changes in the schema to accommodate the new information. Thus, upon encountering an individual who has many features of depression but who is also agitated, we may expand the range of attributes that define the major affective disorder schema. There is always the danger of expanding the schema until it is so all-encompassing as to become almost meaningless. Thus, constructs such as "masked" or "agitated" depression may evolve so that the observed data will continue to fit the existing "depression" schema. More commonly, though, we use the schema to fill in information missing about the particular client.

Scripts

Another higher order mental representation that aids the clinician in performing his or her job is the *script* (Abelson, 1976; 1981). A script is a schema outlining a coherent sequence of events that the individual expects to occur on the basis of prior learning and experience (Schank & Abelson, 1977). Scripts contain rules or suggestions about the probability of particular outcomes in a given situation. As the individual accumulates experience with certain situations, he or she forms a representation of that situation and of behaviors required in it. On subsequent occasions, when the individual encounters elements in the environment resembling the representation formed in earlier situations, he or she will respond with the sequence of behavior associated with it. Well-learned scripts can facilitate a "mindless" state in which individuals no longer actively construct their environment but rather respond automatically with the behaviors expected in the situation (Chanowitz & Langer, 1980). In clinical practice, scripts can be misleading when they become this automatic and therapists are unable to accommodate to change. However, therapy would be impossible if practitioners did not develop some generally agreed upon scripts.

A clinician's script for a typical therapy session might include such elements as the following: (a) client appears at office at predetermined time, (b) minimal interaction between client and therapist initially, (c) client sets tone and agenda for week's session, (d) therapist listens carefully to content of client's remarks, (e) therapist observes any discrepancies between client's verbal and nonverbal behavior, (f) therapist makes insightful interpretations based on a priori theories and observed client behavior. Such a script for a therapy session develops out of past experience, and it is unlikely that a therapist would initiate a session without invoking a skeletal representation of the usual course of events. Therapists are often confused about how to behave when the client does not respond as anticipated by the script (e.g., the client gives the therapist a gift, refuses to pay, or comes to therapy intoxicated).

Confirmation of Hypotheses

One result of information processing guided by knowledge structures like traits, schemas, and scripts is the tendency to seek information that confirms prior hypotheses. Based on theoretical orientation, training, and experience, clinicians develop schemas about clients according to diagnostic categories. In observing behavior in the clinical setting, clinicians are more likely to: (a) observe what they expect to observe (which, in most cases, is pathology); (b) selectively seek theory-confirming information (Snyder, 1981; Snyder & Swann, 1978b; Snyder & Thomsen, this volume); and (c) respond in ways that foster this confirming behavior (Rosenthal & Jacobson, 1968; Snyder & Swann, 1978a). Ambiguous information is particularly vulnerable to this bias. At times, hypothesis confirmation promotes the collection of redundant data. These data tend to bolster confidence in the hypothesis, even though no new information has been garnered (Oskamp, 1965).

Confirmed hypotheses constitute beliefs about clients, and these beliefs tend to persevere, even in the face of contradictory evidence (Ross,

Lepper, & Hubbard, 1975; Ross, Lepper, Strack, & Steinmetz, 1977). For example, in an experiment conducted by Ross et al. (1975), subjects were asked to judge whether suicide notes were fake or real. Following these judgments, subjects were given false feedback about the source of the material they had judged (although in actuality, all of the suicide notes were fake). At the end of the study, the experimenters explained that the suicide notes were not authentic and that the feedback had no factual basis. Yet, subjects' beliefs about their abilities persisted despite this disconfirmation of the information on which they were based. Ross et al. (1975) suggested that subjects had constructed an explanation for their ability upon receiving the false feedback, and they used this explanation, rather than the disconfirmed feedback, as a basis for judgment.

Heuristics

An exhaustive search of all relevant schemas and scripts would be an inefficient way for a clinician to make a decision. Efficient processing of information requires the use of shortcuts or decision rules that cognitive psychologists have termed *heuristics* (Kahneman, Slovic, & Tversky, 1982). Tversky and Kahneman (1973, 1974) have described three commonly used heuristics in clinical decision making: availability, representativeness, and anchoring and adjustment.

Availability. The *availability heuristic* is employed when people estimate the frequency or probability of an event by the ease with which they can recall an instance or an example of that event. For example, people believe that psychotic individuals are prone to extreme violence simply because they can recall more easily an example of a violent psychotic (e.g., Charles Manson, David "Son-of-Sam" Berkowitz), even though the prevalence of violent behavior by emotionally disturbed individuals is actually quite low. Similarly, a clinician who works in a state mental hospital might overestimate the number of paranoid schizophrenics in the clinical population and be more likely to overdiagnose paranoid schizophrenia simply because specific paranoid schizophrenics are so easily called to mind in that setting. Biases due to use of the availability heuristic are quite common, because the ease with which information is brought to mind is influenced by such factors as recency and vividness. For example, if a recent client has committed suicide, the vividness of that event might cause one to overestimate the likelihood that a new client is suicidal.

Representativeness. Another common heuristic, employed when judging how likely a client is to be a member of some diagnostic category, is called "representativeness." The *representativeness heuristic* suggests that decision makers tend to underestimate the importance of base-rate information and focus instead on salient single-case examples (see Einhorn, this volume). Base-rate information gives the likelihood of encountering a category member in the population by chance. In other words, if 20 percent of the population is depressed, a rational decision maker, relying on base rates, would assume that a given client has a 20 percent chance of being depressed. One must consider the probability of encountering someone who fits a particular category and the probability of encountering someone who does not fit this category by chance, given that they both exhibit a specific diagnostic sign. Reliance on the representativeness heuristic might influence a clinician to diagnose a 20-year-old woman living alone as depressed but a 20-year-old man living alone as schizoid. The reason for this potential bias is that young women are more representative in the clinician's mind of "the depressive" than are young men.

Representativeness can lead to the misinterpretation of diagnostic signs. Chapman and Chapman (1967, 1969) found that clinicians believe that certain indicators on the Draw-A-Person test (big eyes, pronounced mouth) are diagnostic of particular disorders (paranoia, dependence), even though research has not validated these relationships. In fact, these "signs" are as likely to be observed in the diagnostic group as in the general population. As Nisbett and Ross (1980) explain, signs that appear to represent some diagnostic category can lead the clinician to generate or confirm a highly reasonable, but very incorrect, theory.

Anchoring and Adjustment. *Anchoring* describes the tendency for decision makers to rely too heavily on early information in the decision process. Initial estimates or predictions, based on preliminary appraisals, serve as the basis for subsequent judgments. Clinicians may fail to see improvement in a client's condition because they are *anchored* to an initial judgment of the client's mental state. Alternatively, clinicians might overvalue information revealed about a client during the intake process (at which point exposure to the client is minimal) and ignore subsequent information revealed during therapy (by which time, knowledge of the client is more extensive and reliable). Meehl (1960) observed that the "image of the patient" formed between the second and fourth session is retained without much change after 24 sessions.

Therapist–Client Interactions

In the course of this chapter, we have examined the influence of information-processing variables on the judgment and decision making of clinicians. But psychotherapy is a *social interaction,* in which the information available and the manner in which it is processed are determined by the interaction. As should be clear, *both* clients and therapists come to therapy with a priori theories, develop expectations, and act in accordance with these preconceived notions. To accurately understand information processing in the course of psychotherapy, we must regard therapists and clients as both perceivers and the objects of perception (see Smith, this volume).

Historically, psychoanalysts have been most aware of the importance of mutual information processing by therapists and clients and have conceptualized this interaction in terms of transference and countertransference (see Singer, this volume). Transference refers to the client's projection of significant others onto the "objectively neutral" therapist. For example, a male client may relate to a therapist as he relates to his father, because this interaction invokes a script concerning appropriate interaction with authority figures. Countertransference refers to the mostly affective responses of the therapist to the client. Many therapists view these feelings as clues to understanding the client's interactions with significant others.

One troubling consequence of the interactive nature of therapy is that therapy may be deemed successful only when the client's conceptual framework and theoretical orientations come to match those of the therapist (Frank, 1974; Scheff, 1966). Because therapists tend to elicit and reinforce statements by clients that confirm their orientations, clients' values come to match those of their therapists over the course of therapy (Rosenthal, 1955). Even the dreams that clients report begin to contain material consistent with their therapists' a priori theories (Whitman, Kramer, & Baldridge, 1963). As another example, Kadushin (1969) observed that the presenting complaints of patients match the orientation of the clinic in which they seek therapy. Applicants to analytic clinics are more likely to add sexual problems to their original set of concerns but drop physical symptoms; applicants to hospital clinics do just the reverse. Clearly, clients do not present their problems irrespective of their perceptions of the therapist. The orientation of the therapist and the setting influence not only how information is processed but also what information is made available by the client (see Snyder & Thomsen, this volume).

The "observational goal" of clinicians serves to focus them on those categories or features of behavior that are relevant to their purpose at the moment. An observational goal is the purpose for which an individual plans to use information gathered from observation of another's behavior. Observational goals thus simplify the perceiver's task, possibly by determining the relative importance of various categories of behavioral information, as well as by providing a structure within which to interpret the information (Cohen, 1981).

In psychotherapy, one observational goal is to identify factors that contribute to the client's presenting problems. Thus, the focus of the interaction is on antecedent factors and the client's idiosyncratic interpretations of information. Correlational information is obtained and often assigned causal significance. Thus, when the client reports, for example, that he first experienced a symptom the night after his father died, the assumption is that the symptom was caused in some way by the father's death. This conjecture by the therapist may lead to a search for historical information concerned with the client's relationship with his father. Further, the therapist may assume that conflicts with the father contributed to the client's current distress and may probe for historical data pointing to this connection. The therapist may begin to fit the client to a schema for passive-aggressive clients with conflictual paternal relationships (Cohen, 1981). Based on the a priori schema for this type of client, the therapist may make certain predictions and may respond to the client in ways that elicit the expected responses for clients of this type.

Therapists send implicit messages to clients about appropriate responses even in the way they ask questions. As Loftus and Palmer (1974) demonstrated, attorneys can obtain the desired responses from witnesses to traffic accidents by framing questions that allow only desired responses. Clinicians learn most of their information about clients by asking questions, and through these questions can communicate expectations and appropriate responses. For example, a different set of expectations is communicated when the therapist asks, "How do your problems interfere with your daily activities?" than when the question is, "What activities do you engage in every day?" When clients respond to what they perceive the therapist wants to hear, they may in time come to internalize these perceived expectations and act to confirm them. Merton (1948) called this phenomenon a *self-fulfilling prophecy*, in which an erroneous conceptualization of the situation evokes new behaviors that make the original false definition come true.

In the process of psychotherapy, following initial assessment, general and specific client observations are used to test therapists' inferences and hypotheses. Ideally, new information will lead to revisions and refinements of case formulation. The assumption is, however, that feedback will serve this corrective function. The research on decision making does not lead us to be excessively optimistic about this (see Snyder & Thomsen, this volume). When therapists attend consistently to important predictive information and apply rational decision-making procedures, then the *probability* of success is increased. Moreover, by analyzing a given decision across many different clients (not just one who springs to mind), we can find out which aspects are important for accurate judgment.

Another difficulty in clinical information processing is provided by the very context in which the client–therapist interaction occurs. In the therapist's office, only the individual is seen and not the situation, and this fact may result in a dispositional bias (the tendency to see problems as residing within the client and a result of inherent traits of the individual). Imagine a client who in each of the first three therapy sessions is nervous, fidgety, and confused. The likely inference on the part of the therapist is that this is a nervous, fidgety, and confused person. But such an inference ignores the possibility that the client's behavior is a reaction to this specific situation—to the unsettling process of seeking help, or perhaps even to the intimidating demeanor of the therapist. False impressions of consistency of behavior can thus result from seeing a person in only one situation (Heider, 1958; see also Jordan, Harvey, & Weary, this volume).

Within the therapeutic encounter, there is an asymmetry of available information. The client is the "figure" and his or her social and physical situation is the "ground" (see Einhorn, this volume). Actors have very different vantage points from observers. As actors, clients tend to focus on situational pressures whereas therapists, as observers, focus on dispositional attributions for the causes of behavior (Jones & Nisbett, 1972; Storms, 1973). Consider the case of a young newlywed described by Valins and Nisbett (1972) who complained of abdominal pains at bedtime. Her psychotherapist interpreted her pains as the expression of sexual anxiety and told her so. Because of this interpretation, the young woman began to worry about her emotional stability. Over time, her anxiety increased, augmenting her negative self-image. She continued to get worse until she visited a relative who suggested that her pain might be an allergic reactions to tomatoes and not a sign of sexual fear. The young woman stopped eating tomatoes and her "sexual fears" disappeared (Valins & Nisbett, 1972).

As Cantor and Kihlstrom (1982) state, "The clinician must get 'inside the head' of the client and see the world as he or she does" (p. 186). But they also point out that this task is fraught with the dangers of misinterpretation and distortion. The therapist might even adopt the client's pathological perspective! Cantor and Kihlstrom see the fundamental task of a therapist as remaining "objective when everything else about the therapeutic enterprise . . . mitigates against objectivity" (p. 189).

What Can Be Done?

Practicing clinicians often must begin an intervention before a thorough behavior analysis has been completed. Elstein, Shulman, and Sprafka (1978) developed a set of heuristics for medical diagnosis that can be translated readily to psychotherapy. The authors counsel the clinician to maintain multiple competing hypotheses, starting with the most probable. Each should be examined and compared with the others for its base-rate likelihood, the availability of appropriate treatment methods, the seriousness of the consequences if treatment fails, and the relative cost of treating versus not treating. After selection of a specific target behavior, clinicians must justify their choice, seek disconfirming evidence, consider multiple targets. and decide which intervention would yield the widest range of targeted versus nontargeted changes. As Cantor (1981) suggests, "everyday" models rather than normative models are appropriate for the clinical situation, since judgments are made under pressure and require quick thinking about complex and unstable events. "Given those conditions (fuzzy stimuli and pressures for hasty cognitions), most optimal decision rules are those that encourage flexibility and continuous revision" (Cantor, 1981, p. 46). In Chapter 10 of this volume, Arnoult and Anderson discuss further a number of specific strategies that may be used by clinicians to reduce some of the sources of bias that can interfere with clinical practice.

To bring about cognitive change, it is necessary to provide individuals, whether clients or therapists, with experiences that facilitate theory revision and the development of new processing heuristics. Yet, cognitive heuristics are quite resistant to change and not readily abandoned (Cantor & Kihlstrom, 1982). We tend to maintain our theories by the journals that we read, the meetings that we attend, the organizations that we join, and the colleagues with whom we associate.

All judgments are not inaccurate, and a priori causal theories are not necessarily wrong. Our emphasis has less to do with accuracy per se than with the correct application of theory, flexibility, and sensitivity to the implications of one's judgments. The fundamental task for therapists regardless of orientation is to remain objective and not be defensive, recognizing that limitations are inherent in *all* human information-processing tasks. The remainder of this volume provides a more detailed discussion of the sources of bias in information processing introduced here as well as strategies for confronting their most egregious consequences.

References

Abelson, R. P. (1981). Psychological status of the script concept. *American Psychologist, 36*. 715–729.

———. (1976). Script processing in attitude formation and decision-making. In J. S. Carroll & J. W. Payne (Eds.), *Cognition and social behavior*. Hillsdale, NJ: Erlbaum.

Asch, S. E. (1946). Forming impressions of personality. *Journal of Abnormal and Social Psychology, 41,* 258–290.

Bandura, A. (1977). *Social learning theory.* Englewood Cliffs, NJ: Prentice-Hall.

______. (1978). The self in reciprocal determinism. *American Psychologist, 33,* 344–358.

______. (1986). *Social foundations of thought and action.* New York: Prentice-Hall.

Bartlett, F. C. (1932). *Remembering.* New York: Cambridge University Press.

Berman, J. S., Read, S. J., & Kenny, D. A. (1983). Processing inconsistent social information. *Journal of Personality and Social Psychology, 45,* 1211–1224.

Bower, G. H. (1978). Contacts of cognitive psychology with social learning theory. *Cognitive Therapy and Research, 2,* 123–146.

Broadbent, D. E. (1958). *Perception and communication.* Oxford, England: Pergamon.

Cantor, N. (1981). A cognitive-social approach to personality. In N. Cantor & J. F. Kihlstrom (Eds.), *Personality, cognition, and social interaction.* Hillsdale, NJ: Erlbaum.

Cantor, N., & Kihlstrom, J. F. (1982). Cognitive and social processes in personality: Implications for behavior therapy. In C. M. Franks & G. T. Wilson (Eds.), *Handbook of behavior therapy.* New York: Guilford Press.

Chanowitz, B., & Langer. E. J. (1980). Knowing more (or less) than you can show: Understanding control through the mindlessness/mindfulness distinction. In J. Garber & M. Seligman (Eds.), *Human helplessness.* New York: Academic Press.

Chapman, L. J., & Chapman, J. P. (1967). Genesis of popular but erroneous psycho-diagnostic observations. *Journal of Abnormal Psychology, 72,* 193–204.

______. (1969). Illusory correlation as an obstacle to the use of valid psychodiagnostic signs. *Journal of Abnormal Psychology, 74,* 271–280.

Cohen, C. E. (1981). Goals and schemata in person perception—making sense from the stream of behavior. In N. Cantor & J. F. Kihlstrom (Eds.), *Personality, cognition, and social interaction.* Hillsdale, NJ: Erlbaum.

Elstein, A. S., Shulman, L. E. & Sprafka, S. A. (1978). *Medical problem solving: An analysis of clinical reasoning.* Cambridge, MA: Harvard University Press.

Frank, J. (1974). *Persuasion and healing* (Rev. ed.). New York: Schocken.

Garner, W. R. (1974). *The processing of information and structure.* Potomac. MD: Erlbaum.

Heider, F. (1958). *The psychology of interpersonal relations.* New York: Wiley.

Jones, E. E., & Nisbett, R. E. (1972). The actor and the observer: Divergent perceptions of the cause of behavior. In E. E. Jones, D. Kanouse, H. H. Kelley, R. E. Nisbett, S. Valins, & B. Weiner (Eds.), *Attribution: Perceiving the causes of behavior.* Morristown, NJ: General Learning Press.

Kadushin, C. (1969). *Why people go to psychiatrists.* New York: Atherton.

Kahneman, D., Slovic, P., & Tversky, A. (1982). *Judgment under uncertainty: Heuristics and biases.* New York: Cambridge University Press.

Kelly, G. A. (1955). *The psychology of personal constructs.* New York: Norton.

Loftus, E. F., & Palmer, J. C. (1974). Reconstruction of automobile destruction: An example of the interaction between language and memory. *Journal of Verbal Learning and Verbal Behavior, 13,* 585–589.

Mahoney, M. J. (1974). *Cognition and behavior modification.* Cambridge, MA: Ballinger.

______. (1977). Reflections on the cognitive-learning trend in psychotherapy. *American Psychologist. 32,* 5–13.

Meehl, P. E. (1960). The cognitive activity of the clinician. *American Psychologist, 15,* 19–27.

Meichenbaum, D. (1977). *Cognitive behavior modification: An integrative approach.* New York: Plenum.

Merluzzi, T. V., Rudy, T. E., & Glass, C. R. (1981). The information processing paradigm: Implications for clinical science. In T. V. Merluzzi, C. R. Glass, & M. Genest (Eds.), *Cognitive Assessment.* New York: Guilford Press.

Merton, R. (1948). The self-fulfilling prophecy. *Antioch Review, 8,* 193–210.

Mischel, W. (1973). Toward a cognitive social learning reconceptualization of personality. *Psychological Review, 80,* 252–283.

Neisser, U. (1967). *Cognitive psychology.* New York: Appleton-Century-Crofts.

Nisbett, R. E., & Ross, L. D. (1980). *Human inference: Strategies and shortcomings of social judgment.* Englewood Cliffs, NJ: Prentice-Hall.

Oskamp, S. (1965). Overconfidence in case-study judgments. *Journal of Consulting Psychology, 29,* 270–276.

Rosenhan, D. L. (1973). On being sane in insane places. *Science, 179,* 250–258.

Rosenthal, D. (1955). Changes in some moral values following psychotherapy. *Journal of Consulting Psychology,* 19, 431–436.

Rosenthal, R., & Jacobson, L. (1968). *Pygmalion in the classroom.* New York: Holt, Rinehart & Winston.

Ross, L., Lepper, M. R., & Hubbard, M. (1975). Perseverence in self-perception and social-perception: Biased attribution processes in the debriefing paradigm. *Journal of Personality and Social Psychology, 32,* 880–892.

Ross, L., Lepper, M. R., Strack, F., & Steinmetz, J. (1977). Social explanation and social expectation: Effects of real and hypothetical explanations on subjective likelihood. *Journal of Personality and Social Psychology, 35,* 817–829.

Schank, R. C., & Abelson, R. P. (1977). *Scripts, plans, goals, and understanding.* Hillsdale, NJ: Erlbaum.

Scheff, T. J. (1966). *Being mentally ill: A sociological theory.* Chicago: Aldine.

Smith, A. F. (1986). *Strategies and structures in selective attention tasks.* Dissertation submitted to Yale University, May 1986.

Snyder, M. (1981). On the self-perpetuating nature of social stereotypes. In D. Hamilton (Ed.), *Cognitive processes in stereotyping and intergroup behavior.* Hillsdale, NJ: Erlbaum.

Snyder, M., & Swann, W. B. (1978a). Behavioral confirmation in social interaction: From social perception to social reality. *Journal of Experimental Social Psychology, 14,* 148–162.

______. (1978b). Hypothesis-testing processes in social interaction. *Journal of Personality and Social Psychology, 36,* 1202–1212.

Storms, M. D. (1973). Videotape and the attribution process: Reversing actors' and observers' points of view. *Journal of Personality and Social Psychology, 27,* 165–175.

Taylor, S. E., & Crocker, J. (1981). Schematic bases of social information processing. In E. T. Higgins, C. P. Herman, & M. P. Zanna (Eds.), *Social cognition: The Ontario symposium in personality and social psychology.* Hillsdale, NJ: Erlbaum.

Tversky, A., & Kahneman, D. (1973). Availability: A heuristic for judging frequency and probability. *Cognitive Psychology, 5,* 207–232.

———. (1974). Judgment under uncertainty: Heuristics and biases. *Science, 185,* 1124–1131.

Valins, S., & Nisbett, R. E. (1972). Attributional processes in the development and treatment of emotional disorders. In E. E. Jones et al. (Eds.), *Attribution: Perceiving the causes of behavior.* Morristown, NJ: General Learning Press.

Whitman, R. M., Kramer, M., & Baldridge, B. (1963). Which dream does the patient tell? *Archives of General Psychiatry, 8,* 277–282.

Wylie, R. (1979). *The self-concept.* Lincoln: University of Nebraska Press.

PART I

Cognition and Decision Making in Clinical Practice

2 Cognitive Processes in Clinical Inference and Decision Making

Arthur S. Elstein

WHEN clinical psychologists think about clinical judgment and reasoning, they generally have in mind diagnostic reasoning in the mental health field. The precedent appears to have been established by early work (Kleinmuntz, 1968; Meehl, 1954) and continues, supported by familiarity with the subject matter and the materials used in research and by ease of access to subjects and settings. Of course, the mental health field is not the only setting for clinical work, and attention has also been paid to diagnostic inference and decision processes in medicine, nursing, and the allied health professions. Contemporary cognitive research in the information-processing tradition has led naturally to studies of experts and novices in several subdomains of these professions, and research on decision making has expanded to examine that function in clinical contexts.

Research on clinical judgment and decision making has been active for about 20 years. From an earlier focus on judgmental accuracy and modeling judgment processes (Slovic & Lichtenstein, 1971), more recent work has shifted to identifying judgmental heuristics and biases and exploring their extent and significance. This shift in thematic emphasis can be dated to the publication of two landmark papers on probability judgment (Kahneman & Tversky, 1973; Tversky & Kahneman, 1974), although it was several years before the viewpoint began to be felt in research on *clinical* judgment and decision making.

This chapter reviews selected work on the psychological characteristics of clinical diagnostic reasoning and decision making. Reference is made to several classical studies of judgment and decision making, but aside from these, studies in which the research subjects were convenient samples of college sophomores or graduate students have been deliverately avoided and replaced by investigations utilizing practitioners or students in one of the health professions as subjects and clinical tasks as the decision environment. This approach will enable us to examine the extent to which broader theories can explain findings derived from studies of the reasoning and decision processes of practitioners in a particular domain. It will also suggest how theories of inference and choice should be modified to account for the effects of specialized content and experience. The chapter thus aims: (1) to place some of the major findings of research on clinical decision making within the framework of a more comprehensive theory of thinking and decision making under uncertainty; (2) to indicate how information-processing theory and behavioral decision theory, which together comprise what may be said to be the "new look" in cognitive psychology, help to describe and explain the reasoning and decision processes of clinicians; and (3) to provide illustrations from clinical environments of cognitive processes first identified in hypothetical settings or experiments.

As is always true, the published literature far exceeds what could be reviewed in the space available. Research employing regression approaches to model and improve upon judgment has been omitted, partly because the general philosophy and approach has already received much attention in clinical and personnel psychology (e.g., Dawes, 1976; Goldberg, 1968, 1970; Meehl, 1957; Slovic & Lichtenstein, 1971). Further, the information-processing and behavioral decision literature has also been selectively reviewed, focusing on studies that address both psychological theory and clinical services. In the interest of focusing on a limited number of topics, this essay also omits newer work dealing with judgment and decision making under ambiguity where the underlying probability distribution is unknown (e.g., Curley, Eraker, & Yates, 1984; Einhorn & Hogarth, 1985), although a crucial feature of many clinical situations may be that they are ambiguous rather than uncertain. The interested reader may wish to consult Christensen-Szalanski's recent overview (1986), as it takes a much different perspective on the problems discussed in this chapter.

The chapter begins with a general overview of information-processing psychology and behavioral decision theory, with special emphasis on their contrasting attitudes to clinical expertise. The following two sections summarize the main features of an information-processing theory of clinical reasoning and the strengths and liabilities identified in clinical inference from this standpoint. The next two sections cover the same ground from the standpoint of decision theory: first, the fundamental principles of decision theory, then the errors and biases identified in clinicians' decision making from this perspective. Questions of research method are then discussed, especially the problem of external validity. The concluding section considers the implications of this research for the education of health professionals and offers some suggestions for future research directions.

General Remarks on Information-Processing Psychology and Behavioral Decision Theory

Research on psychological aspects of clinical reasoning is concerned with the cognitive processes employed by clinicians in reasoning and decision making. The intended application of this research was initially educational: to identify the strategies and knowledge structure characterizing expert performance so as to facilitate instructing novice clinicians (Elstein, Shulman, Sprafka, et al., 1978). With the recent growth of interest in artificial intelligence and medical expert systems (Clancey & Shortliffe, 1984; Szolovits, 1982), psychological research has branched out into detailed specifications of the knowledge structure and cognitive processes to be modeled in an expert system for user-acceptable decision support (Feltovich, Johnson, Moller, & Swanson, 1984; Miller, Pople, & Myers, 1982). The design of these supports is significant because they must capture adequately the complexities of the clinical decision task without becoming so overwhelmed by them as to be impenetrable, and must also take due account of the reasoning capabilities, prior knowledge, and habits of the potential users. In short, this is a classic human factors or man–machine interface problem. To foreshadow a point to be developed later more fully, this research typically begins with the behavior of an expert (or perhaps some novices, for comparison) and moves toward building a model emulating that performance. The prototypical research question, then, is what knowledge structures, cognitive operations, and rule structures are necessary and sufficient to reproduce the observed clinical reasoning.

The information-processing approach rests on close analysis of protocols obtained from problem-solvers, i.e., expert clinicians, as they work out diagnostic problems or make therapeutic decisions. The adequacy of the theoretical formulation of the problem-solving process can be tested in several ways: by comparison with more general cognitive principles to see if the clinical formulation is consistent with them, by the clinical judgment of experts, and by resort to computer simulation (Feltovich et al., 1984; Johnson, Duran, Hasselbrock, Moller, Prietula, Feltovich, & Swanson, 1981; Kunz, Shortliffe, Buchanan, & Feigenbaum, 1984; Miller et al., 1982; Shortliffe, 1976). For this last test, the theory of clinical reasoning is written as a computer program, and if the program runs and solves the problem pretty much as the clinicians did or makes the same mistakes they do, it can be said to be a sufficient representation of the reasoning process.

The aim of research on computerized decision-support systems, such as MYCIN (Shortliffe, 1976) and INTERNIST (Miller et al., 1982), is to create a computer program that emulates an expert clinician. The decision aid should give the same advice or reach the same diagnostic or therapeutic decisions as the expert, and it should be able to explain its reasoning to a user much as expert consultants explain theirs. It is far more important that the system display common sense (e.g., knowing not to consider ectopic pregnancy as a possible cause of abdominal pain in a 25-year-old male) and intuitively clear clinical judgment than that it be quantitative, explicit, and consistent with formal decision theory. It is only natural, given these aims and constraints, that experts are viewed as knowledgeable, intelligent, and flexible, and that their performance and judgment are the criteria by which the computer's performance is assessed. The criterion for validation of the system's advice is the expert's judgment. If the system fails to perform as does the expert being modeled, the rule structure or data base is adjusted until it does. While in principle one could ask if the expert had made a mistake and if the system had improved upon human reason, the more usual approach in systems design is imitative; the objective is not so much to improve upon expert judgment as to make it available to the average practitioner.

In marked contrast to the decision-analytic approach, the form of the reasoning and of the explanation in these expert systems is symbolic and nonquantitative (Fox, 1984; Kunz et al., 1984; Pople, 1982). Published samples of this work (Clancey, 1984) suggest that the explanations are much more concerned with tracing the causes or the temporal course of a disease than with the analysis of risks and benefits so characteristic of decision analysis. Quantitative elements, expressions of informed expert judgments, are involved in both systems (certainty factors in MYCIN; evoking strength, import values, and frequency values in INTERNIST). But these elements are implicit in the programming and are of concern more to the authors of the programs than to the users. They resemble conditional probabilities for they can range from 0.0 to 1.0, but their logical status is far less clear and the design of expert systems does not require that they obey the laws of probability as is necessary in decision analysis (but see Heckerman, 1985; Shortliffe & Buchanan, 1975).

Behavioral decision theory approaches clinical reasoning from the opposite direction: a formal, explicit, quantitative model of inference and decision making is employed as the standard of comparison. This model is statistical decision theory, or expected utility theory, embodied in the procedures and techniques known as decision analysis. Psychological research derived from this model has investigated many questions: the extent to which human decision making corresponds to the model, reasons for observed discrepancies, and the psychological processes employed in carrying out the probability and utility assessments required by decision theory. Beginning with the seminal work of Tversky and Kahneman, psychological studies of decision making have increasingly focused on the conflict between descriptive and normative theories of decision making. Rational decision making should obey the axioms of statistical decision theory, and the properties of preferences would be consistent with those axioms. Yet, there is considerable evidence that certain heuristic principles widely used in human decision making, which seem intuitively reasonable and sensible to many people, may be inconsistent with the normative theory (Lopes, 1981). While most experimental work of this type has not employed expert clinicians as subjects, some studies have. These have also identified systematic errors and biases in information processing and judgment among physicians at various levels of experience (e.g., Elstein, Holzman, Ravitch, Metheny, Holmes, Hoppe, Rothert, & Rovner, 1986; Eraker & Politser, 1982; McNeil, Pauker, Sox, & Tversky, 1982; Politser, 1981; Wolf, Gruppen, & Billi, 1985).

There have been attempts to revise and update the theory (Bell, 1982) and claims that the normative and descriptive theories of decision making are fundamentally irreconcilable (Tversky & Kahneman, 1985). Other investigators (Elstein et al., 1986; Hershey & Schoemaker, 1985) have argued that the errors and biases identified by descriptive studies point out precisely where and why decision support is needed. Consequently, some of the current themes of this research are (1) to develop a more adequate theoretical account of clinical judgment and decision making by obtaining additional relevant data and relating findings to cognitive theory; (2) to clarify the need for decision support systems by assessing more accurately the extent of inefficiencies and biases in everyday clinical judgement; (3) to assess the extent to which implementations of major alternative approaches available for systems design conform to or depart from the thought processes of the experts who will use them; and (4) to develop more effective and useful decision supports.

A central premise shared by both approaches is that of bounded or limited rationality (Newell & Simon, 1972; Simon, 1979). This premise posits that our capacity to carry out rational thought is restricted, in part by the limitations of working memory. As a consequence, problem-solvers are literally required to represent complex problems in simplified problem spaces and to find ways to cut down mental effort and reduce cognitive strain. Information-processing psychology sees experts as adaptive and clever in spite of these limitations on their rationality. They know how to focus on what is critical, disregard the trivial, and put actions in proper temporal sequence (as demonstrated by the saying "we'll cross that bridge when we come to it"), thereby achieving the needed simplification of problem structure. Their opinions and judgments, based upon extensive experience, are therefore viewed as the standard against which other performance, whether human or machine, is to be compared. Despite the fact that human experts made mistakes, expert-systems research esteems clinical judgment so highly that it finds it worthwhile to design computer programs which will mimic such judgments insofar as possible.

Behavioral decision theory takes a much more guarded view of unaided human inference (Hogarth, 1980; Nisbett & Ross, 1980). It argues that the biases and mistakes in information processing, data combination, and inference uncovered by behavioral decision research have been detected both in novices and experts. Since experts are likely to be consulted precisely in situations that are complex and perplexing, the principle of limited rationality implies the possibility that some of their strategies and heuristics will lead to erroneous diagnoses or suboptimal recommendations. Expert systems may thus incorporate biases and inefficiencies as well as true expertise. Errors in the inference process or suboptimal solutions to difficult problems are especially likely if the problem requires the manipulation or estimation of probabilities as well as factual recall from a well-organized memory store. The knowledge representation and heuristic search techniques of the expert who is modeled by the expert system may be subject to the same biases and inefficiencies as plague less expert problem-solvers. Familiarity with the domain does not confer immunity to these biases and they affect both quantitative and categorical judgments (Balla, Iansek, & Elstein, 1985; Christensen-Szalanski, J. J., Beck, Christensen-Szalanski, C. M., & Koepsell, 1983; McNeil et al., 1982). Therefore, even expert performance should be evaluated in the light of a normative model, not because the model is perfect but because it is equally likely that the experts are not perfect either.

Expert-systems research, by contrast, has much more confidence in experts but doubts that the average level of performance meets a demanding standard, mainly because of deficiencies in the knowledge base and representation of nonexperts. The approach concentrates on symbolic, nonquantitative reasoning, while behavioral decision theory examines the domain of everyday reasoning based on statistics or, it might be said, suggests that we view problems we had never thought of as statistical as exactly that. Thus, each approach conveys a different view of clinical expertise and error and suggests a slightly different range of applications for decision support systems.

Clinical Reasoning as Information Processing

A number of investigations have identified hypothetico-deductive reasoning as one basic strategy of diagnostic troubleshooting and inference (Eddy & Clanton, 1982; Elstein et al., 1978; Kassirer & Gorry, 1978; Miller et al., 1982; Pople, 1982). Both experts and novices solve difficult diagnostic problems by generating a set of hypotheses, problem formulations, or schemata based on very limited data and using these formulations to guide subsequent data collection. The workup then functions not simply to gather a complete data base but to test these hypotheses, confirming one or more, discriminating between similar competitors, and reformulating the list along the way if necessary (Kassirer, Kuipers, & Gorry, 1982). Groen and Patel (1985) have recently criticized this mode of analysis on the grounds that expert reasoning in nonproblematic situations does not display explicit hypothesis testing and looks much more like pattern recognition or direct retrieval of needed strategies from a well-organized network of stored information and knowledge. While it is true that expert performance is certainly overlearned and often automatic, the bulk of the literature on this subject suggests that (a) experts explicitly use the hypothetico-deductive method when routine problem recognition methods fail, and (b) if rapid problem recognition is unpacked and dissected, it can be seen to be a mixture of pattern recognition, intuition (whatever that is), and hypothesis testing. Consequently, much can be understood better by recapitulating some features of good clinical reasoning using this strategy:

1. In every domain that has been examined, including clinical medicine, expertise was found to be heavily dependent on a well-organized store of knowledge (Duda & Shortliffe, 1983; Johnson, 1983; Larkin, McDermott, Simon, D. P., & Simon, H. A., 1980; Waldrop, 1984). Of course, experts know more than novices. But more importantly, their greater knowledge is organized, or compiled, so as to be readily retrievable and applicable to new situations. Experts are especially good at developing detailed structures for ill-structured problems (Pople, 1982), an undoubtedly significant component of the reasoning process. A few critical features of a particular case are sufficient to tap into this larger body of knowledge of causes for predictions about the probable course (prognosis of a condition) and for actions that might be taken to improve matters (Carroll, 1980). Experts can develop deep structural models of a particular case that enable them to relate a generic body of knowledge to the unique features of an individual patient (Feltovich & Patel, 1984). Schön (1984) has eloquently argued that the problem-structuring skill of expert practitioners should be viewed as an artistic process making possible the subsequent application of technical rationality; however, in the

nature of the case, this art will not satisfy criteria appropriate to the resolution of well-formed problems, such as utility maximization. Flexibility and adaptability to the task environment are salient characteristics of experts, who do not hesitate to change paths if that seems indicated and are quick to recognize a new problem as a variant of a familiar type. There is an echo here of the Platonic doctrine that knowledge is recollection.

2. The store of expert knowledge contains rules for procedures—what to do next or what to do if certain conditions are met—as well as propositional knowledge of normality and disease (Gagne, 1984). Thus, experts know how to do certain things—they have practical clinical skills—and they know how to determine when these actions should be taken. In other words, a rule structure governs performance, although experts may not routinely be able to state these rules verbally. This implicit rule structure is an important component of "clinical judgment," as it enables one to act in ways that will be judged sensible. Experts often take this knowledge for granted until confronted with the question of why novices stumble, even though they can satisfactorily answer questions about disease mechanisms. Their difficulty makes it clear that planning and procedural skills are not identical with retrospective identification of causal mechanisms and that propositional knowledge does not necessarily imply procedural knowledge.

3. Differences in strategies used by experts and novices are less dramatic than their differences in actual knowledge would imply (Feltovich et al., 1984; Larkin et al., 1980; Neufeld, Norman, Feightner, & Barrows, 1981). A senior clinician with many years of experience treating depressed clients may have a broader store of knowledge about this problem than a new intern. However, they both may use identical strategies for assessing a depressed client. For example, both may ask questions that confirm an initial hypothesis (see Snyder & Thomsen, this volume). In general, experts pursue a hypothesis-testing strategy more efficiently than novices, sometimes so efficiently, it has been argued, that it is an error to assert that they are even using one (Groen & Patel, 1985). Since they have a better sense of the structure of the environment and, therefore, what the reasonably likely diagnostic possibilities are, they can more efficiently generate an early set of plausible hypotheses so as to avoid a fruitless and expensive pursuit of rare diagnoses. Because they are more practiced in history taking and physical diagnosis, experts can focus their efforts on the critical information that must be obtained in any particular encounter (Balla, 1985). For these reasons, experts are generally quicker, more efficient, and more accurate than novices.

4. Good clinical reasoning should also avoid overlooking unusual conditions presenting as common ones or rare conditions that are treatable and potentially harmful if untreated. For example, most headaches

are not caused by benign operable tumors, but a good clinician would not want to miss the few that are. On the other hand, one must avoid false alarms, overcalling relatively rare diagnoses, and wasting money on diagnostic workups that are bound to be futile.

In some of the recent literature on the art of diagnosis (Committee on Evaluation in General Internal Medicine, 1979; Griner, Mayewski, Mushlin, & Greenland, 1981) physicians are called upon not to overlook rare treatable conditions but also not to waste resources in fruitless hunts for nonexistent diseases. Clinical and probabilistic viewpoints are juxtaposed, but, of course, it is impossible to pursue both goals simultaneously to perfection. Some compromise strategy is needed, in the form of a metarule advising when to search for rare conditions (what are the really good indicators that this search will pay off?) and when to work probabilistically. These metarules are not yet formulated, and the choice is left largely to the art of judgment. The rule structure for these puzzles is complex and case-specific and has provided a challenge for emerging decision-support systems and for developing clinical algorithms. In much of the research, the criteria behind the recommendations of experts are implicit and more emphasis is placed on what to do than on justification. Information-processing research employs several concepts to handle this complex task: prototypes, frames, competing hypotheses, lines of reasoning, and deep structural models that relate apparently idiosyncratic or unusual features of a case to deeper underlying principles.

5. The intuitive clinical method is well suited to structuring poorly structured problems (Pople, 1982). Hypotheses are used as flexible cognitive structures that can be easily erected or discarded as evidence accumulates. The clinician is not obligated to pursue a line of reasoning mechanically to the bitter end if subsequent findings suggest that an early hypothesis is a poor candidate for follow-up and a new idea is better. Furthermore, the expert clinician can pay appropriate attention to particularizing features of a case and tailor a set of hypotheses to suit. Laborious processing of quantitative data can be replaced by knowledge-guided problem structuring. However in this process statistical features of the evidence (such as base rates) may be neglected (see section ahead on errors from the standpoint of normative theory).

6. Data collection should be limited and focused. Every clinician recognizes that inexperienced students are more likely than experienced physicians to do unfocused, exhaustive workups. For experts, not everything needs to be explicit; gaps in the data base or the chain of inference can be filled in with informal knowledge or common sense, both of which are often so taken for granted that they are not explicitly mentioned in verbal protocols until a mistake shows that they were not used when they could have been.

7. Quantitative data, both physical findings and laboratory tests, are interpreted on scales in which fairly wide ranges of results are treated as equivalent for practical clinical purposes. For example, body temperature or blood pressure might be encoded as essentially normal, slightly elevated, or seriously elevated. Similarly, masses seen on radiographs are generally encoded on 4- or 5-point scales ranging from definitely abnormal to definitely normal, or some equivalent terminology. Even if measurements of the object visualized are recorded in centimeters or millimeters, the interpretation is processed on a simpler scale. So, while data may be entered on charts as continuous, quantitative measures, they are psychologically coded and processed on 3-, 4-, or (rarely) 5-point scales. This procedure substantially simplifies the problem of representation, eases the information-processing load, and facilitates the management of large amounts of data. One of the main tasks of novice clinicians appears to be learning these coding schemes. This is more difficult than it might seem at first because the coding schemes are largely implicit and their boundaries are fuzzy, ambiguous, and probably vary among experts. Thus, this implicit knowledge—sometimes identified as "common sense" or "tacit knowledge" (Polanyi, 1958)—must be "picked up along the way," a time-consuming process. Detecting and explicating it is a major part of the research agenda in artificial intelligence and cognitive psychology.

Liabilities of Everyday Clinical Inference

Despite its power, this structure for clinical reasoning is not error-proof. One of the unsolved problems in the field is to assess the frequency of errors in actual practice. It is at least possible now to construct a partial catalogue of possible errors so that quantitative research can be directed. Within the framework of the competing-hypothesis model of clinical reasoning, it is convenient to think about errors as falling within the categories of hypothesis generation, data collection, data interpretation, and judgment or information integration. This section begins the task of relating errors or biases identified by behavioral decision research to the information-processing approach to clinical expertise.

A general property of clinical reasoning is that the language employed is vague and ambiguous. From the standpoint of information-processing theory, this may not be a serious problem for the reasoning of the individual clinician, but it does pose serious problems of communication among clinicians. Figure 2–1, adapted from Bryant and Norman (1980), presents some terms widely used in reporting results of radiographs or laboratory tests, and the mean, range, and standard deviation of probability estimates that clinicians attached to these terms.

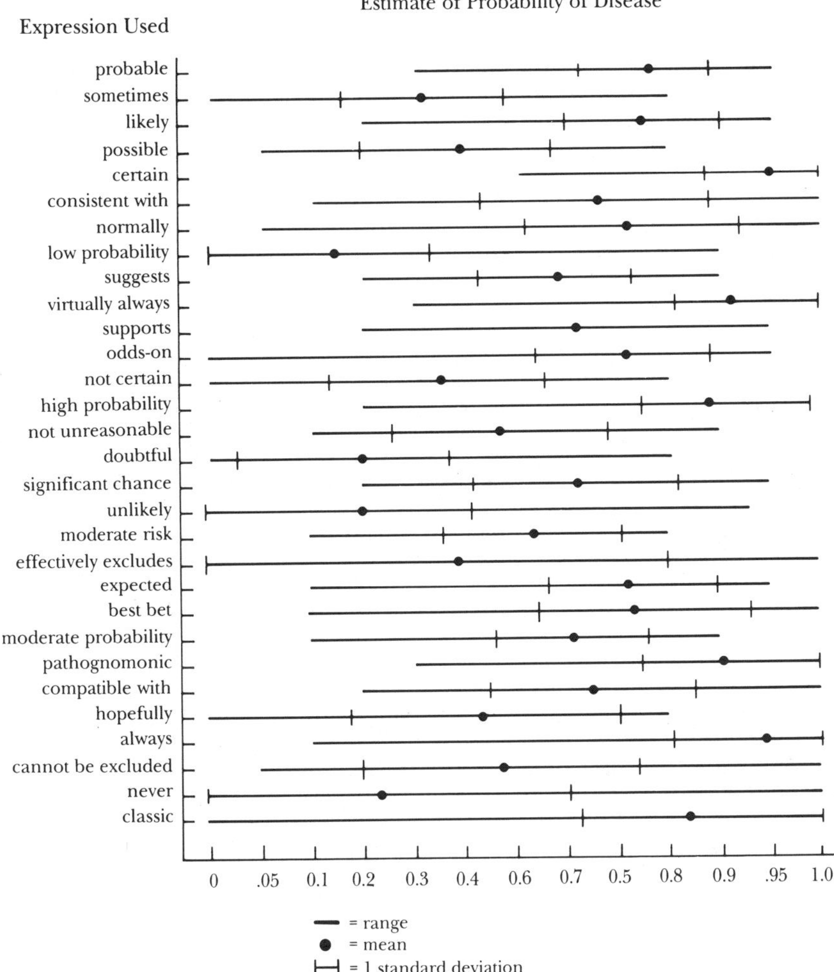

Figure 2–1. Subjective Probabilities of Presence of Disease Judged from Words and Phrases in Common Clinical Use

From Bryant & Norman, 1980. Reprinted by permission of *The New England Journal of Medicine* from vol. 302 (1980), p. 411.

As the graph suggests, the language is exceedingly ambiguous. Bryant and Norman reported that only 9 out of 30 expressions had ranges lower than 0.5 and some had ranges greater than 0.9. Nakao and Axelrod (1983) found similarly wide ranges in the quantitative estimates assigned to commonly used terms, but their data also implied some underlying consensus about a rough ordering of the terms.

Failure to consider the correct hypothesis is a common cause of mistaken diagnosis. Many diagnostic problems are so complex that the correct solution is not contained within the initial set of formulations. Restructuring and reformulating must occur as problem solving proceeds. However, as a problem-solver works with a particular set of hypotheses, psychological commitment takes place and it becomes more difficult to restructure the problem. Ideally, one might want to work purely inductively, reasoning only from the facts, but this strategy is never employed because it is very inefficient and produces high levels of cognitive strain.

For example, a clinician rarely makes a diagnosis by matching every client characteristic to each diagnostic criterion listed under a disorder in DSM-III. Rather, a clinician attends to two or three "prototypic" symptoms for a particular disorder (Horowitz, French, Lapid, & Weckler, 1982). It would be impossible to keep every diagnostic feature in mind simultaneously. As Bartlett (1958) observed, solving unbounded problems requires that they first be structured. Hypotheses provide the needed framework. Early problem formulation is necessary but also potentially biasing.

The emphasis in internal medicine training on formally constructing and analyzing a set of diagnostic alternatives, called the differential diagnosis, is designed to help correct these problems. This is a useful heuristic strategy, rather than one guaranteeing success, for instructions to develop a differential diagnosis generally omit clearly defined rules that state how many alternatives should be on the differential list or what the best alternatives are for a given situation. Everyday clinical reasoning would insist that such rules are too rigid. Thus, the strategy of working through a differential diagnosis can prevent premature closure on a single salient alternative, but it cannot guarantee that the correct diagnostic alternative is included on the list. Of course, the longer and more exhaustive the list, the more likely it is that the correct diagnosis will have been included, but the workup will become correspondingly more expensive and time-consuming.

Several features of human thinking together imply that it will be tempting to search for exotic diseases ("long shots") at the expense of more probable ones. This phenomenon is often observed, and clinicians are regularly urged to alter their behavior, but change has proven to be difficult. Recent cognitive psychological literature suggests several mechanisms underlying this persistence. First, small probabilities tend to be overestimated (Tversky & Kahneman, 1981), and of course the probabilities of rare diseases are very small by definition. Second, because rare conditions are overrepresented in both the clinical literature and in academic training centers, novices, in particular, may tend to overestimate the likelihood of their occurrence in everyday practice. Third, it is difficult for everyday judgment to keep separate accounts for probability and utility. If the rarer disease is more serious, there is a good chance that clinicians will respond to the regret they would feel about missing the diagnosis instead of to a weighted combination of probability and value. Fourth, the anticipated glory that may come from identifying a rare disease that other clinicians have missed may initiate a search that fails to consider more mundane, but possibly correct, diagnoses (Wallsten, 1981).

Expert clinical reasoning should accurately distinguish critical features (signal) from noncrucial aspects of the case (noise) and concentrate on eliciting and weighing findings that are clinically meaningful. Errors can occur in both acquiring and interpreting data. In data acquisition, there is a tendency to seek information that confirms a hypothesis rather than the data that would facilitate logical testing of competing hypotheses (Kern & Doherty, 1982; Wolf et al., 1985). The most common error in weighing findings is to interpret data that should be noncontributory to a particular hypothesis, and that might even suggest a new alternative, as consistent with hypotheses already under consideration. This error of simplification has been called "overinterpretation" (Elstein et al., 1978). The data best remembered tend to be those that support the hypotheses generated. Where findings are distorted in recall, it is generally in the direction of making the facts more consistent with typical clinical pictures. Positive findings are overemphasized and negative findings tend to be discounted (Wason & Johnson-Laird, 1972). The principle of bounded rationality helps us understand the adaptive function of these errors: (1) a problem must be bounded, so hypotheses are required; (2) the problem space must be a simplified representation, so generating more hypotheses and thereby complicating the problem increases cognitive strain. In general, efforts are continually made to keep matters simple and within the capacity of working memory.

Drawing upon Hammond's early work (Hammond, 1971) in using computer graphics to display cue-weighting functions, some recent educationally oriented research has used lens model feedback to help learners acquire and employ more nearly optimal weighting functions (Wigton, Hoellerich, & Patil, 1986). Many other investigators have developed regression equations or discriminant functions as decision supports, not as descriptive models of human judgment.

Thorough data collection is a value taught in all educational programs in the health professions. Only recently, under the pressure created by the need to control the costs of health care, have questions been raised about unnecessary redundancy in diagnostic workups. Both the delay in recognizing this issue and the discomfort felt by clinicians who fear they may not be able to obtain all the data they would like to have point to an enduring issue in clinical inference: More data are collected than are needed, apparently because (1) clinicians are often unaware of the redundancies, and (2) more data increase confidence without increasing accuracy (Oskamp, 1965). So, from an information-processing perspective, we have an organism who has difficulty extracting all the information potentially embedded in a data set and who both needs and likes to add to the store of data despite limited ability to process all of it. In these circumstances, some inefficiency in inference due to information overload is practically inevitable.

Normative and Descriptive Theories of Decision Making

Decision analysis (Keeney, 1982; Raiffa, 1968; Weinstein & Fineberg, 1980; Zarin & Pauker, 1984) consists of a set of techniques for making decisions under uncertainty. The techniques are appropriate for situations in which choices must be made and in which the outcomes of actions are predictable only on the average (in the long run) but not for individual cases. Decision analysis is a tool for analyzing situations where some chance of a poor or less desired outcome exists even if the "right" decision has been made, and where one would wish to distinguish between employing a rational coherent *process* to reach a decision and the achievment of a good *outcome*. The theory can also incorporate problems of the optimal allocation of scarce resources, and of deciding if the incremental benefit of obtaining additional information is worth the cost by weighing the costs and risks associated with data collection and the presumed quality of the information once it is in hand. Clinical interest in decision analysis has grown considerably in recent years, spurred by the growing attention devoted to both ethical and economic issues in health care.

The theoretical foundation of decision analysis is the theory of expected utility (Schoemaker, 1980; Von Neumann & Morgenstern, 1947), a way of ordering preferences for outcomes of action that follows logically and coherently from a few axioms. Because expected utility theory has an axiomatic base, it has had great appeal as the foundation for a rational theory of decision making and choice under certainty.

Decision analysis decomposes any decision problem into discrete components and provides a procedure for synthesizing these components into an overall measure of the attractiveness of alternatives so that the optimal strategy can be selected. Data required are of two types—measures of uncertainty and measures of values. In the vocabulary of decision theory, uncertainties are expressed as probabilities and values as utilities. The criterion for choice is to act so as to maximize expected utility.

Psychological research on decision making (Einhorn & Hogarth, 1981; Kahneman, Slovic, & Tversky, 1982; Slovic, Lichtenstein, &

Fischhoff, in press; Wright, 1984) describes and analyzes the cognitive processes and principles employed in decision making under uncertainty. It is concerned with what people actually do, not with what they should do; the normative theory serves as the standard of comparison. In the early days of this research, the expected utility hypothesis was taken as a fairly good approximation of what people actually do or at least what they would want to do. More recently, the validity of this hypothesis as even a first approximation of actual decision making has come under increasing criticism by psychologists (Fischhoff, 1980; Fischhoff, Goitein, & Shapira, 1982; Kahneman & Tversky, 1979; Lopes, 1981; Schoemaker, 1982; Slovic & Tversky, 1974; Tversky & Kahneman, 1981).

Departures from the normative theory can be demonstrated in each phase of the analytic process: probability estimation, probability revision, utility assessment, and combining the separate estimates to reach a decision. The most troubling psychological problems arise in situations where decision-makers do not obey the expected utility rule and, even after their inconsistency is pointed out to them, insist that they do not want to change their decisions. These conflicts between decisions reached by intuitive processes and by normatively correct procedures cast doubt on the normative status of this major theory of rational decision making and have occasioned much lively debate about the status of the theory and our understanding of what it means to be rational.

In a recent paper, Tversky and Kahneman (1986) assert that the normative and descriptive theories are irreconcilable, because there is no way that consistently identified patterns of behavior can be made to fit the normative model. This means that the normative theory of decision making stands as an ideal and cannot claim to be an account of how people actually make decisions. Lopes (1981) argues that decision principles which make intuitive good sense in the short run are erroneously viewed as suboptimal by the normative approach.

Some of the discrepancies between normative and descriptive theories are caused by bounded rationality, to which reference was made above. That is, because of the requirement that complex problems be represented in simplified spaces that may omit certain aspects of the problem, it will often be the case that different representations are possible, each of which makes different elements salient. To the extent that a decision is guided by its most salient elements, the others being set aside in order to make the problem manageable, different representations will lead to different decisions. But according to the normative theory, choices between formally equivalent problem representations ought not to vary.

It is now clear that the normative theory of decision making does not describe how people actually make decisions, although the extent of departures and their clinical significance are still unanswered questions. The problems with the theory go far beyond difficulties in correctly measuring subjective probabilities and utilities. Whether people ought to make decisions that are consistent with the theory's axioms is another question. I believe the answer to that question is yes, and to support that conclusion, I turn now to a partial catalogue of errors and biases in human decision processes. To some as yet unknown degree, these errors lower the quality of clinical decisions. Therefore, identifying and correcting them is a pressing task for research and teaching in this area.

Errors from the Standpoint of Normative Theory

This section reviews only errors and biases demonstrated to operate in clinicians at various levels of experience. The list is selective, not exhaustive.

Probability Revision

From the standpoint of decision theory, the process of reaching a diagnosis can be conceptualized as probability revision with imperfect information. The formal rule for probability revision with such evidence is Bayes's theorem, which states, in part, that a decision maker must attend to (a) the frequency of occurrence of a diagnostic sign and (b) a disorder in the population being observed (i.e., the "base rates"), as well as (c) the probability that someone with the disorder in question will or will not exhibit the sign, and (d) the probability that normal individuals will also exhibit the sign (see Wiggins, 1973). In the past decade, several studies have been published demonstrating that probability revision in everyday clinical inference does not match the conclusions reached by applying this rule.

The subjects in these studies demonstrated a failure to appreciate the statistical properties of clinical evidence, neglect of Bayes's theorem in revising diagnostic probabilities, and mistaken intuitions about the effects of low base rates on the interpretation of test results (Balla, Elstein, & Gates, 1983; Balla et al., 1985; Berwick, Fineberg, & Weinstein, 1981; Borak & Veilleux, 1982; Casscells, Schoenberger, & Graboys, 1978; Eddy, 1982; Politser, 1984). In particular, the predictive value of a test has been found repeatedly compromised by confusion about test sensitivity and specificity. Test sensitivity refers to the test's accuracy in identifying people who have a disorder; specificity concerns the accuracy of the test in identifying correctly people who do not have the disorder. Unless the problem is structured to call attention to the need

TABLE 2–1
Estimates of 44 Clinicians on Likelihood of Secondary Deposit as Cause of Symptoms in Illustrative Case: 50-year-old man with small-cell carcinoma of the lung

Estimate of Secondary Deposit as Cause of Symptoms (%)	*Number of Clinicians*
<25	29
25–50	7
50–75	5
>75	3

Reprinted from Balla, Iansek, and Elstein, 1985, with permission of *The Lancet* from #8424 (Feb. 9, 1985), p. 327.

Note: Bayesian posterior probability = .9 or greater.

for Bayes's rule, there is a strong tendency to equate test sensitivity with the predictive value of a positive test and test specificity with the predictive value of a negative result.

Some studies have begun to identify the processes clinicians use when revising probabilities that lead to Bayesian violations. For example, base rates are often neglected in favor of individualizing information, presumably because unique case material is more vivid and memorable (Kahneman & Tversky, 1973; Nisbett, Borgida, Crandall, & Reed, 1976). Balla et al. (1985) found that the impact of prior established disease was underestimated and the probability of a new disease overestimated when two conditions were met: the new disease possibility had less ominous prognostic implications, and the probability of obtaining positive findings was greater in the new disease than in the established condition. Base-rate neglect and wishful thinking for a less serious illness combined to yield erroneous probability estimates (see Table 2–1). Wallsten (1981) has also demonstrated errors in probability revision that are systematically linked to cost of mistakes and has thus shown the difficulties experienced in separating assessments of probability from utility (value-induced bias).

Regret and Responsibility

Many clinical decisions seem to be guided by the "minimax principle" (Narragon, 1980): an action is selected because it has the smaller maximum loss. Feinstein (1985) has called minimization of regret the "chagrin factor" and has suggested that it is a major qualitative mechanism in medical decision making, employed instead of quantitative formalisms because it is simpler and hence more intuitively acceptable. The working

TABLE 2–2
Cross-Tabulation of Observed Prescribing Decisions and Recommendations of Decision-Analytic Model

	Decision Analysis			
	Treat	*Toss-up*	*Do Not Treat*	*Total*
Observed decisions				
Treat	97	105	0	202
Toss-up	23	26	0	49
Do not treat	113	224	0	337
Total	233	355	0	588

Reprinted from Elstein et al., 1986, with permission of *The American Journal of Medicine* from vol. 80 (Feb. 1986), p. 252.

Note: Data obtained from 49 physicians.

of this heuristic is illustrated in a recent study of clinicians' decisions concerning estrogen replacement therapy for menopausal women (Elstein et al., 1986). The investigators compared the recommendations of 50 clinicians for 12 hypothetical cases with those of a decision-analytic model that took each physician's subjective probabilities of various risks and benefits and their utilities for each outcome and combined them to arrive at a recommended action.

The findings (Table 2–2) showed that the decision analysis recommended replacement estrogen far more often than the clinicians did. The physicians most frequently preferred not to treat, thereby minimizing outcomes associated with cancer; the decision analysis never recommended this choice. Clinicians also appeared to feel more *responsible* for bad outcomes caused by their direct action (cancers caused by estrogen treatment they had prescribed) than for bad outcomes that "just happen" (spontaneous fractures due to osteoporosis). Their behavior could not be attributed to ignorance of the facts. The majority knew that progesterone with estrogen will reduce cancer risk to about the level of no treatment but they still avoided this regimen. While there were clear individual differences in the accuracy of probability estimates, on the average they were remarkably accurate. Their estrogen replacement decisions hinged on integration of information, not ignorance of specific risks and benefits. If replicated in other studies, this finding would have important implications for programs of continuing medical education.

Overconfidence and the Illusion of Control

The minimax regret principle does not always imply that a therapeutic action should be avoided. In another study, a group of neurosurgeons favored surgery for a congenital arteriovenous malformation that had not bled, while a decision analysis of the situation suggested that conservative medical management of possible seizures was preferable (Iansek, Elstein, & Balla, 1983), since one could always operate later if that proved necessary at no substantial increase in perioperative mortality. Here, again, the operating cognitive principles seem to have been "minimax regret" and overconfidence in one's own skill. The neurosurgeons wished to avoid the worst possible case—death due to hemorrhage of an operable lesion. They appeared not to consider as carefully the relative probabilities of that event and of an unfavorable neurosurgical outcome.

Their decision making may also have been influenced by (1) the availability bias (Tversky & Kahneman, 1974; see also Turk, Salovey, and Prentice, this volume) in that several recent cases of the condition had been successfully operated on at the local hospital, (2) attribution of good surgical outcomes to the skill of the surgeon and the surgical team, and of bad outcomes to chance and just plain bad luck, and (3) wishful thinking, in this case underestimating the risks of surgery and the chances of perioperative complications. Decision analysis can help to minimize these tendencies by requiring decision makers to be explicit about the perceived benefits and risks of all options and by offering a technique for combining competing risks and benefits that does not use the minimax regret principle.

Utility Assessment

In decision analysis, the assessment of utilities is based on the assumption that a preexisting set of reasonably coherent values exists in someone's head and awaits assessment. The problem is thus conceptualized mainly as a measurement task. The techniques used for utility elicitation are supposed to do just that—elicit preferences, not form them. Furthermore, since preexisting preferences are being elicited, assessments ought to be constant over equivalent presentations of the problem.

The evidence for framing and context effects in utility assessment (Eraker & Sox, 1981; McNeil et al., 1982; Slovic, Fischhoff, & Lichtenstein, 1982; Tversky & Kahneman, 1981) seriously challenges this idealized notion of rational choice. For example, McNeil and her colleagues asked patients and physicians about their preferences for alternative therapies for cancer when the outcomes of these therapies were framed as the probabilities of either living or dying within a fixed period of time. These frames are clearly equivalent presentations of the problem, since life and death are complementary outcomes. Nevertheless, patterns of preference showed a marked sensitivity to the wording of the

TABLE 2–3
Effect of Variation in Frame on Physician and Patient Preferences for Alternative Cancer Therapies

	Percent Preferring	
	Surgery	*Radiation*
Survival frame		
Physicians (n = 87)	84	16
Patients (n = 59)	78	22
Mortality frame		
Physicians (n = 80)	50	50
Patients (n = 60)	40	60

Adapted from McNeil et al., 1982. Reprinted by permission of *The New England Journal of Medicine* from vol. 306 (1982), p. 1261.

problem, which is inconsistent with expected utility theory (see Table 2–3). Apparently innocuous changes in the wording of a question can exert powerful effects on our responses to these questions. In addition, different methods of determining utility values yield different numbers (Holmes, Rovner, Holzman, Rothert, Ravitch, & Elstein, 1982; Read, Quinn, Berwick, Fineberg, & Weinstein, 1984; Torrance, 1976). On occasion, these differences may change the recommended course of action, although how often this occurs is not yet clear.

It becomes increasingly difficult to speak of the utility of a particular outcome independent of the language used to describe it and the context of choice. Yet the normative theory per se offers no guidance as to the proper way to word the options. When these questions concern preferences for outcomes, the answers may have consequences for therapeutic decision making. Some of the most interesting questions now on the research agenda in medical decision making concern problems of measuring utilities in the face of framing and context effects. One recommendation for some protection against the bias that may be inherent in a particular frame is to present the options in several different ways and to explore the meaning and significance of variations in the responses. This caution applies not only to clinicians using formal utility-elicitation techniques to involve their patients in decision making, but also to all clinicians who are conscientiously thinking about options and choices on behalf of their patients.

Validity of Research Findings

In discussions of psychological research, a recurrent question is whether and to what degree findings obtained in the laboratory or under experimental conditions will also prevail in the "real world." Are researchers justified in generalizing from behavior elicited in laboratory studies to real life? The question recurs in a variety of guises: Do responses to attitude questionnaires accurately capture behaviorally expressed attitudes? Are respondents telling investigators what they want to hear or what the respondents think they should say? How closely do preelection polls mirror actual voting? Are people trying to mislead survey researchers? In consumer research, will people who say they like a new product really like it once it is marketed? Ebbesen and Konecni (1980) and Christensen-Szalanski (1986) are among those who have argued that the external validity of laboratory experiments using simulated decision tasks is quite limited and that more studies in real-world environments are needed.

With respect to research on the psychological characteristics of clinical reasoning, the problem usually takes the following form: Suppose an investigator has used brief case vignettes (e.g., Holzman, Ravitch, Metheny, Rothert, Holmes, & Hoppe, 1984) or very tightly constructed decision problems (e.g., Tversky & Kahneman, 1981), as is characteristic of much of the research in the judgment/decision-making mode. Suppose, too, that the results are consistent with the operation of certain cognitive biases or are interpreted as showing that the clinicians studied have made suboptimal decisions. Should the results be believed? Perhaps clinicians behave differently with real patients. Motivational, cognitive, and social arguments are generally advanced to support this criticism of the research model.

The motivational argument holds that cases involving hypothetical patients do not motivate clinicians as much as real cases and that performance decrements are experimental artifacts. It is easy to see why actual situations would be more motivating, and this criticism of psychological research is not confined to the clinical domain. When economists were first presented with data from behavioral decision research showing unexpected violations of expected utility theory, for example, the phenomenon of preference reversals, they countered that people behaved contrary to the theory only in hypothetical situations where real money was not at stake but that in the market, things would be different (Grether & Plott, 1981). The criticism of economists thus hinged essentially on the motivational argument. Psychologists then moved on to show that even when subjects played bets for actual gains and losses of modest sums of money, the phenomenon persisted. Similarly, with respect to psychological research on clinical judgment, even if it is conceded that motivation will be higher in actual practice, evidence from studies using clinical simulations suggests that many forms of case simulation are quite engaging. Furthermore, being in a situation that is conceived of as a test is highly motivating, even if the cases are hypothetical.

The cognitive argument holds that hypothetical case studies invariably omit aspects of the total story and that if these were included, observed performance would more closely approximate what is believed to occur in clinical practice. This criticism ignores the problem of cognitive overload and distraction in actual clinical work. Clinicians commonly have to care for and think about more than one patient at a time. In laboratory studies, however, attention can be focused on one case. It can be argued, therefore, that laboratory studies provide an opportunity to display the best of clinical judgment, undistracted by competing demands. From this view, a more focused story should lead to improvements, not declines, in overall performance. The finding that redundant data serve to increase confidence in diagnostic judgments even when the accuracy of judgment does not increase implies that when brief clinical vignettes are used, thereby severely limiting data collection, clinicians' confidence in their judgments will be low, even if their conclusions are essentially the same as they would reach with additional data. Lack of confidence in judgments may be translated into lack of confidence in the conclusions of the research method, particularly when the research is critical of intuitive judgment.

The cognitive argument thus appears to depend also upon an expectation of excellence and consistency in clinical judgment. A study may be suspect because it demonstrates substantial interclinician variability in judgment while clinicians believe that there is little variability in practice, or because it shows that a simple regression equation can account for 75 percent of the variance in what are believed to be highly complicated, individually tailored judgments (Dawes, 1976). But what if we assume instead that there is substantial variability in practice, an assumption shown to be quite plausible in several contexts (Holzman et al., 1984; Wennberg & Gittelsohn, 1973). Then the validity of the clinical vignettes is strengthened, because they can be interpreted as mirroring variation in practice that clinicians did not know existed. If the vignettes validly reflect variability in clinical practice, why not assume that they validly reflect cognitive processes as well? Similarly, work in the heuristics and biases tradition may be discounted, just as were Meehl's arguments about clinical versus statistical prediction, because both health care providers and consumers have substantial psychological commitments to a belief in clinical expertise and much of this work documents errors and inefficiencies that attack that belief. Confidence in the conclusions of psychological research in this tradition may be bolstered by evidence from health services researchers that documents inefficiencies, such as excessive ordering of laboratory tests (Schroeder, 1974). Indeed, the psychological research on excessive data collection suggests reasons for the phenomenon that go beyond economic incentives and may help to suggest how we should go about educating clinicians so as to minimize this waste.

There are essentially two social arguments in the validity controversy. First, social and behavioral research has shown that clinical decisions are often influenced by social variables or factors of which clinicians may be unaware (Crane, 1975; Eisenberg, 1979; Holmes et al., 1982). If these variables are omitted from a case vignette, their role in judgment simply cannot be assessed. One response to this criticism, of course, is to include social variables in the case vignettes. For example, Farber, Bowman, Major, and Green (1984) systematically varied several social factors (e.g., demographic characteristics) in a series of brief case vignettes, and showed statistically significant effects on decisions regarding critical care of the hypothetical patients. It must be acknowledged, however, that these findings do not demonstrate that these social factors would have comparable effects in actual practice, or that factors dependent on social interaction and negotiation can be so readily represented. On the other hand, it can at least be said that brief written cases are not insensitive to the part played by certain social factors in clinical decisions.

The second argument is more subtle. It holds that clinical decisions are an outcome of interaction among providers (working as a team) and/or between providers and consumers and that a research model focusing on individual cognitive processes cannot possibly do justice to these features. It is true that the literature and perspective assessed in this chapter focus on individual decision making. Indeed, over the years comprehensive reviews of the literature on decision making have noted that they were limited to individual decision making and excluded group decision making, voting, bargaining, and negotiation (e.g., Abelson & Levi, 1985; Einhorn & Hogarth, 1981; Shulman & Elstein, 1975). Whether this limitation invalidates the method for the study of all clinical decision making depends on the setting to which the investigator proposes to generalize.

From my perspective, what is striking about clinical decision making is how much is done by solo clinicians and how little is arrived at by jury type of deliberations. Most ambulatory and inpatient health care decisions are individual decisions, involving at most negotiation between a clinician and a consumer/client/patient—not a group effort. Decisions concerning hospitalized patients may involve negotiation and compromise among a group of health professionals, but here, too, the attitudes, preferences, and judgments of individuals can be assessed as part of understanding how consensus is reached. To my knowledge, no investigator has yet used clinical case summaries as a vehicle to obtain and analyze group discussion and deliberation.

It is always possible to heighten the face validity of a set of clinical cases by introducing additional features and adding to the complexity of the simulation. But how will increased complexity upgrade the performance of a clinician operating within the limitations of "bounded rationality"? If cognitive biases and errors can be elicited in simple environments, is there any logical reason to believe that performance will be better when complexity is increased? Simplicity is also a virtue for the researcher trying to analyze the data. The more features a case has, the more difficult it is to determine which were really crucial. Thus, there is an inescapable trade-off between experimental rigor and clinical face validity. Different investigations will strike the balance at different points on the scale, depending on the context of the research, extent of previous work in the area, and the researchers' own preferences, which may themselves change with time.

The argument for cognitive biases in clinical reasoning does not rest on a single study but on a body of studies, executed at different sites by investigators with diverse backgrounds who used subjects with various types and levels of clinical training. Although individual studies have weaknesses, as always, the weight of the evidence is so substantial that the question of external validity ought to be reformulated. The critical research tasks are (1) to specify more precisely the conditions under which a particular cognitive bias or error will be evoked or suppressed; (2) to assess how prevalent and serious the biases and their effects are, by doing more than collecting anecdotes that point to them; (3) to acquaint clinical practitioners with the conditions under which biased assessments are likely to be produced and to develop cognitive strategies minimizing their effects; (4) to motivate clinicians to employ these strategies (rather than to insist they are unneeded); and (5) to begin to design effective decision supports that will help clinicians surmount the effects of the biases in situations where they can be shown, or are believed, to be detrimental. A pervasive problem will be the neglect of statistical principles in everyday clinical inference (Nisbett, Krantz, Jepson, & Kunda, 1983).

In conclusion, experimental materials should include as many relevant features of actual cases as is feasible. On the other hand, the burden of proof is as much on critics to show that brief case vignettes are seriously invalid as it is on proponents to show that they have adequate external validity. In my opinion, the research reviewed in this paper, and the larger body of work on bounded rationality and human decision processes of which it is a part, make quite a convincing case for the operation of cognitive biases that are consistent with the need to simplify complex task environments into workable problem spaces. It is true that many of the clinical studies reviewed do not unequivocally demonstrate the operation of a particular heuristic and bias; rather, the results can be interpreted as an illustration of that heuristic or bias. The more clinically grounded a study is, the more open it is to other interpretations. The more tightly knit an experiment is, the less equivocal will be its interpretation, but the more vulnerable will it be to the criticism that the study lacks external validity. So we pick our way carefully between these hazards, learning what we can.

Educational Implications

In general, professions are defined by a claim to competence in particular areas that are recognized by others and result in the professional being given a license and mandate to practice that profession (Bucher & Stelling, 1969). Nowhere is this definition more clearly exemplified than in medicine. It is the quintessential profession in the sense that there is a highly respected group of individuals who are believed by the society to have substantial knowledge upon which rational practice serving the client's interest is based. The practice of the profession involves both knowing *how* to do certain things and knowing *when* to do them, both of which involve judgment and decision making. Consequently, it should not be too surprising to learn that the research findings summarized in these pages have met at times with some skepticism, for they question the very basis of the profession's claim to competence. Furthermore, the research asks us to become systematically explicit about matters that have traditionally been implicit and covert in clinical work.

Clinicians have traditionally held clinical judgment in understandably high regard and have been suspicious of attempts to become overly explicit about the art-like elements. Apart from automated interpretation of Minnesota Multiphasic Personality Inventory (MMPI) profiles and related tests, information processing in clinical psychology proceeds largely along traditional lines (Wade & Baker, 1977). Yet the message of this review should not be ignored: clinical inference itself has problems and flaws. The principle of limited rationality has been cited and a partial catalog of nearly two decades of psychological research on clinical inference has been assembled. The bulk of this work has shown that despite expertise and substantial accomplishment in clinical judgment and inference, mistakes are made. Further, some of these mistakes are neither random errors nor due to ignorance of the facts. Some are the results of deeply held but erroneous intuitions about the nature of the events observed in clinical practice and about the workings of chance. Others are the results of limitations in our capacity to deal with very complex problems, which leads us to resort to somewhat simplified problem representations. Difficulties are encountered both in problem structuring and in drawing inferences within a problem structure.

The biases and errors identified by psychological research are apparently deeply rooted, intuitive ways of conceiving of the flow of events and of making choices. When one compares how simple these principles are compared to the mental labor involved in decision analysis, their attractiveness and durability become evident. Yet it should not be held that human nature is unchangeable in this regard. In the course of history, we have changed our conception of the world and of our place in it many times, and that process continues. Indeed, it may be said that education consists of coming to see aspects of the world in a new way, which may at times be quite counterintuitive. So it is, in my judgment, with a probabilistic conception of clinical activity.

Apart from automating interpretation of clinical data, what can be done about these problems?

1. Clinical educators must become aware that the problems exist. One cannot begin to correct a problem whose existence is not acknowledged (see Arnoult & Anderson, as well as Salovey & Turk, this volume).

2. Clinicians-in-training should be taught and encouraged to use a probability scale to express their opinions. This will help to reduce the amount of ambiguous language now used to discuss cases, and will provide a framework within which more formal, Bayesian decision making can be carried out (again, see Arnoult & Anderson, this volume).

3. The use of Bayes's theorem to revise diagnostic probabilities as new evidence comes in should be taught. Other quantitative techniques, such as multiple regression or discriminant functions, can be used for aggregating evidence, as appropriate. These techniques are familiar to many psychologists; all that is new is the application setting (see Wiggins, 1973; and Einhorn, this volume).

4. Not all of the ailments that afflict our information processing will be alleviated by knowledge and technique. Framing effects have been described as a type of cognitive illusion. Like optical illusions, they may persist even though we know we are being fooled. In this circumstance, we can deliberately employ multiple perspectives or frames, analogous to the method of multiple competing hypotheses in the differential diagnosis, test if preference is affected by frame change, and ask if it should be (see chapters by Jordan, Harvey, & Weary and by Snyder & Thomsen, this volume).

5. The cognitive biases described in this chapter can make decisions reached using normatively correct procedures seem counterintuitive. The procedures ought not to be dismissed simply because their outputs do not conform to our intuition. Clinical education can and should focus on acquainting clinicians with the psychological characteristics of everyday clinical reasoning and with normatively correct strategies for dealing with probabilistic information. The two activities should proceed together, for without a healthy—but not paralyzing—distrust of clinical intuition, it may be difficult to motivate the acquisition of formal quan-

titative strategies for information processing and judgment. On the other hand, human judgment will continue to be needed, and so clinicians should understand both its strengths and limitations. Efforts along these lines are already under way in the medical domain (Balla, 1985; Cebul, Beck, & Carroll, 1985; Howe, Holmes, & Elstein, 1984; Sackett, Haynes, & Tugwell, 1985; Weinstein & Fineberg, 1980; Zarin & Pauker, 1984; and the series of cases published by Pauker and his co-workers in *Medical Decision Making*). Clinical psychology should also respond thoughtfully and constructively to these ideas, a primary goal of the present volume.

Descriptive studies of clinical decision making that are grounded in significant psychological theory are needed. It is not enough to simply collect data about clinicians' preferences for one act or another. We need to understand the psychological processes by which actions are judged and choices are made. These studies will help to sharpen the contrast between normative models of rational thought and everyday clinical reasoning, and so identify how intuitive problem representations should be revised or reexamined. Moreover, by calling attention to problems in everyday clinical inference and decision making, normative formal principles may gradually become more ingrained in our thinking (Elstein, 1982; Nisbett, Krantz, Jepson, & Kunda, 1983). The most valuable outputs of psychological research in this domain should be greater insight into how we intuitively deal with complex choices and trade-offs, increased awareness of the need for improved techniques for deliberating about these dilemmas, and useful tools for thinking more clearly about increasingly thorny problems.

Acknowledgments

Earlier versions of this chapter were presented at the Conference on Medical Information Sciences held at the University of Texas Health Science Center, San Antonio, July 1, 1985; at the 1985 annual meeting of the Henry J. Kaiser Family Foundation Faculty Scholars in General Internal Medicine; and at a symposium on Medical Understanding and Its Limits held at the American Association of Medical Colleges (AAMC) Conference on Research in Medical Education, October 1985.

The comments of John Barrand, Lionel Bernstein, Marilyn Rothert, Paul Slovic, and Robert Wigton were very helpful. James Dod's thoroughness in checking references and proofreading, and the patience of Sandy Tarter and Anise Brown with repeated drafts, are sincerely appreciated. Preparation of this chapter was supported in part by grants from the Josiah Macy, Jr., Foundation, #B8520004, and from the National Library of Medicine, IM-4583.

References

Abelson, R. P. & Levi, A. (1985). Decision making and decision theory. In G. Lindzey & E. Aronson (Eds.), *Handbook of social psychology* (3rd ed.) (Vol. 1). New York: Random House.

Balla, J. I. (1985). *The diagnostic process: A model for clinical teachers.* New York: Cambridge University Press.

Balla, J. I., Elstein, A. S., & Gates, P. (1983). Effects of prevalence and test diagnosticity upon clinical judgments of probability. *Methods of Information in Medicine, 22,* 25–28.

Balla, J. I., Iansek, R., & Elstein, A. (1985). Bayesian diagnosis in the presence of pre-existing disease. *Lancet,* #8424, February 9, 326–329.

Bartlett, F. C. (1958). *Thinking.* New York: Basic Books.

Bell, D. E. (1982). Regret in decision making under uncertainty. *Operations Research, 30,* 961–980.

Berwick, D. M., Fineberg, H. V., & Weinstein, M. C. (1981). When doctors meet numbers. *American Journal of Medicine, 71,* 991–998.

Borak, J., and Veilleux, S. (1982). Errors of intuitive logic among physicians. *Social Science and Medicine, 16,* 1939–1947.

Bryant, G. D., & Norman, G. R. (1980). Expressions of probability: Words and numbers. *New England Journal of Medicine, 302,* 411.

Bucher, R., & Stelling, J. (1969). Characteristics of professional organizations. *Journal of Health and Social Behavior, 10,* 3–15.

Carroll, J. S. (1980). Analyzing decision behavior: The magician's audience. In T. S. Wallsten (Ed.), *Cognitive processes in choice and decision behavior.* Hillsdale, NJ: Erlbaum.

Casscells, W., Schoenberger, A., & Graboys, T. B. (1978). Interpretation by physicians of clinical laboratory results. *New England Journal of Medicine, 299,* 999–1001.

Cebul, R. D., Beck, L. M., & Carroll, J. G. (1985). *Teaching clinical decision making.* New York: Praeger.

Christensen-Szalanski, J. J. (1986). Improving the practical utility of judgment research. In B. Brehmer, H. Jungermann, P. Lourens, & E. G. Sevon (Eds.), *New directions in research on decision making.* New York: Elsevier-North Holland.

Christensen-Szalanski, J. J., Beck, D. E., Christensen-Szalanski, C. M., & Koepsell, T. D. (1983). Effects of expertise and experience on risk judgments. *Journal of Applied Psychology, 68,* 278–284.

Clancey, W. J. (1984). Acquiring, representing and evaluating a competence model of diagnostic strategy. Stanford University Heuristic Programming Project.

Clancey, W. J., & Shortliffe, E. H. (Eds.). (1984). *Readings in medical artificial intelligence: The first decade.* Reading, MA: Addison-Wesley.

Committee on Evaluation in General Internal Medicine. (1979). *Clinical competence in internal medicine.* Philadelphia: American Board of Internal Medicine.

Crane, D. (1975). *The sanctity of social life.* New York: Russell Sage Foundation.

Curley, S. P., Eraker, S. A., & Yates, J. F. (1984). An investigation of patients' reactions to therapeutic uncertainty. *Medical Decision Making, 4,* 501–511.

Dawes, R. M. (1976). Shallow psychology. In J. S. Carroll & J. W. Payne (Eds.), *Cognition and social behavior.* Hillsdale, NJ: Erlbaum.

______. (1979). The robust beauty of improper linear models in decision making. *American Psychologist, 34,* 571–582.

Duda, R. O., & Shortliffe, E. H. (1983). Expert systems research. *Science, 220,* 261–268.

Ebbesen, E. B., & Konecni, V. J. (1980). On the external validity of decision-making research: What do we know about decisions in the real world? In T. S. Wallsten (Ed.), *Cognitive processes in choice and decision behavior.* Hillsdale, NJ: Erlbaum.

Eddy, D. M. (1982). Probabilistic reasoning in clinical medicine: Problems and opportunities. In D. Kahneman, P. Slovic, & A. Tversky (Eds.). *Judgment under uncertainty: Heuristics and biases.* New York: Cambridge University Press.

Eddy, D. M., & Clanton, C. H. (1982). The art of diagnosis: Solving the clinicopathological exercise. *New England Journal of Medicine, 306,* 1263–1268.

Einhorn, H. J., & Hogarth, R. M. (1981). Behavioral decision theory: Processes of judgment and choice. *Annual Review of Psychology, 32,* 53–88.

______. (1985). Ambiguity and uncertainty in probabilistic inference. *Psychological Review, 92,* 433–461.

Eisenberg, J. M. (1979). Sociological influences on decision-making by clinicians. *Annals of Internal Medicine, 90,* 957–964.

Elstein, A. S. (1982). Comment on "Errors of intuitive logic among physicians." *Social Science and Medicine, 16,* 1945–46.

Elstein, A. S., Holzman, G. B., Ravitch, M. M., Metheny, W. A., Holmes, M. M., Hoppe, R. B., Rothert, M. L., & Rovner, D. R. (1986). Comparison of physicians' decisions regarding estrogen replacement therapy for menopausal women and decisions derived from a decision analytic model. *American Journal of Medicine, 80,* 246–258.

Elstein, A. S., Shulman, L. S., Sprafka, S. A., et al. (1978). *Medical problem solving: An analysis of clinical reasoning.* Cambridge, MA: Harvard University Press.

Eraker, S., & Politser, P. E. (1982). How decisions are reached: Physician and patient. *Annals of Internal Medicine, 97,* 262–268.

Eraker, S. A., & Sox, H. C. (1981). Assessment of patients' preferences for therapeutic outcomes. *Medical Decision Making, 1,* 29–39.

Farber, N. J., Bowman, S. M., Major, D. A. & Green, W. P. (1984). Cardiopulmonary resuscitation (CPR): Patient factors and decision making. *Archives of Internal Medicine, 144,* 2229–2232.

Feinstein, A. R. (1985). The "chagrin factor" and qualitative decision analysis. *Archives of Internal Medicine,* 145, 1257–1259.

Feltovich, P. J., Johnson, P. E., Moller, J. H., & Swanson, D. B. (1984). LCS: The role and development of medical knowledge in diagnostic expertise. In W. J. Clancey & E. H. Shortliffe (Eds.), *Readings in medical artificial intelligence: The first decade.* Reading, MA: Addison-Wesley.

Feltovich, P. J., & Patel, V. L. (1984). *The pursuit of understanding in clinical reasoning.* Paper presented at the American Educational Research Association, April.

Fischhoff, B. (1980). Clinical decision analysis. *Operations Research, 28,* 28–43.

Fischhoff, B., Goitein, B., & Shapira, Z. (1982). The experienced utility of expected utility approaches. In N. T. Feather (Ed.), *Expectations and actions: Expectancy value models in psychology.* Hillsdale, NJ: Erlbaum.

Fox, J. (1984). Formal and knowledge-based methods in decision technology. *Acta Psychologia, 56,* 303–331.

Gagne, R. (1984). Learning outcomes and their effects: Useful categories of human performance. *American Psychologist, 39,* 377–385.

Goldberg, L. R. (1970). Man versus model of man: A rationale, plus some evidence, for a method of improving on clinical inferences. *Psychological Bulletin, 73,* 422–432.

———. (1968). Simple models or simple processes? Some research on clinical judgments. *American Psychologist, 23,* 483–496.

Grether, D. M., & Plott, C. R. (1981). Economic theory of choice and the preference reversal phenomenon. *The American Economic Review. 69,* 623–638.

Griner, P. F., Mayewski, R. J., Mushlin, A. I., & Greenland, P. (1981). Selection and interpretation of diagnostic tests and procedures: Principles and applications. *Annals of Internal Medicine, 94,* 553–600.

Groen, G. J. & Patel, V. L. (1985). Medical problem-solving: Some questionable assumptions. *Medical Education, 19,* 95–100.

Hammond, K. R. (1971). Computer graphics as an aid to learning. *Science, 172,* 903–908.

Heckerman, D. (1985). Probabilistic interpretations for MYCIN's certainty factors. AAAI/IEEE Workshop on Uncertainty and Probability in Artificial Intelligence. Los Angeles, August.

Hershey, J. C., & Schoemaker, P. J. H. (1985). Probability versus certainty equivalence methods in utility measurement: Are they equivalent? *Management Science, 31,* 1213–1231.

Hogarth, R. M. (1980). *Judgment and choice.* New York: Wiley.

Holmes, M. M., Rovner, D. R., Holzman, G. B., Rothert, M. L., Ravitch, M. M., & Elstein, A. S. (1982). Factors affecting laboratory utilization in clinical practice. *Medical Decision Making, 2,* 471–482.

Holzman, G. B., Ravitch, M. M., Metheny, W. A., Rothert, M. L., Holmes, M. M., Hoppe, R. B. (1984). Physicians' judgments about estrogen replacement therapy for menopausal women. *Obstetrics and Gynecology, 63,* 303–311.

Horowitz, L. M., French, R., Lapid, J. S., & Weckler, D. (1982). Symptoms and interpersonal problems: The prototype as an integrating concept. In J. C. Anchin & D. J. Kiesler (Eds.), *Handbook of interpersonal psychotherapy.* Oxford, England: Pergamon.

Howe, K. R., Holmes, M., & Elstein, A. S. (1984). Teaching clinical decision making. *Journal of Medicine and Philosophy,* 9, 215–228.

Iansek, R., Elstein, A. S., & Balla, J. I. (1983). Application of decision analysis to cerebral arteriovenous malformation. *Lancet, 21,* 1132–1135.

Johnson, P. E. (1983). What kind of expert should a system be? *Journal of Medicine and Philosophy, 8,* 77–97.

Johnson, P. E., Duran, A. S., Hassebrock, F., Moller, J., Prietula, M., Feltovich, P., & Swanson, D. B. (1981). Expertise and error in diagnostic reasoning. *Cognitive Science, 5,* 235–285.

Kahneman, D., Slovic, P., & Tversky, A. (Eds.). (1982). *Judgment under uncertainty: Heuristics and biases.* New York: Cambridge University Press.

Kahneman D., & Tversky, A. (1973). On the psychology of prediction. *Psychological Review, 80,* 237–251.

———. (1979). Prospect theory: An analysis of decision under risk. *Econometrica, 47,* 263–291.

Kassirer, J. P., & Gorry, G. A. (1978). Clinical problem solving: A behavioral analysis. *Annals of Internal Medicine, 89,* 245–255.

Kassirer, J. P., Kuipers, B. J., & Gorry, G. A. (1982). Toward a theory of clinical expertise. *American Journal of Medicine, 73,* 251–259.

Keeney, R. L. (1982). Decision analysis: An overview. *Operations Research, 30,* 803–836.

Kern, L., & Doherty, M. E. (1982). "Pseudodiagnosticity" in an idealized medical problem-solving environment. *Journal of Medical Education, 57,* 100–104.

Kleinmuntz, B. (1968). The processing of clinical information by man and machine. In B. Kleinmuntz (Ed.), *Formal representation of human judgment.* New York: Wiley.

Kunz, J. C., Shortliffe, E. H., Buchanan, B. G., & Feigenbaum, E. A. (1984). Computer-assisted decision making in medicine. *Journal of Medicine and Philosophy, 9,* 135–160.

Larkin, J., McDermott, J., Simon, D. P., & Simon, H. A. (1980). Expert and novice performance in solving physics problems. *Science, 208,* 1335–1342.

Lopes, L. L. (1981). Decision making in the short run. *Journal of Experimental Psychology: Human Learning and Memory, 7,* 377–385.

McNeil, B. J., Pauker, S. G., Sox, H. C., & Tversky, A. (1982). On the elicitation of preferences for alternative therapies. *New England Journal of Medicine, 306,* 1259–1262.

Meehl, P. E. (1954). *Clinical versus statistical prediction: A theoretical analysis and a review of the evidence.* Minneapolis: University of Minnesota Press.

———. (1957). When shall we use our heads instead of the formula? *Journal of Counseling Psychology, 4,* 268–273.

Miller, R. A., Pople, H. E., Jr., & Myers, J. D. (1982). Internist-I, an experimental computer-based diagnostic consultant for general internal medicine. *New England Journal of Medicine, 307,* 468–476.

Nakao, M. A. and Axelrod, S. (1983). Numbers are better than words: Verbal specifications of frequency have no place in medicine. *American Journal of Medicine, 74,* 1061–1065.

Narragon, E. A. (1980). Decision analysis. In E. A. Narragon (Ed.), *A study manual for operations research.* Education and Examination Committee, Society of Actuaries and Casualty Actuarial Society, Printing Department, University of Chicago.

Neufeld, V. R., Norman, G. R., Feightner, J. W., & Barrows, H. S. (1981).

Clinical problem-solving by medical students: A cross-sectional and longitudinal analysis. *Medical Education, 15,* 315–322.

Newell, A. & Simon, H. A. (1972). *Human problem solving.* Englewood Cliffs, NJ: Prentice-Hall.

Nisbett, R. E., Borgida, E., Crandall, R., & Reed, H. (1976). Popular induction: Information is not always informative. In J. S. Carroll & J. W. Payne (Eds.), *Cognition and social behavior, 2,* 227–236.

Nisbett, R. E., Krantz. D. H., Jepson, C., & Kunda, Z. (1983). The use of statistical heuristics in everyday inductive reasoning. *Psychological Review, 90,* 339–363.

Nisbett, R. E. & Ross, L. (1980). *Human inference: Strategies and shortcomings of social judgment.* Englewood Cliffs, NJ: Prentice-Hall.

Oskamp, S. (1965). Overconfidence in case study judgments. *Journal of Consulting Psychology, 29,* 261–265.

Polanyi, M. (1958). *Personal knowledge.* Chicago: University of Chicago Press.

Politser, P. E. (1981). Decision analysis and clinical judgment: A re-evaluation. *Medical Decision Making, 1,* 361–389.

———. (1984). Explanations of statistical concepts: Can they penetrate the haze of Bayes? *Methods of Information in Medicine, 23,* 99–108.

Pople, H. E. (1982). Heuristic methods for imposing structure on ill-structured problems: The structuring of medical diagnostics. In P. Szolovits (Ed.), *Artificial intelligence in medicine.* Boulder, CO: Westview Press.

Raiffa, H. (1968). *Decision analysis: Introductory lectures on choice under uncertainty.* Reading, MA: Addison-Wesley.

Read, J. L., Quinn, R. J., Berwick, D. M., Fineberg, H. V., & Weinstein, M. C. (1984). Preferences for health outcomes: Comparison of assessment methods. *Medical Decision Making, 4,* 315–329.

Sackett, D. L., Haynes, R. B., & Tugwell, P. (1985). *Clinical epidemiology: A basic science for clinical medicine.* Boston: Little, Brown.

Schoemaker, P. J. H. (1980). *Experiments on decisions under risk: The expected utility hypothesis.* Boston: Martinus Nijhoff.

———. (1982). The expected utility model: its variants, purposes, evidence and limitations. *Journal of Economic Literature, 20,* 529–563.

Schön, D. A. (1984). The crisis of professional knowledge and the pursuit of an epistemology of practice. Harvard Business School 75th Anniversary Colloquium on Teaching by the Case Method. Cambridge, MA: Harvard Business School.

Schroeder, S. A. (1980). Variations in physican practice patterns: A review of medical cost implications. In E. J. Carels, D. Neuhauser, & W. B. Stason (Eds.), *The physician and cost control.* Cambridge: MA: Oelgeschlager, Gunn & Hain.

Schroeder, S. A. (1974). Variation among physicians in use of laboratory tests: Relation to quality of care. *Medical Care, 12,* 709–713.

Shortliffe, E. H. (1976). *Computer-based medical consultations: MYCIN.* New York: Elsevier.

Shortliffe, E. H., & Buchanan, B. G. (1975). A model of inexact reasoning in medicine. *Mathematical Biosciences, 23,* 351–379.

Shulman, L. S., & Elstein, A. S. (1975). Studies of problem solving, judgment and decision making: Implications for educational research. In F. N. Kerlinger (Ed.), *Review of Research in Education, 3,* 3–42.

Simon, H. A. (1979). Information processing models of cognition. *Annual Review of Psychology, 30,* 363–396.

Slovic, P., Fischhoff, B., & Lichtenstein, S. (1982). Response mode, framing, and information-processing effects in risk assessment. In R. M. Hogarth (Ed.), *New directions for methodology of social and behavioral science: Question framing and response consistency,* No. 11. San Francisco: Jossey-Bass.

Slovic, P., & Lichtenstein, S. (1971). Comparison of Bayesian and regression approaches to the study of information processing in judgment. *Organizational Behavior and Human Performance, 6,* 648–744.

Slovic, P., Lichtenstein, S., & Fischhoff, B. (in press). Decision making. In R. C. Atkinson, R. J. Herrnstein, G. Lindzey, & R. D. Luce (Eds.), *Stevens' handbook of experimental psychology* (2nd ed.). New York: Wiley.

Slovic, P., & Tversky, A. (1974). Who accepts Savage's axiom? *Behavioral Science, 19,* 368–373.

Szolovits, P. (Ed.) (1982). *Artificial intelligence in medicine.* Boulder, CO: Westview Press.

Torrance, G. W. (1976). Social preferences for health states: An empirical evaluation of three measurement techniques. *Socio-Economic Planning Science, 10,* 129–136.

Tversky, A., & Kahneman, D. (1974). Judgment under uncertainty: Heuristics and biases. *Science, 185,* 1124–1131.

———. (1981). The framing of decisions and the psychology of choice. *Science, 211,* 453–8.

———. (1986). Rational choice and the framing of decisions. *Journal of Business, 59,* 5251–5278.

Von Neumann, J. & Morgenstern, O. (1947). *Theory of games and economic behavior.* Princeton: Princeton University Press.

Wade, T. C., & Baker, T. B. (1977). Opinions and use of psychological tests: A survey of clinical psychologists. *American Psychologist, 32,* 874–882.

Waldrop, M. M. (1984). The necessity of knowledge. *Science, 223,* 1279–1282.

Wallsten, T. S. (1981). Physician and medical student bias in evaluating information. *Medical Decision Making, 1,* 145–164.

Wason, P. C., & Johnson-Laird, P. N. (1972). *Psychology of reasoning: Structure and content.* Cambridge, MA: Harvard University Press.

Weinstein, M. C., & Fineberg, H. V. (1980). *Clinical decision analysis.* Philadelphia: Saunders.

Wennberg, J., & Gittelsohn, A. (1973). Small area variations in health care delivery. *Science, 182,* 1102–1108.

Wiggins, J. S. (1973). *Personality and prediction: Principles of personality assessment.* Reading, MA: Addison-Wesley.

Wigton, R. S., Hoellerich, V. L., & Patil, K. D. (1986). How physicians use clinical information in diagnosing pulmonary embolism: An application of conjoint analysis. *Medical Decision Making, 6,* 2–11.

Wolf, F. M., Gruppen, L. D., & Billi, J. E. (1985). Differential diagnosis and the competing hypotheses heuristic: A practical approach to judgment under uncertainty and Bayesian probability. *Journal of the American Medical Association, 253,* 2858–2862.

Wright, G. (1984). *Behavioural decision theory.* New York: Penguin.

Zarin, D., & Pauker, S. G. (1984). Decision analysis as a basis for medical decision making: The tree of Hippocrates. *Journal of Medicine and Philosophy, 9,* 181–213.

3 Diagnosis and Causality in Clinical and Statistical Prediction

Hillel J. Einhorn

I BEGIN with the following clinical prediction: the clinical versus statistical prediction controversy (Dawes, 1979; Meehl, 1954; Sawyer, 1966) will intensify as the use of personal computers continues to grow. The reason is simple; more people will learn about, have access to, and in some cases, be required to use computers to perform a variety of tasks, including the making of complex judgments and decisions. Furthermore, as pointed out in a recent report to the National Academy of Sciences (Simon, 1986), the use of "expert systems" and "artificial intelligence" will become more widespread, raising many questions about how, or if, human and machine intelligence should be combined.

The purpose of this chapter is to understand the roots of the controversy. Three basic arguments are advanced: (1) Clinical *and* statistical prediction rest on diagnostic processes that are causal and constructive. Such processes result in a model of the phenomenon, from which predictions are made. (2) The lack of awareness that predictions depend on prior diagnostic inference can lead to incorrect assessments of forecast accuracy, overconfidence, and the confusion of diagnostic and prognostic probabilities. (3) The clinical and statistical approaches differ with respect to what is considered an acceptable level of accuracy in prediction. In particular, the statistical approach accepts error as inevitable while the clinical approach does not. After discussing these issues, a decision analysis is introduced to examine the costs and benefits of subscribing to each position.

Diagnostic Inference in Clinical Judgment

In attempting to predict behavior, the clinician first looks backwards in time to understand the determinants of current behavior. Thus, symptoms, signs, and the like, are seen as manifestations of a causal process and the diagnostic task is to use backward inference to connect observable effects to prior causes. It is contended that diagnostic, backward inference depends on skills of construction based on causal thinking. Such skills include hypothesis formation and change, identifying relevant causal variables, linking those variables in causal chains or scenarios, assessing the strength of those chains, and evaluating alternative explanations. The clinician, like the historian, has much latitude (or degrees of freedom) in reconstructing the past to make the present seem most likely (a kind of maximum likelihood approach). However, the specific processes by which hypotheses are first generated from data are poorly understood (cf. Elstein, Shulman, & Sprafka, 1978; Gettys & Fisher, 1979). Nevertheless, it seems likely that they involve the use of analogy, metaphor, and other aspects of similarity. Thus, in attempting to explain a phenomenon that is not understood, a search is made for one that is and that has similar features. Bronowski (1978) has put this well by noting that

> every act of imagination is the discovery of likeness between two things which were thought unlike. And the example I gave was Newton's thinking of likeness between the thrown apple and the moon sailing majestically in the sky. A most improbable likeness, but one which turned out to be (if you will forgive the phrase) enormously fruitful. (pp. 109–110)

It is interesting to note that hypothesis formation is not well handled within formal statistical systems. Indeed, Suppes (1966) points out that the Bayesian view of statistical inference cannot deal with the generation of entirely new concepts from data, since there is no mechanism for concept formation. Furthermore, an important aspect of hypothesis generation is that hypotheses can be enlarged, narrowed, and otherwise modified to provide a causal model that accounts for the data of interest. This process is therefore constructive in nature. However, in most formal approaches, evidence affects the probability of given hypotheses without changing the hypotheses themselves. To see the difference, consider Agatha Christie's *Murder on the Orient Express.* After a murder is committed aboard the train, Inspector Poirot seems to start with 12 mutually exclusive and exhaustive suspects. As we discover to our surprise, all 12 did it! Alternatively, consider a therapist who holds several hypotheses regarding what disorder a client has and arrives at a diagnosis in which the client has disorder A with complications due to disorder B. Such creative syntheses of hypotheses into new, more complex entities are not well handled by formal models. In the first case, it might be argued that Inspector Poirot considered all possible combinations of hypotheses in advance but this is clearly stretching information-processing requirements, even for the remarkable Poirot. In the second example, it is clear that an a priori enumeration of all possible combinations of diseases is impossible. Thus, changing hypotheses rather than changing the probabilities of hypotheses is involved.

The need to enlarge and form complex hypotheses has important implications for formal inferential methods, especially with regard to the practical problems of defining sets of mutually exclusive and exhaustive hypotheses. For example, consider the hypotheses that a patient has schizophrenia (H) or not (~H). It is clear that having schizophrenia and not having schizophrenia cannot coexist. However, of what exactly does ~H consist? Does it include other disorders such as mental retardation, Korsakoff's psychosis, or a drug-induced psychosis? Does it also include conjunctions of these other disorders? Can it include complex disorders in which schizophrenia is a conjunct? The last alternative of these other disorders may *also* be schizophrenic. Furthermore, if ~H contains other disorders, then the intersection of H with, say, drug-induced psychosis is no longer null since a patient could have both. That is, a patient being treated for a drug-induced psychosis may actually have a long history of schizophrenia. Such difficulties pose major problems in developing formal models of hypothesis construction and change that adhere to the usual canons of statistical theory. In any event, the modeling of constructive processes in diagnosis remains a major challenge for future research.

Cues-to-Causality as Constraints on Hypothesis Construction

Since diagnostic inference is essentially causal, it is necessary to discuss the relevant aspects of causal inference as they relate to hypothesis construction. Einhorn and Hogarth (1986) have recently proposed that judgments of probable cause are made up of four components: (1) probabilistic indicators of causal relations, called "cues-to-causality"; these include temporal order, covariation, contiguity in time and space, and similarity of cause and effect; (2) a causal field or context in which judgments of probable cause are made; (3) judgmental strategies used for combining the causal field with the cues-to-causality; and (4) the discounting of causal strength by alternative explanations. The first three aspects are briefly considered here.

The construction of a causal model goes hand in hand with the assessment of the strength of that model. Both involve cues-to-causality such as temporal order (causes precede effects in time), contiguity in time and space (one typically seeks causes that are close to the effect in time and space), covariation (causes tend to covary with effects), and similarity of cause and effect (including physical similarity, analogy and metaphor, and congruity of length and strength between cause and effect). The cues serve two related functions. First, they indicate likely directions in which to seek relevant variables. Second, they constrain the number of causal scenarios or chains that can be constructed to link causal candidates to their supposed effects.

To illustrate, consider that you are interested in predicting outbreaks of mass hysteria. You first note the following tendency: Six months before an outbreak, increased sunspot activity often occurs (a related hypothesis about the business cycle and sunspots was in fact advanced by the eminent 19th-century economist Jevons [1984]). Note that several cues-to-causality are engaged here; temporal order and covariation are both consistent with a causal relation, while low contiguity in time and space are not. In addition, there does not seem to be a way of directly linking the two events. At this point, one must construct a causal chain that bridges the spatial and temporal gap. If such a chain cannot be constructed, no causal relation will be seen. Hence, causal relations must be "achieved" in the sense that prior knowledge and imagination are needed to construct a schema, scenario, or chain, to link cause and effect. Now imagine the following chain: Sunspots affect weather conditions, which affect agricultural production, which affects diet, which leads to mass hysteria about gastrointestinal disease. The construction of this chain is constrained both by the cues of contiguity in time and space and by congruity (length and strength of cause and effect). Consider the role of contiguity in time and space. In order to link sunspots and mass hysteria, the spatial and temporal gaps must be bridged by positing a change in weather, etc. Imagine, however, that mass hysteria occurs immediately after sunspot activity, rather than six months later. The closeness in time between the two events precludes the weather–diet scenario since that chain requires a time delay between cause and effect. Hence, to link sunspots and mass hysteria, one would have to construct another story that is consistent with high contiguity in time. Similarly, imagine taking up smoking and getting lung cancer the next week. It seems highly unlikely that smoking is the cause since a causal chain with high contiguity in time is not easy to construct.

Now consider the incongruity between cause and effect; that is, small causes–big effects or big causes–small effects. To account for this, the causal chain must involve some type of "amplification" in the first case and "dampening" in the second. For example, consider the incongruity between germs and illness, as exemplified in the germ theory of disease. When Pasteur advanced this theory it must have seemed incredible to his contemporaries that invisible creatures caused death, plagues, and so on.

Without knowledge of how germs enter the body, multiply, disseminate through the system, and are communicated to others, there was no causal chain that could amplify such small causes to produce the large effects.[1]

[1]Although the diagnostic process involves the construction of causal chains, the strength of those chains is an important consideration in judging the adequacy of a causal hypothesis. Recently, Einhorn and Hogarth (1986) have proposed the following model to account for the strength of a causal chain. Let c_j be the absolute size of the correlation of variables at the *j*th link in the chain ($j = 1, 2, \ldots, J$), and let Q_L denote the strength of the chain. It is assumed that (a) if one cannot construct a causal chain, the hypothesis or explanation is given no attention and $Q_L = 0$; (b) the construction of a causal chain is constrained by the cues of contiguity (in time and space), and congruity between cause and effect; and (c) the strength of a chain can be modeled by the equation,

$$Q_L = \prod_{j=1}^{J} c_j \qquad (j = 1, \ldots, J) \tag{1}$$

By assuming a multiplicative function, equation (1) implies the following: (a) The strength of a chain is equal to its weakest link. Thus, if c_1 has the lowest link strength in the chain, Q_L is at best equal to C_1 (if all other links are 1). Indeed, note that if any $c_j = 0$, $Z_L = 0$, regardless of the strength of the other links; (b) Because c_j is between 0 and 1, the longer the chain (J), the lower the strength of the whole chain (since one is multiplying fractions). This makes clear why the sunspot–business cycle scenario is implausible on the basis of Q_L. Since $J = 4$ in that chain, even if all $c_j = .5$, for example, Q_L is still only .065 (i.e., $.5^4$). Therefore, longer chains are generally weaker than short ones. However, equation (1) also implies that if all the C_j's are high, the length of the chain is less important in affecting Q_L. Indeed, if $c_j = 1$ for all j, the length of the chain is irrelevant.

To illustrate how the cues-to-causality can reduce the number of explanations for an event, consider an analogous situation involving the perception of a scene that contains k cues (Hogarth, 1982). In viewing such a scene, one can pay attention to any combination of i cues ($i = 1,2,\ldots, k$). For example, if only one cue is used, there are k possible perceptions based on each cue. If two cues are used, ${}_kC_2$ combinations of cues are possible, and so on. If one considers all possible combinations of i cues out of k, there are m combinations, where m is given by,

$$m = \sum_{i=1}^{k} ({}_kC_i) \tag{2}$$

If the order in which the cues are processed affects the perception of the scene, there are $i!$ (i factorial) permutations or orders in which the cues can be processed. Therefore, the total number of different combinations and permutations of cues can be given by,

$$n = \sum_{i=1}^{k} [({}_kC_i)\,(i\,!)] \tag{3}$$

To appreciate the above, note that for a scene with only 10 cues ($k = 10$), $n = 9{,}864{,}100$.

When a clinician is confronted with just 10 pieces of information, people cannot evaluate the almost 10 million different possible diagnoses based on the nearly 10 million different combinations of these data. Instead, by attending to the cues-to-causality, they are able to reduce the number of possible interpretations to manageable proportions. To illustrate, in the above example, consider that 3 cues can be ignored because of constraints having to do with lighting conditions ($k = 7$). Moreover, if the cues must follow a particular order (as in the construction of a causal chain or scenario), the number of possible interpretations is reduced to 127. Since other cues also constrain the type of causal chain, the number of possible interpretations is reduced further.

Presuppositions and the Causal Field

The idea of a causal field was introduced by the philosopher Mackie (1965, 1974), to account for why some variables are considered to be casually "relevant" while others are not. Mackie argued that judgments of causal relevance are related to the degree that a variable is a "difference-in-a-background." This means that factors that are part of some presumed background or causal field are judged to be of little or no causal relevance. For example, does birth cause death? Although birth is both necessary and sufficient for death (and therefore covaries perfectly with it), it seems odd to consider one the cause of the other. Rather, because death presupposes birth, birth is part of the causal field and its causal relevance is low. The concept of a causal field has three important implications for clinical judgment: (1) What events/outcomes trigger causal reasoning? (2) How are causes distinguished from conditions? and, (3) How do shifts in the causal field affect causal relevance? (See also the chapter by Smith, this volume, for further discussion of the difficulties in perceiving elements in a complex context or field like the clinic.)

1. Much psychological research indicates that processes of perception and judgment are sensitive to differences or deviations from present states and reference points (e.g., Helson, 1968; Kahneman & Tversky, 1979; Smith, this volume). Therefore, diagnostic curiosity is usually triggered by noting that something is abnormal or unusual. Indeed, in reviewing research on spontaneous causal reasoning, Weiner (1985) found that the search for a causal explanation is typically elicited by an unexpected event: for example, a win by an underdog, suicide by an individual not obviously depressed, more or less profits than expected, and so on. Thus, one rarely seeks the cause of why one feels "average," why traffic flowed normally, or why some accident is typical. To be sure, the need for causal explanations can be aroused vis-à-vis normal events. However, this is most likely to occur when the events violate expectations and are therefore seen as unusual after all. For example, we might want to know why traffic flowed normally if major highway improvements were just completed, or why we feel average after hearing about a death in the family.

2. It is important to note that not all differences-in-a-background are seen as causally relevant. In particular, one must distinguish between causes and conditions. Consider diseases that are confined to particular segments of the population; for example, Alzheimer's disease is generally found in old people. It seems strange to say that old age causes Alzheimer's disease. Rather, old age is seen as a condition that when conjoined with some other event(s) such as exposure to a virus, toxic substance, or bacteria, produces the disease. The distinction between causes and conditions is highly dependent on some assumed context. However, as Mackie argued (1974), perceptions of causes are typically

distinguished from conditions in that (i) events are more causal than standing conditions (viruses are more causal than being old); (ii) intrusive events are more causal than events that usually occur; (iii) something abnormal or wrong is more causal than what is normal and right (e.g., the car accident was caused by the person veering to the left, not by the other person who drove straight ahead).

3. The causal field helps to explain why variables considered as causally relevant at one level of analysis are not relevant at a different level. For example, at one level it could be said that turning on a switch causes a light bulb to be lit. At a lower level of analysis, it might be stated that the light was caused by electricity flowing into the bulb and heating the filament (Cook & Campbell, 1979). Since causal relevance is at least a difference-in-a-field, a cause at one level will not necessarily be relevant at another. Furthermore, the appropriate level at which to infer causality depends on one's purposes and the extent of one's presumed knowledge of the phenomenon in question. For example, a clinician interviewing a distressed woman may assume that her difficulties are rooted in her husband's inattention to her. Hence, inattention is seen as the first link in the causal chain. But what if the husband has few skills for coping with a stressful work situation and is preoccupied by job demands and anxiety? At this more microscopic level, the cause of this woman's distress might be her husband's coping deficiencies. Indeed, an important distinction between clinical and statistical approaches concerns the level of causal analysis that is viewed as desirable. Specifically, the clinical approach seeks a more complete (reductionistic) explanation involving "root causes" and complex causal chains. However, one consequence of seeking explanations at more microscopic levels is that the number of links in the chains connecting X to Y increase (e.g., the links between the husband's problem and the wife's marital distress as noted above). Note that such chains are not necessarily weaker than those at more global levels *if* the association between links in the chain at the lower levels are considerably higher and thus compensate for the greater number of links. Indeed, when the links at the fine-grained level are strong (i.e., the associations between links are all high), the length of the chain is less important in affecting causal strength. On the other hand, if the lower-level links are not well established, the increased complexity of the chain makes the resulting scenario implausible and far-fetched. In simple terms, the finer grained the causal analysis, the more links there are in the causal chain, and the less likely that the first link in this chain will have much power in predicting the final outcome.[2]

[2]In Einhorn and Hogarth (1986), we specify this relationship more formally in terms of how the causal background and the cues-to-causality combine in determining the strength of an explanation (X). This is given by the model,

$$s(X,Y) = Q_T Q_B Q_L \, (\lambda_C Q_C + \lambda_S Q_S) \qquad (4)$$

where $s(X,Y)$ represents the strength of X for explaining Y; Q_T represents the cue of

Although the causal processes that I have been describing apply equally to judgments involving physical and clinical processes, there is an important distinction. The difference lies in the fact that human behavior is assumed to result from goal-oriented factors of some type. Thus, outcomes are frequently explained by unobservable constructs such as motivations, intentions, goals, or "personalities" of actors. Moreover, the presumed existence of such causes affects the cues-to-causality such that beliefs that a given factor causes a particular outcome are increased. For example, note that a motive or intention exists prior to the taking of action and is thus consistent with the temporal order cue; that is, depression is presumed to cause suicidal ideation. Furthermore, high contiguity in time and space, as well as high congruity between motives and actions, results in a short and direct causal chain linking outcomes to goals, intentions, or motives. Thus, in distinguishing between causal candidates, studies of causal attributions in the clinical domain typically depend on two cues, covariation and salience, as represented by the degree to which there is a difference-in-a-background—for example, the actor–observer phenomenon in attribution theory (for a description see Nisbett and Ross, 1980, as well as Jordan, Harvey, & Weary, this volume).

Diagnostic Inference in Statistical Modeling

The process by which statistical models are constructed for prediction purposes also relies on backward inference. In particular, why are certain variables chosen as "relevant" to predicting some phenomenon while others are not? This issue is central to all prediction problems and is highlighted by the succinct conclusion of Dawes and Corrigan (1974, p. 105) on the superiority of equally weighted linear models (in a regression equation) for prediction: "The whole trick is to decide what variables to look at and then know how to add." Assuming that we can add, how do we decide what variables to look at? On this point, we have little

---

where $s(X,Y)$ represents the strength of X for explaining Y; Q_T represents the cue of temporal order ($Q_T = 0,1$); Q_B measures the extent to which X is a difference in the causal background ($0 \le Q_B \le 1$); Q_L denotes the strength of the causal chain ($0 \le Q_L \le 1$); Q_C represents the covariation between X and Y ($0 \le Q_C \le 1$); Q_S refers to physical similarity; and the λ_i's are attentional weights (where $\lambda_C + \lambda_S = 1$). From the present perspective, the importance of (4) is that for an explanation to have nonzero strength, temporal order ($Q_T = 1$) must be correct, X must be a difference-in-a-background ($Q_B > 0$), and a plausible causal chain must be constructed between X and Y ($Q_L > 0$). Note that if any of these cues is zero, $s(X,Y)$ will also be zero. Moreover, because (4) is defined as a multiplicative function of these three cues, even if all are moderately high, their product could still be low. Finally, although $s(X,Y)$ may not be zero, X may nevertheless be ignored if $s(X,Y)$ is below some threshold level. Indeed, the concept of a threshold that varies as a function of specific factors in a task (for example, time pressure, costs of making an error in diagnosis, and so on) is an appealing idea that is similar to the notion of a changing criterion/cut-off point in signal-detection theory (Green & Swets, 1966).

guidance other than some ill-defined notions of experience, intuition, feeling, and so forth. From the perspective of this discussion, one must have some hypothesis or theory for selecting relevant from irrelevant variables. Indeed, relevance can only be understood in relation to some model of what generates the variable to be predicted. Therefore, even statistical prediction depends on backward inference that involves both the construction of hypotheses to interpret the past and the choosing of relevant from irrelevant variables in that construction.

Diagnosis and Prediction

Awareness that predictions are dependent on prior diagnosis is important for three reasons: (1) Diagnosis is necessary in choosing among competing models; (2) a causal model of how outcomes are generated is needed to assess the accuracy of predictions; and, (3) Confusion of diagnostic and prognostic information can lead to serious errors in judgment. The following examples illustrate each of these points.

1. Imagine that you have been asked to evaluate the scholarly output of a colleague being considered for promotion. Your colleague has produced 11 papers; of these the first nine represent competent, albeit unexciting scholarly work. On the other hand, the last two papers are quite different; they are innovative and suggest a creativity and depth of thought absent from the earlier work. What should your recommendation be? As someone who is aware of regression fallacies, you might consider the two outstanding papers as outliers from a stable generating process and thus predict regression to the mean. Alternatively, you might consider the outstanding papers as extreme responses that signal (or are diagnostic of) a change in the generating process. If this were the case, you should be predicting future papers of high quality. If one asks what is the nature of the signaling in this case, it is obvious that the chronological order of the papers is crucial for making the diagnosis. Indeed, imagine that the outstanding papers were the first two that were written; or, consider that they were the second and sixth. In the former case, one might attribute the quality of the work to the thesis advisor and committee. In the latter case, the diagnosis may suggest an erratic researcher who generally does mundane work but who produces outstanding research on occasion. In either case, it is clear that the diagnosis of the process can affect the prediction. What is less well understood is that the diagnosis *should* affect the prediction.

2. The determination of predictive accuracy would seem to be a simple and noncontroversial matter. However, diagnoses and predictions are generally made for taking action; i.e., diagnoses determine treatments, and predictions determine who gets preferred actions (e.g., whether to prescribe medication, whether to hospitalize). The following

examples illustrate the difficulties of assessing predictive accuracy when action is taken based on diagnoses or predictions: (a) Following the Challenger space shuttle catastrophe, psychologists, predicting an increase in emotional distress for NASA employees, reacted by offering preventive counseling. Clearly, action is taken to intervene in the process and the resulting outcomes are a joint function of the factors on which the prediction is based and the action taken. Under these circumstances, the meaning of predictive accuracy is ambiguous; in fact, one can imagine that predictive accuracy is not desirable. For example, the more effective the preventive counseling in changing the process, the less accurate the initial prediction will have been. Or, imagine the prediction is inaccurate, but the counseling had a boomerang effect that actually caused psychological difficulties (i.e., it sensitized NASA workers to *potential* problems). In many cases of this type, without knowledge of the joint effects of the prediction and the treatment, assessing the accuracy of the prediction is problematic. (b) People in a small town hear a rumor that the bank is about to fail. They think that if this prediction is accurate, they had better withdraw their money as fast as possible. Accordingly, they go to the bank to close their accounts and by the end of the day the bank *has* failed. This case differs from (a) in that the action taken leads to confirmation of the initial prediction (demonstrating the so-called "self-fulfilling prophecy" effect). What is particularly disturbing about these cases is that awareness of the effects of actions on outcomes is low and can lead to overconfidence in predictions that are of low or even zero accuracy (see Einhorn, 1980; Einhorn & Hogarth, 1978; Snyder & Thomsen, this volume).

3. The lack of awareness of a difference between diagnosis and prognosis can lead to serious errors in judgment. In particular, people often have difficulty in distinguishing between probabilities of the form, $p(Y|X)$ and $p(X|Y)$ (i.e., the probability of outcome Y, given event X, versus the probability of outcome X, given event Y). To illustrate, consider the case of mammography and breast cancer (Eddy, 1982). For women with breast cancer (C), the probability of a positive mammogram (M) is .79 (i.e., $p(M|C) = .79$). Eddy reports that most physicians misinterpret the statements about the test and estimate the probability of breast cancer given a positive test to be approximately .75 (i.e., $p(C|M) = .75$). He points out that

> When asked about this, the erring physicians usually report that they assumed that the probability of cancer given that the patient has a positive X-ray . . . was approximately equal to the probability of a positive X-ray in a patient with cancer. . . . The latter probability is the one measured in clinical research programs and is very familiar, but it is the former that is needed for clinical decision making. It seems that many if not most physicians confuse the two. (p. 254)

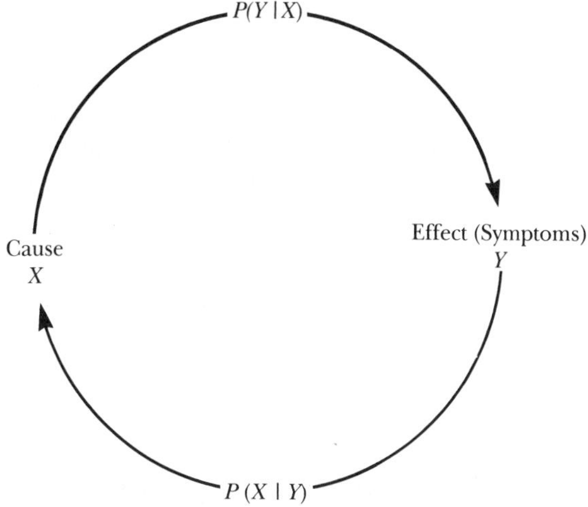

Predict back in time

Figure 3–1. Looplike Structure in Confusion of Predictive and Diagnostic Probabilities

The confusion is particularly serious in this case. To see why, please refer to note 3 below.

Under what conditions is the confusion described in note 3 most likely to occur? First, note that cancer causes the positive test result and not vice versa. Therefore, denote cancer as the cause that temporally precedes the test as an effect. However, the test result is known first in time and is used to predict the cause. The peculiarity here is that the test predicts a prior state (cancer) that presumably existed before the test and that caused the test result itself. Hence, this situation has a looplike structure that makes the temporal order of events particularly confusing. This looplike structure is shown in Figure 3–1. Note that the causal probability of a positive mammography in someone with cancer is not

[3]The probability of cancer given a positive mammography is equal to the probability of a cancer and a positive mammography divided by the probability of a positive mammography. However, the probability of a positive mammography in a patient with cancer takes this same numerator but divides it by the probability of cancer, as depicted in formula 5.

$$p(C|M) = p(C \cap M)/p(M) \text{ and, } p(M|C) = p(C \cap M)/p(C) \qquad (5)$$

Although both conditional probabilities have the same numerators, they differ with respect to their denominators, which are the base rates of having a positive mammogram [$p(M)$] and having cancer [$p(C)$], respectively. Since the base rate of having a positive mammogram is considerably larger than that of breast cancer, this means that, $p(C|M) < p(M|C)$. Therefore, if physicians confuse the two types of probabilities, they are likely to diagnose too many women as having cancer on the basis of a positive mammogram. Furthermore, if action is then taken on the basis of the prediction, as in performing a mastectomy, too many unnecessary surgeries will be performed.

predictive in the usual sense; that is, whereas having cancer predicts the test, this is irrelevant to the practical issue. On the other hand, the test (which is known first in time), is used to predict the disease that preceded it. Therefore, there are two temporal order cues in problems of this type: causes precede effects, but effects are seen first and are used to predict their prior causes. Under such conditions, confusion of diagnostic and prognostic probabilities is quite understandable.

Clinical Versus Statistical Prediction

While clinical and statistical models are developed via diagnostic reasoning, there are three important differences in the way each deals with prediction problems. These differences involve: (a) the domain of prediction; (b) the complexity and level of detail in the causal model; and, (c) the treatment of "random error."

a. Statistical concepts such as probability, average, variability, and so on, clearly indicate that the domain to which inferences are made are aggregates of some sort. Therefore, one is concerned with the general case or with classes of cases. Indeed, the importance of set theory for defining statistical concepts emphasizes that individual cases are to be considered as members of sets or subsets of like members. Moreover, when this cannot be easily accomplished, as when considering one-of-a-kind events, controversy exists regarding the meaning and meaningfulness of probability statements (cf. Shafer & Tversky, 1985). Now consider the domain of the clinician. Here prediction is done on a case-by-case basis—what caused Mr. X's breakdown? Will Mrs. Y be depressed again? While appeal can be made to general laws or principles in answering such questions, the relevance of such evidence is often questioned on the grounds that the specific case is not a member of this or that class. Indeed, it is not uncommon to hear that certain events and people are considered "in a class by themselves."

b. At a recent conference of decision theorists, military personnel, and State Department officials, the ambassador to a Central American country stated during one of the discussions, "I'm an essayist, not a statistician!" This statement captures much of the difference between clinical and statistical thinking; the clinician/essayist is involved in constructing complex causal scenarios that are rich in detail and rely almost exclusively on the particular content in the situation. From this perspective, the statistician's emphasis on base rates, regression equations, and the like, is bloodless, abstract, and essentially uninteresting (to non-statisticians). On the other hand, from the statistician's viewpoint, the clinician is seen to be lost in a morass of details, without hope of discerning the general patterns and laws that apply to the particular case. To give some idea of the difference between the two approaches, imagine the following hypothetical "analyses" and predictions concerning a dissolving marriage.

Clinician: The couple fights over money, control of the children, and has problems of intimacy. The husband is domineering and refuses to listen to his wife's opinion. She, on the other hand, resents giving up her career to stay home and take care of the children. The hostility in the relationship needs to be aired since both partners have difficulty in expressing anger. Indeed, the husband is an only child with a very domineering mother, making it difficult for him to. . . Therefore, a divorce is likely. (Obviously, this is only a very brief outline of the scenario the clinician can construct.)

Statistician: Let P = probability of a divorce, F = number of fights per week, and I = number of times the couple has sexual intercourse per week (with each other). Then assume the model,

$$P = f(F - I) \quad (6)$$

and thus, the larger the positive difference between F and I, the greater the probability of a divorce.

The above model (derived from Howard & Dawes, 1976), is abstract, general, and deals with aggregates. Moreover, the "game" in the statistical approach is to build a model with as few variables and parameters as possible. Hence, parsimony and simplicity are important concerns. On the other hand, the clinical scenario is rich in detail, with long and complex causal chains that connect present behavior with past actions. Indeed, the degree of parsimony achieved in the statistical approach is generally eschewed by clinicians. Thus, a common reaction to statistical models is that they ignore the complexity of human behavior and are thus "simpleminded."

c. The clinical approach to diagnosis and prediction can be characterized by its strong reliance on attempting to explain all the data. Indeed, a significant feature of diagnostic thinking is the remarkable speed and fluency that people have for generating explanations to explain any result. For example, "discussion sections" in journal articles are rarely at a loss to explain why the results did not come out as predicted (cf. Slovic & Fischhoff, 1977); psychotherapists are quick to point out that a patient's suicide should have been anticipated; and commissions, panels, committees, and the like, place blame on administrators for not knowing what is "obvious" in hindsight. As Fischhoff (1975) has pointed out, the past has few surprises but the future has many (p. 296). Why should this be so?

One consequence of the fluency of causal reasoning and the lack of awareness that backward and forward inference are different is that diagnostic models are used as the basis for extrapolating to the future via processes such as the "representativeness" heuristic (Kahneman & Tversky, 1973; Turk, Salovey, & Prentice, this volume). Such predictions are subject to a variety of errors that have been well documented and discussed in the literature; for example, nonregressiveness of predictions, insensitivity to base rates, and sample size, overconfidence, and so on (see Hogarth & Makridakis, 1981, for a review). In fact, a useful analogy of this process is provided by multiple regression analysis. In deriving a model (backward inference), one seeks the combination of variables and parameters that maximizes some measure of fit. One can continually add more variables and parameters to the equation so that the fit of the model improves. However, such overfitting of the model leads to the following surprise: When the model is used to predict new cases, it does a poor job since the fitting procedure accounts for all the variance, including the "noise" in the system. On a new set of cases, the noise is not the same, and the equation is useless. Hence, it is often the case that the power of post hoc explanations is matched by a paucity of predictive accuracy.

When deviations between predictions and outcomes occur, the clinical and statistical approaches diagnose the situation quite differently. These differences have much to do with the meaning and significance of "random error" or "noise." While the concept of randomness is complex and difficult to define (Lopes, 1982), it suggests an irreducible unpredictability and disorder of outcomes. The basic question then becomes, how much of behavior is random and how much systematic? The answer to this depends on what is meant by randomness. For example, consider trying to predict the outcome of a roulette wheel. Since this is a simple physical system, the final position of the ball should be derivable from well-known physical laws. However, even if one grants that this system is totally deterministic in principle, in practice it is only predictable in a probabilistic sense. Indeed, I suspect that the gambling games which use simple physical systems (e.g., dice, slot machines, and roulette) owe much of their popularity to the belief that something so simple and mechanical must be manipulable and thus predictable. Consider a different example, the prediction of stock market prices. One leading theory of stock prices posits that they fluctuate randomly. While most people have not heard of this theory, many have had first-hand experience with its implications. Do stock prices vary randomly? To date, the market is difficult to predict on a consistent basis. However, does that mean that it is impossible to do so? Imagine that there is a seven-way interaction that predicts price changes, but no one has yet induced it from the mass of complex and noisy data that is available. If there is hidden systematicness, one's gamble in trying to induce a predictive rule may pay off. On the other hand, such an interaction may not exist, despite the fact that there are experts selling advice on what stocks to buy. Thus, if prediction error is due to our lack of knowledge and randomness is only a label for our current ignorance, at least two reactions are possible. The first is characteristic of the clinical approach; it says that the goal of perfect predictability, while difficult to attain, is not impossible. Moreover, this goal may be useful in itself since it can motivate the search for improved predictability via increased effort and attention. The second reaction is characteristic of the statistical approach and emphasizes the possibility of a futile search for a perfectly predictable world.

Although the clinical approach rests on the worthy and optimistic goal of perfect predictability, it is a goal that can have negative consequences (see below). The statistical approach, on the other hand, accepts error. This acceptance can occur in several ways. First, one may believe that the world is inherently uncertain. In this case, probabilistic knowledge is the best one can hope for and random error cannot be reduced by greater knowledge. Second, one can maintain a causal determinism but believe that our knowledge will always be fragmentary and hence uncertain. In this case, randomness is due to ignorance, but the goal of perfect predictability is abandoned as being too unrealistic. Third, the use of any equation or algorithm, with its limited number of variables and mechanical combining rule, can never capture the richness and full complexity of the phenomenon it is meant to predict (recall Meehl's discussion of "broken leg cues," 1954, p. 25). Thus, models are simplifications of reality that must lead to errors in prediction (cf. Chapanis, 1961).

Let us now consider how the acceptance of error can lead to less error. To do so, recall the research on probability learning done several years ago (e.g., Edwards, 1956; Estes, 1962). In these studies, either a red or green light is illuminated on each of a number of trials, and subjects are asked to predict which light will go on. If the prediction is correct, subjects are given a cash payoff; if the prediction is wrong, there is no payoff. However, unbeknownst to the subject, the lights are programmed to go on according to a binomial process with a given proportion of red and green, say 60 percent red and 40 percent green. Thus, the process is random although subjects do not know this. The major result of these experiments is "probability matching"; i.e., subjects respond to the lights in the same proportions as they occur. For example, in the above case, subjects predict red 60 percent of the time and green 40 percent. The expected payoff for such a strategy can be calculated as follows: since the subject predicts red on 60 percent of the trials and red occurs on 60 percent, the subject will be correct (and receive the payoff) on 36 percent of the trials. Similarly for green; the subject predicts green on 40 percent of trials and green occurs on 40 percent. Hence, 16 percent of the trials will be correctly predicted. Therefore, over both predictions, subjects will be correct on 36 percent + 16 percent = 52 percent of the trials. Now consider how well subjects would do by using a simple rule that said always predict the most likely color. Note that such a strategy accepts error; however, it also leads to 60 percent correct predictions (i.e., I always say red and red occurs 60 percent of the time). Since 60 percent is greater than 52 percent, subjects would make more money if they accepted error and consistently used a simple rule. Indeed, such a rule maximizes their wealth in this situation. However, most are trying to predict perfectly and are engaged in a futile attempt to see patterns in the data that are diagnostic of the (nonexistent) rule that they believe determines the onset of the lights.

While the idea of accepting error may be surprising, there are several other advantages of the statistical approach that deserves mention. First, the statistical approach demands that empirical evidence, rather than authority, be the deciding factor in determining the predictive accuracy of any device. Hence, the statistical approach is suspicious—it trusts no one and takes little on faith. In fact, Armstrong's (1978) notion of a "seersucker theory of prediction" captures the attitude of the statistical approach to all undocumented claims of expertise. The theory has only one axiom: for every seer there is a sucker. A second issue concerns inconsistency in judgment due to fatigue, boredom, memory and attentional limitations, and so on. Such inconsistency is not, in general, useful. Indeed, if someone has a valid rule which is inconsistently applied, predictive accuracy will suffer. However, clinical judgment can be improved by techniques such as "bootstrapping," in which a model of the clinical thought processes predicts more accurately than the person from whom the model was developed (Goldberg, 1970). Such models have been developed in many fields and the results are encouraging (see Camerer, 1981, for a review and theoretical discussion).

A Decision Analysis

The choice between clinical and statistical prediction, like most choices, has advantages and disadvantages associated with each alternative. To analyze these, consider Figure 3–2, which shows a decision matrix with choices as rows and states of the world as columns. For the sake of simplicity, only two choices and states are shown. First consider the choice alternatives: one can decide that a phenomenon of interest is systematic and thus capable of being predicted; or, one can decide that the phenomenon is random and not predictable. Now consider the possible states of nature. In the first column, the phenomenon is systematic, while in the second it is random. The intersection of rows and columns

		States of Nature	
		Systematic	Random
Choices	Systematic	Hit	Myth, magic, illusion of control
	Random	Lost opportunity, illusion of no control	Hit

Figure 3–2. Decision Matrix for Deciding Between the Clinical and Statistical Approaches

results in four possible outcomes; the "hits," shown in the diagonal, and the errors, shown in the off-diagonal. Note that there are two kinds of errors. If one decides that a phenomenon is systematic and it is random, the error that results is manifested in myths, magic, superstitions, and illusions of control (Langer, 1975). This error is most likely to characterize the clinical approach, which seeks causal explanations for all behavior. Moreover, there are numerous examples of this type of error that have been discussed in the behavioral decision theory literature (for a review, see Einhorn & Hogarth, 1981; Nisbett & Ross, 1980).

Let us now consider the other error, which is more likely to characterize the statistical approach. In this case, one decides that a phenomenon is random when it is systematic. This error results in lost opportunities and illusions of the lack of control. For example, consider the state of knowledge of the movement of heavenly bodies after Copernicus but before Kepler. The Copernican revolution put the sun at the center of the solar system with the planets revolving in circular orbits. This model of planetary motion gives reasonably accurate predictions. However, we know that the orbits are not circular; they are elliptical, and errors in prediction occurred. If probabilism were around in the time of Copernicus, one might have explained planetary motion as consisting of circular orbits *plus a random error term.* While such a probabilistic model would explain most of the variance, it would represent a lost opportunity to better understand the true nature of the phenomenon. Of course, success in explaining all the variance of behavior is dramatic. However, dramatic failures also exist. Recall Einstein's famous statement, "God does not play dice with the world," His unsuccessful attempts to disprove quantum theory illustrate the futility of adhering to the goal of perfect predictability.

What conclusions can be drawn from the above? First, the choice between clinical and statistical prediction in any given situation will depend on: (a) One's beliefs regarding the probabilities of the states of nature. While I have only considered two states, there are many states representing various levels of systematicness and random error. Hence, one's prior beliefs about these various states will greatly affect the choice of strategy; (b) The relative costs of the two types of errors. For example, to what degree is superstition an appropriate price to pay for not missing an opportunity to predict more accurately? (c) The relative payoffs for the hits, or correct choices. Hence, the choice between the clinical and statistical approaches can be seen as a special case of decision making under uncertainty; each has its associated risks and potential benefits. At the least, this conceptualization demonstrates why the controversy will never be resolved. Researchers and practitioners will "place their bets" differently, whether the field be clinical psychology or particle physics.

Conclusion

The controversy regarding the predictive superiority of clinical versus statistical methods is both real and apparent. On the one hand, there *is* a basic conflict concerning the predictability of behavior and the level of error that is considered tolerable. On the other hand, both approaches rest on diagnostic inferences that are causal and constructive. Without such inferences, there would be no models (clinical or statistical) from which to base predictions in the first place.

While the empirical evidence is clear and convincing that the statistical approach does a better overall job of prediction, the clinical approach is not without its virtues. Indeed, from the present viewpoint, the clinical approach can be seen as a high-risk strategy—i.e., the chance of predicting all the variance of behavior (or even a substantial amount), is very low, but the payoff is correspondingly high. On the other hand, the acceptance of error to make less error is likely to be a safer and more accurate strategy over a wide range of practical situations. Thus, the statistical approach leads to better performance on average. For a statistician like myself, this is crucial. However, to paraphrase Oscar Wilde, one shouldn't take averages to extremes.

Acknowledgment

This work was supported by a contract from the Office of Naval Research.

References

Armstrong, J. S. (1978). *Long-range forecasting: From crystal ball to computer.* New York: Wiley.

Bronowski, J. (1978). *The origins of knowledge and imagination.* New Haven: Yale University Press.

Camerer, C. (1981). General conditions for the success of bootstrapping models. *Organizational Behavior and Human Performance, 27,* 411–422.

Chapanis, A. (1961). Men, machines, and models. *American Psychologist, 16,* 113–131.

Cook, T. D., & Campbell, D. T. (1979). *Quasi-experimentation: Design and analysis for field settings.* Chicago: Rand McNally.

Dawes, R. M. (1979). The robust beauty of improper linear models in decision making. *American Psychologist. 34,* 571–582.

Dawes, R. M., & Corrigan, B. (1974). Linear models in decision making. *Psychological Bulletin, 81,* 95–106.

Eddy, D. M. (1982). Probabilistic reasoning in clinical medicine: Problems and opportunities. In D. Kahneman, P. Slovic, & A. Tversky (Eds.), *Judgment under uncertainty: Heuristics and biases.* New York: Cambridge University Press.

Edwards, W. (1956). Reward probability, amount, and information as determiners of sequential two-alternative decisions. *Journal of Experimental Psychology, 51,* 177–188.

Einhorn, H. J. (1980). Learning from experience and suboptimal rules in decision making. In T. S. Wallsten (Ed.), *Cognitive processes in choice and decision behavior.* Hillsdale, NJ: Erlbaum.

Einhorn, H. J., Hogarth, R. M. (1975). Unit weighting schemes for decision making. *Organizational Behavior and Human Performance, 13,* 171–192.

______. (1978). Confidence in judgment: Persistence of the illusion of validity. *Psychological Review, 85,* 395–416.

______. (1981). Behavioral decision theory: Processes of judgment and choice. *Annual Review of Psychology, 32,* 53–88.

______. (1982). Prediction, diagnosis, and causal thinking in forecasting. *Journal of Forecasting, 1,* 23–36.

______. (1986). Judging probable cause. *Psychological Bulletin, 99,* 3–19.

Elstein, A. S., Shulman, L. E., & Sprafka, S. A. (1978). *Medical problem solving: An analysis of clinical reasoning.* Cambridge, MA: Harvard University Press.

Estes, W. K. (1962). Learning theory. *Annual Review of Psychology, 13,* 107–144.

Fischhoff, B. (1975). Hindsight ≠ foresight: The effect of outcome knowledge on judgment under uncertainty. *Journal of Experimental Psychology: Human Perception and Performance, 1,* 288–299.

Gettys, C. F., & Fisher, S. D. (1979). Hypothesis plausibility and hypothesis generation. *Organizational Behavior and Human Performance, 24,* 93–110.

Goldberg, L. R. (1970). Man versus model of man: A rationale, plus some evidence, for a method of improving on clinical inferences. *Psychological Bulletin, 73,* 422–432.

Green, D. M., & Swets, J. (1966). *Signal detection theory and psychophysics.* New York: Wiley.

Helson, H. (1964). *Adaptation-level theory.* New York: Harper and Row.
Hogarth, R. M. (1982). On the surprise and delight of inconsistent responses. In R. M. Hogarth (Ed.), *Question framing and response consistency.* San Francisco: Jossey-Bass.
Hogarth, R. M., & Makridakis, S. (1981). Forecasting and planning: An evaluation. *Management Science, 27,* 115–138.
Howard, J. W., & Dawes, R. M. (1976). Linear prediction of marital happiness. *Personality and Social Psychology Bulletin, 2,* 478–480.
Jevons, W. S. (1984). Commercial crises and sun-spots. In H. S. Foxwell (Ed.), *Investigations in currency and finance.* London: Macmillan.
Kahneman, D., & Tversky, A. (1973). On the psychology of prediction. *Psychological Review, 80,* 237–251.
———. (1979). Prospect theory: An analysis of decision under risk. *Econometrica, 47,* 263–291.
Langer, E. J. (1975). The illusion of control. *Journal of Personality and Social Psychology, 32,* 311–328.
Lopes, L. L. (1982). Doing the impossible: A note on induction and the experience of randomness. *Journal of Experimental Psychology: Human Learning and Memory, 8,* 626–636.
Mackie, J. L. (1965). Causes and conditions. *American Philosophical Quarterly, 2,* 245–264.
———. (1974). *The cement of the universe: A study of causation.* Oxford, England: Clarendon Press.
Meehl, P. E. (1954). *Clinical versus statistical prediction: A theoretical analysis and review of the literature.* Minneapolis: University of Minnesota Press.
Nisbett, R. E., & Ross, L. D. (1980). *Human inference: Strategies and shortcomings of social judgment.* Englewood Cliffs, NJ: Prentice-Hall.
Sawyer, J. (1966). Measurement *and* prediction: Clinical *and* statistical. *Psychological Bulletin, 66,* 178–200.
Shafer, G., & Tversky, A. (1985). Language and designs for probability judgment. *Cognitive Science, 9,* 309–339.
Simon, H. A. (1986). Report of the research briefing panel on decision making and problem solving. *Research Briefings 1986, National Academy of Sciences.* Washington, D.C.: National Academy Press.
Slovic, P., & Fischhoff, B. (1977). On the psychology of experimental surprises. *Journal of Experimental Psychology: Human Perception and Performance, 3,* 544–551.
Suppes, P. (1966). Probabilistic inference and the concept of total evidence. In J. Hintikka & P. Suppes (Eds.), *Aspects of inductive logic.* Amsterdam: North-Holland.
Weiner, B. (1985). "Spontaneous" causal thinking. *Psychological Bulletin, 97,* 74–84.

PART II | Sources of Bias

4 | Perceiving the Client

Albert F. Smith

One of the principal tasks of the clinician is to make judgments, and the description of the ways in which clinicians make judgments as well as prescriptions about how they should are the topic of many of the chapters of this volume. In particular, recent interest has focused both on the cognitive processes used by clinicians as they make judgments and on ways in which those reasoning strategies may lead to judgmental outcomes that deviate from the optimum. Such analyses place special emphasis on ways in which clinicians store knowledge and on the ways in which they retrieve and utilize this knowledge. It is important, however, to recognize that there is another important starting point from which to consider clinical judgment and reasoning, and that is the stimulus about which the clinician makes judgments and about which the clinician reasons. That stimulus is the client.

The purpose of this chapter is to present a framework within which to consider the therapist's perception of the client. Just what is it that clinicians perceive when they perceive a client? In what way does the perceptual input initiate the judgments that are made by clinicians and the reasoning that they carry out? A premise of the chapter, as of much of contemporary psychology, is that various cognitive processes may be initiated either externally, through perception, or internally, through imagery or expectations. Whereas several of the chapters in this volume emphasize the latter, it is the purpose of this chapter to review what is known about the former.

The following general strategy will be pursued: First, the notion of a person as a stimulus will be reviewed. The fundamental point—one that is hardly new—is that persons, and, in particular, clinical clients, may be conceived as bundles of attributes. Mental decomposition of the client into his or her attributes is in fact a common clinical approach. Second, the idea that attributes, or properties, interact in perception will be discussed, and the consequences of such interactions for clinical perception will be considered. Given this seemingly reasonable way of approaching the problem of conceptualizing the person as stimulus and acknowledging that attributes of people—like attributes of other phenomenon—interact in perception, the third concern of the chapter will be to consider just what the attributes of people in general and of clients in particular might be. It is in this section that some of the difficulties in arriving at neutral, objective descriptions of people will become clear. Finally, the ways in which perceived information is organized into representations of the client will be described.

It is essential to bear in mind while reading this chapter that the emphasis on perception is not intended to deny the significance of the thoughtful—if sometimes errorful—cognitive processes that others emphasize. Rather, this chapter asserts that clinical judgment and reasoning are the outcome of interactions between stimulation from the world—the client—and an organized mind, and that analysis of the former can contribute significantly to a more complete understanding of the nature of clinical reasoning and judgment.

The Client as Stimulus

The stimulus for the clinician is the client, and, as noted earlier, the client can be considered a bundle of properties. Of what properties people consist—in a sense meaningful for clinical cognition—is not clear; a description of some possibly meaningful properties comes later. To assert that people consist of attributes is essentially to assert that they are defined in this way: Some cluster of attributes comprises the definition of any person, and hence the concept of that person. It is with the mental representation, or concept, of the client that the clinician deals.

For the time being it is necessary only to accept the basic idea, and to remain relatively neutral concerning the sorts of properties involved. One of the objectives of some clinical approaches is to decompose the client into his or her attributes. For example, administration of the Minnesota Multiphasic Personality Inventory (MMPI) yields a score for the client on a variety of scales, each of which may be considered to represent an attribute of the client. Administration of any personality scale may be viewed as a means of identifying a single attribute of the client. Systematic manifestation of a particular behavior, or systematic response on the part of a client to a class of stimulus situations, may be considered an attribute of the client. If a child beats his mother, or if a person is afraid of heights—these are attributes of those people.

These examples yield several messages for the general conceptualization of people as bundles of attributes. First, any person is composed of infinitely many attributes (see Garner, 1974, lecture 8; Smith, 1986), and a variety of factors may lead to any particular attribute's being more or less discernible. Second, there may be different points of view concerning what attributes of the person are relevant to the clinician. Some clinicians may consider behaviors to be relevant attributes, whereas others may emphasize more abstract attributes such as MMPI scale values. Third, some clinicians may have as their goal the identification and analysis of a single attribute of the client—a particular class of behaviors or an aspect of personality that is represented by a single scale—whereas others may be interested in many attributes.

What attributes are perceived, and what attributes are perceivable, is the puzzle of person perception. If perceived people are infinitely complex in terms of attribute structure, what can be said about the attributes that are perceived? This question can be answered at several levels. Specific answers concerning the nature of people's attributes are deferred to a later point of this chapter, but even at a more general level, it is important to address the question of what attributes are perceived.

Two important aspects of the problem warrant consideration. First, perceived attributes depend on contextual factors. A variety of empirical studies (e.g., McGuire & McGuire, 1982; Smith, 1986; Tversky & Gati, 1978) have demonstrated that the particular reference set of stimuli with respect to which a particular stimulus is perceived influences the attributes that are perceived in that context. This has been demonstrated for people as well as for other sorts of stimuli. McGuire and McGuire showed, for example, that children's self-conceptions, measured by their descriptions of themselves, are influenced by the particular reference set of people that they infer at the time of the measurement (e.g., family or schoolmates). It is important to recognize that stimuli—whether they be visual patterns or people—are composed of attributes, various subsets of which may be extracted by a perceiver, and that the particular subset of attributes that is extracted from the stimulus depends on the reference context.

The potential instability of the definition of the client in terms of the extracted set of attributes leads to the second general concern about the nature of perceived attributes. The particular set of attributes that is available to clinicians and that will serve as the basis of their reasoning will likely be sensitive to the way in which that attribute information is presented. There are, for example, many ways in which a client may be introduced to a clinician. The clinician may obtain information about a client or a potential client in ways that range from examining the numerical results of a battery of psychological tests to conducting a face-to-face interview. Surely the nature and availability of information about the attributes of the client differ in these situations. The range of situations in which clinicians may collect information about clients makes salient two points about the nature of judgment situations. First, the clinician really has two tasks to carry out with these attributes that have been the focus of this discussion. These tasks may be labeled *analysis* and *synthesis*. Analysis involves extraction of attribute information from the stimulus client, whereas synthesis involves assembling extracted attributes into a unified mental representation of that client. Thus, second, certain formats in which information about a client might be presented (e.g., numerical results of psychological tests, or reports by an intake interviewer in a clinic) restrict substantially the nature of the mental representation of the client that may be synthesized by the clinician.

The notion that each person consists of an infinitude of attributes has been described. Because people are highly sensitive to explicitly presented information, to have a particular set of attributes about the client made available may result in substantial restriction of variety in the nature of the mental representation of the client that the clinician forms. This is a potential result of leaving decisions about what attributes of the client are relevant to someone external to the clinician who will actually make judgments about that client. Two clinicians may come to quite different conclusions about a potential client if they observe the individual behaving freely in his or her environment, but to quite similar conclusions if each studied a report about the individual that was prepared by someone else. (This issue will receive further attention below.) Although there is a degree to which different perceivers agree on the level of particular attributes that they assign to people about whom they make judgments, perceivers—presumably including clinicians—vary substantially in what particular attributes serve as the frameworks within which they organize their perceptions of and judgments about people (Dornbusch, Hastorf, Richardson, Muzzy, & Vreeland, 1965; Park, 1986).

Perceptual Interactions of Attributes

Faced with the prospect of a client who is defined as the composition of an infinitude of attributes, what is the clinician to do? To address this question requires some attention to the relation between the task of the clinician and the attributes of the client. It was suggested in the previous section that identifying attributes of the client was an important part of the clinical task. This is relatively clear when the types of judgments that clinicians make about clients are considered.

Clinicians classify, infer, and predict. Classification involves assigning clients to diagnostic categories based on either an explicit or an implicit measurement of one or more attributes. For example, clients might be classified as depressed either on the basis of a score on a depression inventory or on the basis of their manifesting a particular behavior (e.g., staying in bed for weeks at a time). A somewhat more complicated classification would involve assigning clients to diagnostic categories on the basis of several attributes. For example, a group of clients in a psychiatric hospital might be classified according to their MMPI profiles; the MMPI yields values on a number of scales, and these may be considered jointly. Inferences about what properties characterize a client frequently depend on those that have already been perceived, and predictions about a client's prognosis depend on the way the client has been classified. The operation of the representativeness heuristic in clinical reasoning, for example, depends on an initial classification of the client that itself depends on the identification of one or more attributes of the client. There is a sense in which perception of attributes drives the whole cognitive system.

If the properties of people were available to the clinician as a list, or as a set of numerical indices, then given some notion of which properties were relevant to the various judgments that might be made, clinical perception might be reduced to checking an individual's value on various properties and carrying out an appropriate treatment. However, as described earlier, the attributes of the individual tend not to be neatly laid out, as in a list, and this is particularly true for the most ecologically valid of clinical stimuli, the client encountered in a face-to-face interview. When faced with such an individual, the clinician must mentally untangle various attributes, sorting the relevant from the irrelevant, in order to identify properties that bear on the sorts of judgments that need be made.

The problem of mentally untangling attributes is essentially a problem of selective attention, and the nature of the problem is best conveyed by an example. The fundamental point to be made is that there are differences in how different combinations of attributes interact in perception. These differences influence the ease with which the clinician utilizes particular attributes that may be considered critical to classification or judgment. Figure 4–1 shows a set of four individuals defined on two attributes, family membership and having been the victim of sexual assault. The four individuals represented in Figure 4–1 are two sets of identical twins (from two families). Therefore, the twins from each family should be considered identical in every respect except having been the victim of a sexual assault or being the sister of someone who was the victim of sexual assault. Assuming that these individuals present themselves for treatment at a rape crisis center, within each family the two twins should be differently classified on the basis of the one attribute that distinguishes them. When the set of four individuals is considered,

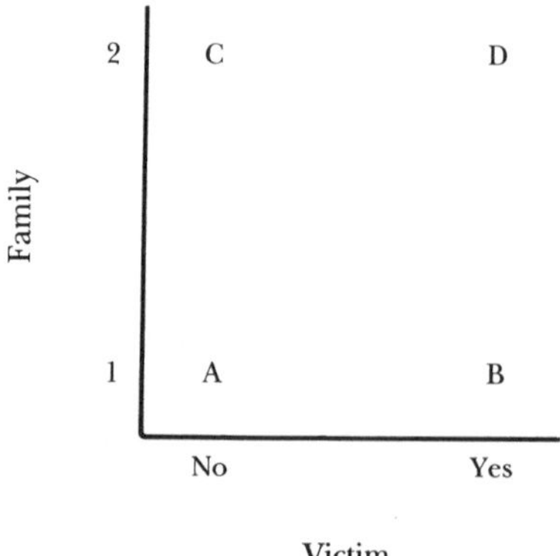

Figure 4–1. Four People Defined by Family Membership and by Experience as a Victim of Sexual Assault. The Members of Each Family Are Identical Twins, Who Thus Differ Only in Whether They Have Been Victims of Assault.

the problem is to classify the two individuals who have been victims of sexual assault into a treatment group and the two who have not suffered the trauma into a different group. This is described as a problem in selective attention because, as indicated in Figure 4–1, these four individuals vary in two respects, family membership and experience as a victim, and classification should depend only on the latter. In this example, experience as a victim of sexual assault is the attribute that is *relevant* for classification, and family membership is *irrelevant.* Note that this is the case even if, overall, each individual is more similar to her identical twin sister than to the other member of the diagnostic class to which she is being assigned.

Given this basic notion of relevant and irrelevant attributes, a somewhat more complicated example will illustrate the notion of perceptual interactions of attributes. The set of 16 individuals schematized in Figure 4–2 are based on an example suggested by Bieri, Atkins, Briar, Leaman, Miller, and Tripodi (1966), who were among the first clinical investigators to consider seriously how the perceiving clinician might deal with the multiattribute client. The attributes of importance for this example are aggressiveness and dependence, as shown in Figure 4–2a, and the 16 individuals vary among themselves as shown in these two attributes. It should be assumed that the attributes are measured by psychometrically appropriate instruments and that scores on the instruments are uncorrelated in the population. Thus, Person A is characterized by low dependence and low aggressiveness, and Person D is characterized by high dependence and the same low value of aggressiveness as Person A. Assume that, for purposes of receiving

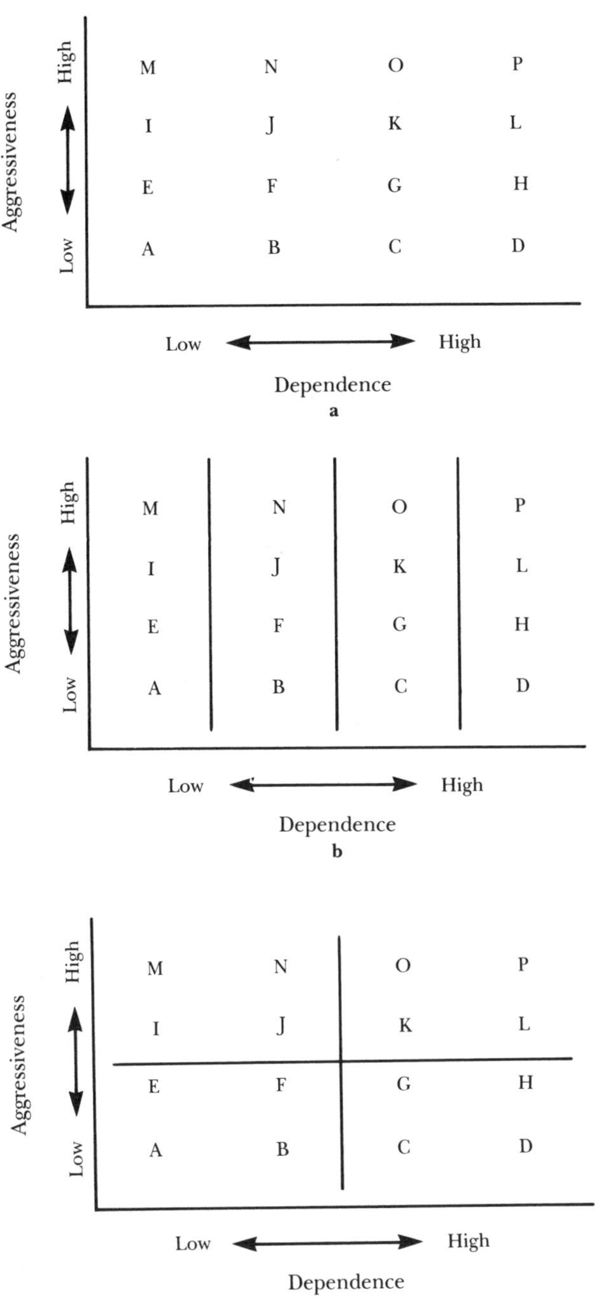

Figure 4–2. (a) Sixteen People Defined by Various Degrees of Dependence and Aggressiveness. (b) Classification into Four Groups of Four According to Levels of Dependence. (c) Classification into Four Groups of Four According to Overall Similarity Defined on Both Attributes.

therapies, the clinician is to classify these 16 individuals into four groups of four people each. Obviously, the clinician must base this classification on some criterion of similarity—some rule for determining what people will appropriately receive the same therapy. Although there are over 63 million ways to classify 16 people into four groups of four, it is the two ways that are shown in Figures 4–2b and 4–2c that are of interest for this example. Each of these is a reasonable classification of the 16 individuals, but different similarity criteria have been used.

The classification shown in Figure 4–2b is strictly according to the "values" of the 16 individuals on one attribute—dependence. This classification implies that the attribute of dependence can be discerned by the classifying clinician; that is, that the clinician can *attend* to it without interference from the client's value on the aggressiveness attribute. The clients in each of the four classes of Figure 4–2b are perceived as similar in dependence without regard to their level of aggression. When attributes interact in a way that makes it easy to use a similarity criterion that groups clients according to their value on one attribute without regard to their values on another, the nature of the interaction is called *separable* (Garner, 1976).

A second way of classifying the 16 individuals of Figure 4–2a into four groups of four individuals each is shown in Figure 4–2c. The similarity criteria used in this classification take into account the values of the 16 individuals on both the attributes of dependence and aggressiveness. If this classification is due to the *inability* of the classifying clinician to discern the individuals' values on the two attributes separately, then the nature of the interaction of the attributes is called *integral.* Although arguments might be made for the theoretical existence of the attributes, for purposes of perception it is not strictly correct to speak of them (see, e.g., Garner, 1976). To reiterate, attributes or properties are said to interact integrally in perception when it is either impossible or extremely difficult to use the attributes independently in making judgments.

The distinction between these two ways in which attributes may be said to interact clarifies two additional points. The first, made earlier, is that the particular way in which information about a client is made available, or is obtained, by the judging clinician will have significant consequences for the kind of judgments that will be made, because it will influence the very definition of the client. For example, if information about the 16 clients described in Figure 4–2 were presented as ordered pairs of numbers indicating levels of dependence and aggressiveness, classification of these individuals according to the system shown in Figure 4–2b would be relatively easy, and this would be the appropriate classification if one wanted to treat dependence and regarded aggressiveness as irrelevant. On the other hand, if information about the clients was collected during an unstructured interview, it would probably be much more difficult to separate information about dependence from information about aggressiveness, and classification of the 16 individuals into groups along the lines of Figure 4–2c would much more likely result.

The second point is that, historically, much of the research concerned with clinical information processing and clinical judgment has focused on the ways in which clinicians integrate multiple sources of information to come to a judgment (e.g., Einhorn, Kleinmuntz, D. N., & Kleinmuntz, B., 1979). Studies of this sort present clinicians with information about a number of client attributes and ask them to use this attribute information to form an integrated judgment (e.g., a classification). This is the synthesis task described above. However, less attention has been given to where the attribute information comes from in the first place; that is, how the therapist analyzes the clinical stimulus. The preceding discussion of Figure 4–2 suggests that knowing how a clinician would use information about aggressiveness and dependence to classify an individual tells little if there is no information about how the clinician extracts reliable information from the client about his aggressiveness and dependence.

This discussion about the ways in which properties of people are perceived to interact, and the significance of these interactions for clinical perception, would be incomplete without discussion of yet a third kind of interaction—the *configural* interaction (Garner, 1976; Smith, 1986). Properties interact configurally when the stimulus objects of which those properties are characteristics are marked by emergent features. An example of such an interaction arises when there is some embedded relationship among the attributes, so that the notion of congruence of attributes, or, for the particular case of person attributes in clinical psychology, "normality," makes sense. For example, one can imagine a set of people characterized by a value on each of two attributes, where no particular level of either attribute would necessarily be considered maladaptive but the combination of levels might indicate a maladaptive condition. Such dimensions of personality as extroversion and assertiveness may be considered to interact configurally. An assertive extrovert, or a nonassertive introvert, are in some sense "normal"—that is, expected. It is the assertive introvert—the introvert characterized by an atypically high level of assertiveness—who is considered asocially hostile and the nonassertive extrovert who is considered insecure or fraudulent.

The Properties of People

The discussion in this chapter has referred repeatedly to the properties of people without specifying exactly what those properties are. Despite decades of formal and centuries of less formal interest in the properties of people, there exists no solid theory or taxonomy of these properties. Properly defining the stimulus in person perception has always been a problem (see, e.g., Taguiri, 1969). In part, this is because there is a degree of instability in the attribute structure of people. The particular goals of a clinician within the diagnostic or therapeutic situation can shape, or define, the attributes that the client will manifest (e.g., Jones & Thibaut, 1958; Snyder & Thomsen, this volume; Swann, 1984).

As noted earlier, much research has involved studying the integration of piecemeal information about target people into unified impressions (e.g., Anderson, 1981; Asch, 1946; Bruner, Shapiro, & Taguiri, 1958), and much of that research used trait adjectives (e.g., "generous," "friendly") as the units of information given to judges. However, traits are surely not attributes of people in the sense of being raw, directly perceivable information (although see McArthur, 1982, and Berry & McArthur, 1986, for another view): traits are more appropriately considered judgments or inferences. It is useful at this point to distinguish sharply between data that can be obtained from the world, that is, by directly observing the client, and judgments that are made about that data. The two categories of person attributes that may be observed directly are physical properties and behaviors. It is of some interest to know how these sorts of perceived attributes contribute to clinical judgments.

Raw Attributes

Physical Attributes. When people are simply asked to describe other individuals, a significant part of the content of the descriptions is information about the physical appearance of the target person (see, e.g., Fiske & Cox, 1979). The important issue for clinical perception is whether the physical characteristics of people influence the judgments that are made about them. Numerous studies have shown that the perceived attractiveness of an individual strongly influences judgments that are made about him or her (see Maruyama & Miller, 1982, for many citations to the extensive literature on perceived attractiveness). For example, Secord (1958; Secord & Muthard, 1955) reported that subjects systematically associated personality traits with people whose photographs they viewed, and Berry and McArthur (1986) reported systematic relations between such physically identifiable attributes of faces as forehead size and the degree to which subjects attributed such psychological qualities as maturity to the owners of those faces. These studies leave open the question of precisely what physical attributes contribute to perceived attractiveness but underscore the point that physical properties cannot be neglected in studies of person perception.

More practically, the course of interpersonal interactions may be modified or determined by the perceived attractiveness of a target person. For example, Snyder, Tanke, and Berscheid (1977) demonstrated that, in phone conversations, men formed more positive impressions of women they believed to be attractive than of women they believed to be unattractive. Furthermore, independent raters, who listened to tapes of the conversations and were unaware of the men's beliefs about the attractiveness of their conversation partners, rated the women thought to be more attractive as more attractive. In general, initial judgments of attractiveness can influence the subsequent course of a relationship. This may well be the case for clinical relationships. Barocas and Black (1974), for example, showed that attractive people are referred for therapy more often than are unattractive people and that attractive people receive more favorable clinical prognosis. Maruyama and Miller (1982) concluded that an individual's appearance, by way of its effects on other people, can affect the development of the characteristics of that individual's personality.

The perceived physical properties of an individual evidently influence judgments of that person. Whether these judgments are biased or are normatively correct deserves further attention, as do the ways physical features interact with each other to influence the behavior of others. Physical properties are an important, directly observable class of personal attributes that probably play a significant, if underrecognized, role in clinical judgment.

Behaviors. People can be observed as they behave in the environment. Their motor acts are publicly accessible; thus, these behaviors constitute a class of attributes of the people manifesting them that should be of interest for a formal analysis of person perception. As was the case in the previous section, the objective of an analysis of person perception is to understand how perceived behaviors influence judgments made about the people who exhibit those behaviors.

A special subcategory of behaviors are reports by individuals of their thoughts, feelings, and experiences. These self-reports constitute much of the informational base available to the clinician. The clinician may either assess and analyze the information or accept the data at face value, but in either case, the attribute information and the structure of the judgment situation must be understood as a subset of the total possible pool of information, a subset that the client has chosen to provide.

How to observe, measure, and analyze behavior is a classic problem in psychology. It has often struck investigators of person perception as being so formidable that they have used as stimulus information such substitutes for direct observation as trait adjectives. The clinician does not have this luxury.

In reality, the distinction between behaviors as raw data and traits inferred from those behaviors is vague. Rarely, it seems, are behaviors described in a neutral, noninterpretive fashion. Some recent research on the implication of traits by behaviors will be described below; for the present, it is sufficient to say that when asked to list a set of behaviors exhibited by another person, people tend to use words describing traits rather than behaviors, and many of the behaviors listed tend to be expressed in a way indicating that they have been interpreted. So, for example, whereas such behaviors as "played football in the snow at night," "slept through morning classes," "masturbated in the bed above me," and "left clothes all over the room" are phrased in a relatively neutral manner, such other descriptions of behaviors as "stormed away from the table," "lost control during sex," and "trapped someone under the mistletoe" are somewhat more judgmental.

In principle, it seems reasonable to argue that behaviors are an important class of personal attributes or features; in practice, it is difficult to know whether, within the domain of *interpersonal* behaviors—behaviors pertaining to relations between people—it is possible to obtain theory- or judgment-free descriptions. For example, such a description of behavior as "he pounded the man on the back" might describe an act of aggression or altruism, friendship or hostility. In describing interpersonal behaviors, it seems very difficult for people not to be interpretive.

Inferred Attributes: Traits

Traits are systematic tendencies for people to behave in certain ways, behavior that may be described conveniently with a single adjective. Although much research on person perception and impression formation has involved presenting lists of trait adjectives to subjects and asking them to evaluate the target person or to predict other aspects of the target person's personality, it has been argued above that traits can at best be inferred from other sources of information. Neither the status of traits nor the basis for their assessment and judgment is generally agreed on; for example, standard psychometric assessments of traits usually do not yield consistent measures for individuals (e.g., Mischel, 1968). Nevertheless, traits require some attention as attributes of people because the perception of traits or the assignment of trait labels appear to be a compelling aspect of interpersonal interaction (Nisbett, 1980). This is demonstrated by the tendency of people to interpret behaviors that was discussed at the end of the last section. Not only laypersons but clinicians as well characterize people in trait terms (e.g., aggressive, demanding, needy), and these characterizations, in addition to being judgments about the people described, are likely to contribute to further judgments and predictions about them.

Several empirical efforts have been concerned with the way in which people make trait judgments on the basis of information about behaviors manifested by a target individual. An example of such research, which foreshadowed many later investigations, was reported by Bieri (1962), who looked at the strength of trait judgments as a function of the consistency of the behaviors described. Although seemingly elementary, the importance of this study was its recognition that trait labels are assigned on the basis of observed behaviors, and that the psychological processes involved are of some interest.

More recently, other investigators have pursued the relationship between trait labels and manifested behaviors. For example, Buss and Craik (1980, 1981, 1983) found that subjects agree substantially about the centrality of particular behaviors to particular trait categories. After asking one group of subjects to list behaviors that represented various interpersonal traits, Buss and Craik found that independent raters agreed substantially about the degree to which those listed behaviors were good examples of behaviors typifying that trait. For example, subjects agreed that such a behavior as "he forbade her to leave the room" better exemplifies dominance than does "he walked ahead of everybody else."

Understanding how observed behaviors are collected and synthesized into trait judgments appears to be an important aspect of the analysis of clinical cognition, and the approach of Buss and Craik appears to be a promising initial step. An obvious weakness, of which Buss and Craik are themselves aware, is that whereas their results are informative concerning the cognitive status of behaviors within particular dispositional categories, they are less so concerning the more general problem of how any particular behavior would be categorized (but see Borkenau, 1986). As noted earlier, behaviors do not imply traits unambiguously. If behaviors were to be classified without the benefit of a small number of trait categories that have been labeled a priori, the problem of making such classifications would be considerably more complex.

Mental Representations of Clients

What happens to the perceived information about attributes? The ultimate goal of clinical person perception is to form an attribute-based mental representation of the client. After information about relevant attributes has been extracted from the clinical stimulus, whether this be a report about a prospective client or an interview with that individual, a mental representation can be synthesized. During recent years, personality and social psychologists have given some attention to the nature of such representations; it is likely that this will continue to be a focus of empirical research.

The mental representation of any thing or person, or of any class of things or persons, may be called a *concept;* research and theorizing about the structure of concepts may be informative about the nature of the mental representation of the client. Traditional psychological thinking held that concepts were well defined, so that whether any object was a member of a concept could be determined by consulting a list of properties that constituted criteria for membership in that concept (cf. Smith & Medin, 1981). For example, the features that are necessary and sufficient for an object to be a square are four equal sides and four right angles; any object that satisfies this description is a square, and any object that fails to satisfy it is not a square. More recent thinking (e.g., Rosch & Mervis, 1975) holds that the membership of concepts is not well-defined: There are no attributes that are necessary or sufficient to determine whether any object is a member of a concept; rather, if an object has some subset of a loosely defined set of properties, it may be a member of the concept. Cantor, Smith, French, and Mezzich (1980) demonstrated that psychodiagnostic categories were ill-defined concepts. In particular, there is no set of attributes that is shared by all clients that are given any particular diagnosis.

A second aspect of this contemporary notion about the mental representation of concepts is that concepts are hierarchically structured and that the "basic level" of a category is cognitively the most useful and accessible (Rosch, Mervis, Gray, Johnson, & Boyes-Braem, 1976). It appears that this approach might usefully describe the mental representation that is formed of the individual client. The clinician may well develop a hierarchically structured mental representation of the client. The most general attributes of the client may define the superordinate level of a hierarchical conceptual structure, with each situation in which the individual appears or each behavior in which the individual engages considered instances of the category. This approach is compatible with the notion of the individual having multiple selves and is compatible with the notion of cognitive complexity (e.g., Bieri, 1961; Linville, 1982).

To summarize, the mental representation of the client synthesized by the clinician on the basis of collected attribute information might range from being quite simple to being quite complex. The complexity of the mental representation will probably depend on the quantity of information that is extracted from the client and the degree to which the attributes involved are contingent on such factors as the situation in which the client appears. For example, a client may report that he is dependent in one class of situations and independent in another class of situations; each class of situations, along with the attributes defining the client in those situations, may be considered instances of the more general concept of the client. The objective of the clinician is to use the available information to synthesize an accurate representation of the client.

Summary

Much contemporary interest in clinical information processing focuses on the reasoning processes of clinicians, including the organization of their knowledge and the strategies that they use to deal with information. This chapter addresses the question of just what that information consists of by considering the perception of the clinician's stimulus—the client.

Consistent with a number of clinical approaches, the chapter proposed that the client may be conceptualized as a bundle of properties, and that the task of the clinician is to engage in a perceptual analysis of the client which will extract properties relevant to the diagnostic or therapeutic goal. That the properties of people may be perceived as interacting was discussed, and several of the ways in which properties may interact was illustrated. These notions provided a framework within which to consider the attributes of clients in the clinical setting and led to a consideration of what those attributes might be. Answers to the question of what people's attributes are were neither conclusive nor satisfactory, but it was proposed that a taxonomy of person attributes must include at least raw attributes, which are directly accessible to perception, and inferred attributes, which are judgments based on raw attributes and other inferred attributes. The former category includes physical properties and behaviors; the latter includes trait labels. The final section described one sort of mental representation that might result from the perceptual attribute analysis of the client. This proposal about mental representations relied both on contemporary thinking regarding the structure of concepts and recent research on the structure of the self.

A complete understanding of clinical information processing calls for an understanding of the stimulus and of how it is perceived as well as of the clinician's reasoning processes. The approach represented by this chapter is that an understanding of how the clinician perceives the client requires an understanding of the "structure" of the client. Although it is difficult at this point to specify precisely what the attributes of the client are, it is important to understand that they are the raw data of clinical judgment. Future research on clinical information processing must therefore focus on a detailed analysis of the raw data of clinical judgment.

Acknowledgment

Preparation of this chapter was supported in part by a Biomedical Research Support Grant from the National Institutes of Health to the Research Foundation of the State University of New York.

I appreciate the comments of Deborah Prentice and Peter Salovey on earlier drafts of a more complex version of this chapter (Smith, 1987), and the assistance of Kathryn Murphy in preparing that manuscript.

References

Anderson, N. H. (1981). *Foundations of information integration theory.* London: Academic Press.

Asch, S. E. (1946). Forming impressions of personality. *Journal of Abnormal and Social Psychology, 41,* 258–290.

Barocas, R., & Black, H. K. (1974). Referral rate and physical attractiveness in third grade children. *Perceptual and Motor Skills, 39,* 731–734.

Berry, D. S., & McArthur, L. Z. (1986). Perceiving character in faces: The impact of age-related craniofacial changes on social perception. *Psychological Bulletin, 100,* 3–18.

Bieri, J. (1961). Complexity-simplicity as a personality variable in cognitive and preferential behavior. In D. W. Fiske & S. R. Maddi (Eds.), *Functions of varied experience.* Homewood, IL: Dorsey.

———. (1962). Analyzing stimulus information in social judgments. In S. Messick & J. Ross (Eds.), *Measurement in personality and cognition.* New York: Wiley.

Bieri, J., Atkins, A. L., Briar, S., Leaman, R. L., Miller, H., & Tripodi, T. (1966). *Clinical and social judgment.* New York: Wiley.

Borkenau, P. (1986). Toward an understanding of trait interrelations: Acts as instances for several traits. *Journal of Personality and Social Psychology, 51,* 371–381.

Bruner, J. S., Shapiro, D., & Taguiri, R. (1958). The meaning of traits in isolation and in combination. In R. Taguiri & L. Petrullo (Eds.), *Person perception and interpersonal behavior* Stanford, CA: Stanford University Press.

Buss, D. M., & Craik, K. H. (1980). The frequency concept of disposition: Dominance and prototypically dominant acts. *Journal of Personality, 48,* 379–392.

———. (1981). The act frequency analysis of interpersonal dispositions: Aloofness, gregariousness, dominance, and submissiveness. *Journal of Personality, 49,* 174–192.

———. (1983). The act frequency approach to personality. *Psychological Review, 90,* 105–126.

Cantor, N., Smith, E. E., French, R., & Mezzich, J. (1980). Psychiatric diagnosis as prototype categorization. *Journal of Abnormal Psychology, 89,* 181–193.

Dornbusch, S. M., Hastorf, A. H., Richardson, S. A., Muzzy, R. E., & Vreeland, R. S. (1965). The perceiver and the perceived: The relative influence on the categories of interpersonal cognition. *Journal of Personality and Social Psychology, 1,* 434–440.

Einhorn, H. J., Kleinmuntz, D. N., & Kleinmuntz, B. (1979). Linear regression and process tracing models of judgment. *Psychological Review, 86,* 465–485.

Fiske, S. T., & Cox, M. G. (1979). Person concepts: The effect of target familiarity and descriptive purpose on the process of describing others. *Journal of Personality, 47,* 136–161.

Garner, W. R. (1974). *The processing of information and structure.* Potomac, MD: Erlbaum.

______. (1976). Interaction of stimulus dimensions in concept and choice processes. *Cognitive Psychology, 8,* 98–123.

Jones, E. E., & Thibaut, J. W. (1958). Interaction goals as bases of inference in interpersonal perception. In R. Taguiri & L. Petrullo (Eds.), *Person perception and interpersonal behavior.* Stanford, CA: Stanford University Press.

Linville, P. (1982). Affective consequences of complexity regarding the self and others. In M. S. Clark & S. T. Fiske (Eds.), *Affect and cognition.* Hillsdale, NJ: Erlbaum.

Maruyama, G., & Miller. N. (1982). Physical attractiveness and personality. *Progress in Experimental Personality Research, 10,* 117–166.

McArthur, L. Z. (1982). Judging a book by its cover: A cognitive analysis of the relationship between physical appearance and stereotyping. In A. H. Hastorf & A. M. Isen (Eds.), *Cognitive social psychology.* New York: Elsevier.

McGuire, W. J., & McGuire, C. V. (1982). Significant others in self-space: Sex differences and developmental trends in the social self. In J. Suls (Ed.), *Psychological perspectives on the self.* Hillsdale, NJ: Erlbaum.

Mischel, W. (1968). *Personality and assessment.* New York: Wiley.

Nisbett, R. E. (1980). The trait construct in lay and professional psychology. In L. Festinger (Ed.), *Retrospections on social psychology.* New York: Oxford University Press.

Park, B. (1986). A method for studying the development of impressions of real people. *Journal of Personality and Social Psychology, 51,* 907–917.

Rosch, E., & Mervis, C. B. (1975). Family resemblance studies in the internal structure of categories. *Cognitive Psychology, 7,* 573–605.

Rosch, E., Mervis, C. B., Gray, W., Johnson, D., & Boyes-Braem, P. (1976). Basic objects in natural categories. *Cognitive Psychology, 8,* 382–439.

Secord, P. F. (1958). Facial features and inference processes in interpersonal perception. In R. Taguiri & L. Petrullo (Eds.), *Person perception and interpersonal behavior.* Stanford, CA: Stanford University Press.

Secord, P. F., & Muthard, J. E. (1955). Personalities in faces: II. Individual differences in the perception of women's faces. *Journal of Abnormal and Social Psychology, 50,* 238–242.

Smith, A. F. (1986). *Configurations and dimensions in pattern perception.* Unpublished manuscript, State University of New York, Binghamton, NY.

______. (1987). *The perception and organization of information about people.* Unpublished manuscript, State University of New York, Binghamton, NY.

Smith, E. E., & Medin, D. L. (1981). *Categories and concepts.* Cambridge, MA: Harvard University Press.

Snyder, M., Tanke, E. D., & Berscheid, E. (1977). Social perception and interpersonal behavior: On the self-fulfilling nature of social stereotypes. *Journal of Personality and Social Psychology, 35,* 656–666.

Swann, W. B. (1984). Quest for accuracy in person perception: A matter of pragmatics. *Psychological Review, 91,* 457–477.

Taguiri, R. (1969). Person perception. In G. Lindzey & E. Aronson (Eds.), *The handbook of social psychology* (Vol. 3). Reading, MA: Addison-Wesley.

Tversky, A., & Gati, I. (1978). In E. Rosch & B. B. Lloyd (Eds.), *Cognition and categorization.* Hillsdale, NJ: Erlbaum.

5 Attributional Biases in Clinical Decision Making

John S. Jordan
John H. Harvey
Gifford Weary

ATTRIBUTION theory began with Fritz Heider's (1944; 1958) seminal analyses of how people perceive and explain the actions of others. Although Heider addressed many facets of social perception (e.g., how one person thinks and feels about another person, what one expects another to do or think, how one reacts to the actions of another), the bulk of attribution research follows from his notions about the "commonsense," implicit theories people use in understanding the causes of events they observe in their daily lives.

Put simply, attributions are inferences—inferences about the characteristics of persons, objects, events, and behavior or of the causal relationships among them. Note what a broad array of perceptual and cognitive activities the phrase "attributional processes" encompasses. Some have argued that the term attribution has been used indiscriminately, overinclusively, and oversimplistically (cf. Antaki & Brewin, 1982; Ostrom, 1981). Nevertheless, the seminal value of the concept of attribution in the recent history of psychological theory and research cannot be underestimated.

Clinicians and Attributions: Why and When

The need to understand, organize, and form meaningful perspectives about the myriad events we encounter is considered to be a major goal of attributional processes. By developing and testing hypotheses about human behavior, we develop an understanding of our social world that presumably renders it more predictable and controllable (Harvey & Weary, 1981; G. Kelly, 1955).

Virtually all clinical endeavors, diagnostic and therapeutic, have attributional processes at their core. Implicitly or explicitly, clinicians make frequent causal judgments. The following questions are illustrative. What caused this patient's headache? What brought the client to therapy at this time? What contributes to the patient's marital conflict? Why is this patient better or worse, late or early, smiling or sad today? How have I helped this patient?

The clinician's conceptual framework—whether behavioral, dynamic, or humanistic—is a set of systematic attributions for the causes of human behavior. Clinicians' implicit causal theories direct the information search and hypothesis-testing strategies that are part of diagnostic and therapeutic endeavors. As will be discussed, psychodiagnostic and therapeutic decisions sometimes reveal more about the clinician's hypotheses or preconceptions of psychopathology than about the actual status of the patient (Alloy, 1985).

Some Caveats Regarding the Current State of Attribution Theory and Research

Heider's (1958) work provided a general conceptual framework with which to understand perceptions of causality. The value of his work was not fully appreciated, however, until the mid-1960s when Edward Jones, Harold Kelley, and their colleagues developed, largely from Heider's ideas, more systematic theoretical statements on attributional processes. Many have observed that during the 1970s social psychology research was dominated by research in attributional processes. While much has been learned, the reader should be aware that there is no monolithic attribution theory, no coherent logical network that ties together general conclusions regarding attributional processes (cf. Harvey & Weary, 1981; Kelley, 1978).

Although many types of attributions may be of potential interest (e.g., inferences about individuals' personalities, religious beliefs, intelligence, likableness), the bulk of attribution research has addressed specifically the phenomena of *causal* judgment. In practice, the term "attribution" has often been used synonymously with "causal attribution." Hence, in the present exploration of attributional biases in clinical decision making, we will concern ourselves primarily with biases in causal judgment.

We must caution the reader about the term "bias" as it applies to attribution research. Ultimately, attribution researchers must be concerned with the accuracy of the explanations people offer for their own and other's behavior. However, the development of *defensible* criteria of accuracy represents a serious challenge for psychology. As Kelley and

Michela (1980) noted, "Since the entire enterprise of psychology is directed toward specification of the true causes of behavior, and since the causes and their relative magnitudes are not yet known, it may be impossible to design a study to test unequivocally the accuracy of attribution" (p. 479; cf. Batson, O'Quin, & Pych, 1982).

There also has been much debate about the basic nature of bias in attributional judgments. Perhaps because attribution theorists have emphasized the fundamentally cognitive nature of mechanisms involved in self- and interpersonal perception, most writers have stressed the importance of informational as opposed to motivational sources of bias (Weary, 1981). Some (e.g., Ross, 1977) even have advocated that motivational concerns be abandoned in the search for potential mediating causes of attributional bias. There is, however, a substantial body of literature that has demonstrated apparent self-serving or ego-defensive biases (see review by Weary Bradley, 1978; Weary & Arkin, 1981). Under most circumstances, nondepressed individuals are prone to take credit for good acts and deny blame for bad outcomes, thereby enhancing or protecting their self-esteem.

In most instances, motivational and cognitive sources of attributional bias are probably complexly intertwined. In this chapter, we will adopt the perspective that particular clinical judgment biases may be described as primarily "motivational" in nature, primarily "cognitive," or as representing an interaction of cognitive–motivational processes. We recognize, however, that even this scheme may be an oversimplification.

Considerable research has examined possible biases in attributional judgment, but virtually none of it has addressed directly attributional biases in clinical judgment. Hence, by necessity, this chapter must be largely speculative and exploratory. Often it will be necessary to extrapolate from data collected from "naive" (i.e., nontrained) participants—subjects in psychology experiments drawn from introductory psychology classes and subjects recruited from the community. Fortunately, such generalizations may be warranted. It appears that the attribution processes employed by trained clinicians are fundamentally the same as those employed by everyone else (Cantor, 1982). As will be seen in the next section, clinical training certainly does not make one immune from attributional bias and, in many cases, may augment it.

Sources of Attributional Bias

Divergent Perspectives: Actor–Observer Differences

People with different perspectives frequently diverge in their causal attributions for the same behavior. The alcoholic blames his consumption of alcohol on his stressful life circumstance, whereas his therapist sees his drinking as a manifestation of an underlying personality disorder. An obese man ordering a double fudge banana split complains to another about his "metabolism" problem.

Jones and Nisbett (1972) hypothesized that actors and observers are likely to differ systematically in the causal attributions they make for the same behavior because they differ in their foci of attention and background knowledge. Jones and Nisbett assert that actors tend to attribute causality for their behavior to situational influences, whereas observers are prone to attribute causality for the same behavior to stable dispositions possessed by the actors. Observers may often lack information about the distinctiveness or consistency of the actor's behavior, whereas actors may be influenced by their recollection that their behavior has shown variance in similar situations in the past. While the hypothesized actor–observer bias may not be quite as pervasive as Jones and Nisbett originally suggested, it has received considerable empirical confirmation (cf. Harvey, Harris, & Barnes, 1975; Monson & Snyder, 1977).

Trained clinicians, like naive observers, may be biased in the direction of attributing others' behaviors to stable dispositions. For example, many personality theorists consider personality traits to be psychological properties of people that function as causes of behavior (e.g., Allport, 1966; Cattell, 1950). These trait-based beliefs persist despite the poor cross-situational consistency in individual differences on various trait dimensions (e.g., Bem & Allen, 1974; Mischel, 1968). By weaving what seem to be disparate and variable patient behaviors into a common, stable thread, clinicians create at least an illusion of understanding, predictability, and control.

Particularly to the nonpsychologically trained observer, it may seem incredible that extremes in patient behavior can be readily incorporated into the same diagnostic label or personality construct. For example, both a complete absence of speech and loud, bizarre speech may be labelled "typically schizophrenic." A client may exhibit agitation or, conversly, psychomotor retardation and in both cases be diagnosed as depressive.

Of course, clinicians do not invariably perceive stable dispositions as the causes of all patient behaviors. We will consider how clinicians' theoretical perspectives and aspects of patient behavior may each affect the likelihood of such bias.

Theoretical Perspective. With nonclinical observers, Storms (1973) found that when observers' attention was focused on the actors' environment, they attributed the actors' behavior more to situational causes than when their attention was directed to other aspects of the actor. Clinicians' theoretical perspective may lead them to focus selectively on situational *or* dispositional factors. For example, whereas behavioral clinicians stress the importance of environmental cues and consequences as determinants of behavior, dynamic clinicians emphasize intrapsychic factors. Consequently, given the same presenting patient problem, dynamic clinicians will likely search for intrapsychic causes while behaviorists will search for situational determinants. Both are likely to find what they are looking for (Snyder, 1981).

Aspects of Patient Behavior. Responsibility for behaviors that are intense, changing, complex, novel, and/or "unit-forming" is more likely to be attributed to the actor (patient) than subdued, ordinary, simple, static, and/or fragmented behaviors (see McArthur, 1981). For example, Orvis, Cunningham, and Kelley (1975) found that low-consensus behaviors (i.e., behaviors rarely exhibited by other people) were more often attributed to the actor than to the situation. Most psychiatric behaviors are anything but subdued or ordinary. In fact, some have argued (e.g., Braginsky, Braginsky, & Ring, 1969) that behaviors labeled "psychiatric" are those deemed "unusual" (nonnormative, unacceptable) by a given society (hence, the large psychodiagnostic discrepancies between cultures and over time). It follows that the more intense, changing, or novel a patient's behavior is, the more likely an attribution of causality to the patient becomes.

Egocentric or Self-serving Biases

There is considerable evidence that people accept more responsibility for success than for failure (Miller & Ross, 1975). This seems equally true for clinicians. Books, journal articles, workshops and symposia exalt (often uncritically) particular treatment techniques; failures are rarely emphasized. One notable exception is Foa and Emmelkamp's edited volume on behavior therapy failures (1983) in which many failures are ascribed to clinician errors (e.g., patient misclassification, inadequate treatment trial, lack of specific relapse prevention, poor therapeutic relationship). More characteristically, however, failures are attributed to factors "beyond the control" of the clinician.

A patient's poor success is often attributed to "resistance," "defensiveness," or "unwillingness." Such attributions are even satirized in popular humor: "Question: How many psychologists does it take to change a light bulb? Answer: One, but the light bulb really has to want to change." After a treatment failure, patient characteristics are "discovered" retrospectively that presumably rendered the patient "unsuitable" from the outset. Sometimes clinicians may blame powerful "secondary gains" (e.g., extra attention from a spouse or pending disability payments) for treatment failure. The patients who are most recalcitrant to treatment may get labeled "borderline" or be seen as having some other fundamental (i.e., untreatable) "characterological defect." All of the above judgments serve to shift the burden of responsibility for treatment failure away from the clinician.

Clinicians may be biased in the degree of positive influence they perceive themselves as having on patients. Schopler and Layton (1972) have examined some of the behaviors that may facilitate perceptions of influence. First, several studies with teachers (e.g., Beckman, 1970; Johnson, Feigenbau, & Weiby, 1964) have demonstrated that we are more likely to infer influence over others when they have succeeded rather than failed. Second, in accord with Kelley's principle of covariance (1972), the more a patient behaves in new or unexpected ways, the more we are likely to perceive influence. Clinicians are likely to perceive therapy as being the "distinctive" or "noncommon"—and therefore causal—element in patients' lives. Other changes in a patient's life circumstances, or changes internal to the patient not attributable to therapy, may be overlooked completely or diminished in importance.

Similarly, clinical researchers may be biased in attributing greater success to their favored intervention. For example, psychotherapy outcome studies in which the assessment of therapeutic outcome has a potential for bias (i.e., raters are not "blinded" to treatment condition), tend to show that the favored therapy works best. In contrast, studies with unbiased assessment of therapy outcomes are likely to show no differences among the therapies compared (Alloy, 1985). Similarly, the popularity of clinical biofeedback in the treatment of many medical disorders (e.g., headaches, hypertension, chronic pain) has risen sharply in the last decade. While many biofeedback proponents have attributed their success to use of the biofeedback machines, controlled research repeatedly demonstrates that biofeedback per se usually is not the essential ingredient—various other methods of relaxation training seem to produce equally good results (e.g., Biofeedback Society of America, 1978; Surwit & Jordan, 1987; Turk, Meichenbaum, & Berman, 1979).

Publicly accepting responsibility for success and denying responsibility for failure may not always yield a positive social reaction. When there is a "social norm of responsibility" that dictates who is supposed to be held responsible for failures, clinicians (and patients) may be motivated to make "counterdefensive" attributions (i.e., accepting responsibility for failure). In contrast to the two previously mentioned studies of "self-serving" teacher attributions for pupil success and failure, Ross, Bierbrauer, and Polly (1974) and Tetlock (1980) found that experienced teachers were likely to blame themselves publicly for pupil failure, perhaps because there is a social norm that experienced teacher have internalized stating that pupils should not be blamed for classroom failures.

We have observed that clinicians are much less cautious (and less modest) in taking credit for treatment success, blaming external factors for treatment failure and affirming the certainty of their diagnostic (i.e., causal) formulations, when future invalidation is less likely (cf. Weary Bradley, 1978). After a patient has terminated therapy or has been discharged from the hospital such judgments often can be made with impunity. In clinical teaching conferences, it seems that predictions are made more ardently when the future course of the patient will not be followed (in this connection, Meehl's 1973 paper, "Why I Do Not Attend Case Conferences," is particularly worthy of review).

Defensive Attributions: Blaming the Victim

There is considerable evidence that victims are often blamed for the negative circumstances that befall them (e.g., Walster, 1966). Such blame attributions are presumed to serve a defensive function: By blaming a characteristic or behavior of the victim, you can feel more secure that the same consequences will not befall you by chance. Giving help to a victim may be mediated by perceptions of the victim's degree of control (cf. Weiner, 1980).

Weiner, Graham, and Chandler (1982) have provided evidence that people feel pity for others who are in trouble for reasons over which they are perceived to have no control, but will feel anger toward others in trouble for reasons perceived to be controllable. For example, mothers of enuretic children are more angry toward and less tolerant of their children if they perceive the causes to be controllable by the child (e.g., child is older, perceived as lazy or "getting back" at parent; Butler, Brewin, & Forsythe, 1985).

Similarly, patients who are perceived to be "victims" of uncontrollable events may be treated very differently from patients who are perceived to have been "willing victims" or responsible for their fate. Medical students have been found to be more willing to prescribe psychotropic medications for patients whom they view as experiencing "uncontrollable" as opposed to "controllable" life events (Brewin, 1984), even though this judgment about the controllability of the life situation may be based on superficial information. What determines a clinician's perception of controllability? Extrapolation from Shaver's (1970) research on causal attributions made about accident victims suggests that the more similar a victim is to a clinician (e.g., in age, personality, personal history, physique), the more likely it may be that the clinician will attribute negative events in the patient's life to external factors.[1]

[1]The reader may wish to compare these ideas to Murray's (1938, 1962) notions of complementary and supplementary projection.

Biased Covariation Assessment

Several researchers (e.g., Chapman & Chapman, 1967, 1969; Golding & Rorer, 1972; Starr & Katkin, 1969) have demonstrated "illusory" correlation effects with the Rorschach, Draw-a-Person, and Incomplete Sentences tests. Naive students and experienced clinicians hold erroneous beliefs about the relationship between test responses and particular psychosocial problems (e.g., "eyes" relate strongly to "suspiciousness").

Alloy (1985) contends that the illusory correlation effects, as well as the labeling and therapy outcome biases described in previous sections, are all instances of erroneous or biased covariation assessments. Covariation refers to the co-occurrence of events—the degree to which one event occurs more often in the presence than in the absence of another event. For accurate diagnosis, a clinician must be able to accurately detect which symptoms covary together and which symptoms are associated with which diagnostic categories.

Alloy and Tabachnik (1984) proposed that two sources of information jointly determine covariation perception: the objective contingency between the events and the individual's prior beliefs or expectations about the event covariation. The degree to which the subjective judgment of covariation matches the objective contingency depends on (1) the relative strength of prior expectations; and (2) current situational information. Strength of situational information has to do with relative availability and ambiguity (i.e., the distinctiveness and consistency of the information and the consensus regarding it). Expectations may come from clinical training.

There are four basic combinations of situational and expectational strength:

		Situation	
		Weak	*Strong*
Expectations	*Weak*	*1*	*3*
	Strong	*2*	*4*

Among trained clinicians, making judgments in their areas of presumed expertise, expectational strength would typically seem very high. In the face of weak situational evidence (Cell 2), judgments are predicted by Alloy and Tabachnik to be a direct reflection of a priori expectations. Accuracy will be determined by the accuracy or appropriateness of the individual's extant beliefs.

In Cell 4 situations, both expectations and situational information are strong. If both sets of information are congruent, individuals tend to make covariation judgments in which they have extreme confidence more accurately. If, however, generalized beliefs and situational information are incongruent and imply different perceptions of contingency, the perceiver is faced with a "cognitive dilemma" (Metalsky & Abramson, 1981). The empirical evidence reviewed by Alloy and Tabachnik suggests that in this situation, people tend to make covariation assessments biased in the direction of their initial expectations unless there is substantial or particularly salient contradictory evidence (e.g., Coppel & Smith, 1980; Crocker & Taylor, 1978; Dickinson, Shanks, & Evenden, 1984).

A clinician's preconceptions can produce error in any of the cognitive steps that may lead to subjective estimates of contingency, including: how much and what kinds of information are relevant; selecting or sampling information from available evidence; classifying selected instances as confirming or disconfirming; recalling and estimating the relative frequency of confirming and disconfirming information; and combining the information obtained into a judgment (Alloy & Tabachnik, 1984; Crocker, 1981). In short, one resolution of this cognitive dilemma is to interpret or recall the situational evidence in line with one's prior beliefs (e.g., Kayne & Alloy, in press).

Schematic Processing Errors

Attribution theories have been criticized for their assumption that individuals routinely operate like intuitive scientists in a highly deliberate and "mindful" manner. Abelson (1976) and Langer (1978) have presented provocative accounts of how people may often operate in a highly scripted or automatic ("mindless") way in carrying out certain complex or familiar sequences of actions.[2] Among the situations that Langer (1978) suggests are likely to require more mindful and deliberative thinking are novel situations (for which there are no scripts); situations in which scripted behavior is interrupted; and situations where scripted behavior becomes effortful.

Most clinicians seem to gravitate toward specialty practices based on type of clinical problem (e.g., headache, depression), patient characteristics (e.g., adolescent, lesbian), or type of clinical service (e.g., neuropsychological assessment, relaxation training). Presumably, repeated experiences working with patients with common features enhances (at least a perception of) the clinician's competence. The clinician can engage in (hopefully accurate) ongoing covariation assessments of diag-

[2]See Kelley's (1972) book on causal schemata and Nisbett and Wilson's (1977) paper on a priori causal theories for extended discussions of concepts related to scripts.

nostic and treatment outcomes that result in improved clinical efficacy, efficiency (and satisfaction) for the clinician.

Presumed familiarity with a particular clinical problem, patient type, or procedure may also lead to increasingly scripted thinking and behavior by the clinician. Implicitly or explicitly, clinicians develop formulas (or "clinical heuristics") for conceptualizing or approaching particular cases. Given the high service demands placed on most clinicians today (by both patients and administrators), developing cognitively efficient strategies may be an essential task for the clinician.

While scripted behavior in many ways may be more efficient, it also may be more subject to inaccuracy. If it is only the novel case or the one for which routine procedures do not produce the expected results that elicits a more "mindful" approach from the clinicians, then causal beliefs may reflect more about their scripts than about the patient. In one study, traditional therapists who were expecting to observe a "patient" evaluated the person as more disturbed than those who were expecting to observe a "job applicant" (Langer & Abelson, 1974). As will be discussed in the next sections, once faulty causal attributions (or diagnostic labels) are made, contradictory (accurate) information may be discounted; self-fulfilling prophecies may then confirm the faulty diagnosis, and treatment may proceed inappropriately.

Biased Hypothesis Testing

Snyder (1981) cites evidence suggesting that judgments about the causes of individuals' behavior are frequently biased or inaccurate because only confirmatory hypothesis-testing strategies are employed. Competing hypotheses and contradictory information are often overlooked. "Having diagnosed the client's 'problem,' the therapist may selectively and preferentially solicit confirming evidence. This activity may be guided by a hypothesis about what kinds of 'backgrounds' lead up to what kinds of current 'problems'" (Snyder, 1981, p. 294).

For example,

> The psychiatrist who believes (erroneously) that adult gay males had bad childhood relationships with their mothers may meticulously probe for recalled (or fabricated) signs of tension between their gay clients and their mothers, but neglect to so carefully interrogate their heterosexual clients about their maternal relationships. No doubt, any individual could recall some friction with his or her mother, however minor or isolated the incidents. (Snyder, 1981, p. 274)

Renaud and Estess (1961), after examining the life histories of 100 healthy, occupationally, maritally, and psychologically well-adjusted men, concluded that they would have had no trouble finding evidence of the "background factors" that supposedly predispose individuals to any number of problems (e.g., colitis, ulcers, phobias, work inhibitions). "As long as one only probes into the backgrounds of 'troubled' adults, it will be all too easy to blame any and all contemporary problems on whatever 'pathogenic' background is demanded by one's hypothesis that links current symptoms and historical causes" (Snyder, 1981, p. 295).

Self-fulfilling Prophecies

Merton (1957) defined a self-fulfilling prophecy as "a *false* definition of the situation evoking a new behavior which makes the originally false conception come *true*" (p. 423). The work by Rosenthal and colleagues (1966, 1968) demonstrated that teachers and experimenters actually elicit from students and subjects what they want and expect to observe. This observation is no less applicable in psychotherapy.

There has been considerable concern regarding the extent to which clients' behaviors come to match the conceptual framework and theoretical orientations of their therapists (e.g., Frank, 1974; Scheff, 1966). Somehow, therapists elicit from their clients values, historical data, and even dream material that confirm their own views (cf. Bandura, Lipsher, & Miller, 1960; Frank, 1973; Whitman, Kramer, & Baldridge, 1963). "Psychiatrists, as doctors, can without much difficulty convert patients into accepting their diagnostic impressions and induce them to accept the illness and concurrent symptoms and traits associated with these prescribed impressions" (Keisner, 1985, p. 435; cf. Schur, 1971).

Reducing Clinicians' Attributional Errors

A thorough consideration of training strategies that may reduce the possibility of the various clinical inferential errors discussed above is beyond the scope of this chapter; for an in-depth discussion, see Arnoult and Anderson, this volume. However, it may be useful at this point to consider briefly several of the more effective strategies for minimizing attributional errors in the clinical setting.

Our consideration of the sources of attributional bias indicates that, for a variety of reasons, clinicians often may err in the direction of making too many dispositional attributions (cf. Batson et al., 1982). How might we reduce the likelihood of such errors through our clinical training? Two possibilities suggest themselves, both involving changes in the process of perceiving client behavior.

First, research by Storms (1973) suggests that altering the visual perspective of the clinician may reduce the likelihood of dispositional attributions. In a study of divergent actor–observer differences, Storms reversed the point of view of subjects by using a videotape. He found that when observers were provided with an actor's visual perspective of dyadic interaction, observers made fewer dispositional attributions for the actor than did the actor herself. Since clinical training often involves the videotaping of assessment and therapy activities, it would seem possible to change the clinician's typical focus of attention and attributional tendencies by focusing the camera on him or her, rather than on the client. Training in empathy may also produce a similar reversal in the clinician's perspective (Regan & Totten, 1975). Of course, this is not to invalidate the informational value of nonverbal cues garnered by clinicians when they take the perspective of the observer. Rather, taking the actor's and the observer's perspective during clinical interactions should contribute to the making of valid judgments.

Second, the way in which clinicians organize their clients' behaviors may also affect the likelihood of dispositional attributions. Research by Newtson (1973) found that subjects made more dispositional attributions about others and were more confident in their attributions when they were instructed to segment videotaped, "free" behavior sequences into fine units. Since clinicians typically scrutinize small segments of clients' behaviors, they may be more likely than lay observers to organize perceptual information into fine units and to arrive at dispositional attributions (Brehm, 1976). Although, at times, dispositional explanations may be appropriate, these behaviors by clinicians may blind them to potential situational explanations for clients' behaviors. With practice, clinicians may well be able to learn to make large-unit analyses of ongoing behavioral sequences and reduce attributional errors.

A third strategy for reducing attributional errors in clinical settings focuses not so much on the perceptual activities as on the inferential processes of the clinician. In an earlier section, we argued that clinical judgments about the causes of clients' behaviors may frequently be biased or inaccurate because clinicians (like lay observers) primarily use confirmatory hypothesis-testing strategies. Is there a way to force clinicians to avoid the tendency to solicit evidence whose presence confirms a given hypothesis? Interestingly, research indicates that the only procedure that successfully induces individuals to avoid confirmatory information search strategies is one that gives them *no* hypotheses to test (Snyder, 1981). Since it would be hard to conceive of a clinical situation in which no hypotheses were being tested, such a procedure does not seem useful in the present context. Instead, we would suggest that clinicians learn how to search for disconfirming information and how to formulate and test competing hypothesis.

Summary and Future Research Directions

In this chapter, we have argued that most major endeavors carried out by the clinician involve attributional processes. Broadly construed, such processes include inferences about the patient, such as situational and dispositional attributions for behavior, attributions about the patient's environment, and attributions about the self with respect to interaction with the patient. Either explicitly or implicitly, clinicians engage in such attributions from the moment of meeting the patient (or before) to the end of therapy (and beyond). Despite the pervasiveness of attributional activities in the clinical arena, there has been little empirical work designed to address systematically these activities, their consequences and correlates.

Given the paucity of available empirical literature, a great number and variety of questions await research on clinical attributional judgment. We need work on a better articulation of clinicians' actual decisional processes, such as on criteria used in diagnosis and in decisions about changes in therapy regimen. Most of our analysis has been based on extrapolation from theory and research in other contexts. Therefore, the meaningfulness of attributional concepts in the area of clinical judgment also needs to be addressed. More specifically, we greatly need work designed to probe motivational and cognitive biases in the attributions of clinicians—both for different types of patients and by different types of clinicians. Conceivably, for example, the attributions of novice and experienced therapists may reflect different tendencies. While some of this work might be done using simulation and analogue techniques, the most informative data probably will emerge from correlational–descriptive studies that involve multivariate analyses of patient–therapist interaction over extended periods of time.

References

Abelson, R. P. (1976). A script theory of understanding, attitude, and behavior. In J. S. Carroll & J. W. Payne (Eds.), *Cognition and social behavior.* Hillsdale, NJ: Erlbaum.

Alloy, L. B. (1985). *Clinician biases in covariation assessment.* Paper presented at the convention of the American Psychological Association, Los Angeles.

Alloy, L. B., & Tabachnik, N. (1984). Assessment of covariation by humans and animals: The joint influence of prior expectations and current situational information. *Psychological Review, 91,* 112–149.

Allport, G. W., (1966). Traits revisited. *American Psychologist, 21,* 1–10.

Antaki, C., & Brewin, C. R. (Eds.). (1982). *Attributions and psychological change: Applications of attributional theories to clinical and educational practice.* London: Academic Press.

Bandura, A., Lipsher, D. H., & Miller, P. E. (1960). Psychotherapists approach-avoidance reactions to patients' expressions of hostility. *Journal of Consulting Psychology, 24,* 1–8.

Batson, C. D., O'Quin, K., & Pych, V. (1982). An attribution theory analysis of trained helpers' inferences about clients' needs. In T. A. Wills (Ed.), *Basic processes in helping relationships.* New York: Academic Press.

Beckman, L. (1970). Effects of students' performance on teachers' and observers' attributions of causality. *Journal of Educational Psychology, 61,* 76–82.

Bem, D. J., & Allen, A. (1974). On predicting some of the people some of the time: The search for cross-situational consistencies in behavior. *Psychological Review, 81,* 506–520.

Biofeedback Society of America. (1978). B.S.A. Task Force Report, *Biofeedback and Self-Regulation, 3.*

Braginsky, B. M., Braginsky, D. D., & Ring, K. (1969). *Methods of madness: The mental hospital as a last resort.* New York: Holt, Rinehart & Winston.

Brehm, S. S. (1976). *The application of social psychology to clinical practice.* New York: Wiley.

Brewin, C. R. (1984). Perceived controllability of life events and willingness to prescribe psychotropic drugs. *British Journal of Social Psychology, 23,* 285–287.

Butler, R. J., Brewin, C. R., & Forsythe, W. I. (1985). *Maternal attributions and tolerance for nocturnal enuresis.* Unpublished paper, Institute of Psychiatry, London.

Cantor, N. (1982). "Everyday" versus normative models of clinical and social judgment. In G. Weary and H. L. Mirels (Eds.), *Integrations of clinical and social psychology.* New York: Oxford University Press.

Cattell, R. B. (1950). *Personality: A systematic theoretical and factual study.* New York: McGraw-Hill.

Chapman, L. J., & Chapman, J. P. (1967). Genesis of popular but erroneous psychodiagnostic observations. *Journal of Abnormal Psychology, 72,* 193–204.

______. (1969). Illusory correlation as an obstacle to the use of valid psychodiagnostic signs. *Journal of Abnormal Psychology, 74,* 271–280.

Coppel, D. B., & Smith, R. E. (1980). Acquisition of stimulus-outcome and response-outcome expectancies as a function of locus of control. *Cognitive Therapy and Research, 4,* 179–188.

Crocker, J. (1981). Judgment of covariation by social perceivers. *Psychological Bulletin, 90,* 272–292.

Crocker, J., & Taylor, S. E. (1978). *Theory-driven processing and the use of complex evidence.* Paper presented at the meeting of the American Psychological Association, Toronto, Canada.

Dickinson, A., Shanks, D., & Evenden, J. (1984). Judgment of act-outcome contingency: The role of selective attribution. *Quarterly Journal of Experimental Psychology, 36,* 29–50.

Foa, E. B., & Emmelkamp, P. M. (Eds.). (1983). *Failures in behavior therapy.* New York: Wiley.

Frank, J. D. (1973). *Persuasion and healing.* Baltimore: Johns Hopkins University Press.

Golding, S. L., & Rorer, L. G. (1972). Illusory correlation and the learning of clinical judgment. *Journal of Abnormal Psychology, 80,* 249–260.

Harvey, J. H., Harris, B., & Barnes, R. D. (1975). Actor-observer differences in the perceptions of responsibility and freedom. *Journal of Personality and Social Psychology, 32,* 22–28.

Harvey, J. H., & Weary, G. (1981). *Perspectives on attributional processes.* Dubuque, IA: Brown.

Heider, F. (1944). Social perception and phenomenal causality. *Psychological Review, 51,* 358–374.

———. (1958). *The psychology of interpersonal relations.* New York: Wiley.

Johnson, T. J., Feigenbau, R., & Weiby, M. (1964). Some determinants and consequences of the teacher's perception of causation. *Journal of Educational Psychology, 55,* 237–246.

Jones, E. E., & Nisbett, R. E. (1972). The actor and the observer: Divergent perceptions of the causes of behavior. In E. E. Jones, D. E. Kanouse, H. H. Kelley, R. E. Nisbett, S. Valins, & B. Weiner (Eds.), *Attribution: Perceiving the causes of behavior.* Morristown, NJ: General Learning Press.

Kayne, N. T., & Alloy, L. B. (in press). Clinician and patient as aberrant actuaries: Expectation-based distortions in assessment of covariation. In L. Y. Abramson (Ed.), *Attribution processes and clinical psychology.* New York: Guilford.

Keisner, R. H. (1985). Self-fulfilling prophecies in psychodynamic practice. In G. Stricker & R. H. Keisner (Eds.), *From research to clinical practice.* New York: Plenum.

Kelley, H. H. (1972). *The process of causal schemata and the attribution process.* Morristown, NJ: General Learning Press.

———. (1978). A conversation with Edward E. Jones and Harold H. Kelley. In J. H. Harvey, W. Ickes, & R. F. Kidd (Eds.), *New directions in attribution research* (Vol. 2). Hillsdale, NJ: Erlbaum.

Kelley, H. H., & Michela, J. L. (1980). Attribution theory and research. *Annual Review of Psychology, 31,* 457–501.

Kelly, G. (1955). *The psychology of personal constructs* (Vols. 1 & 2). New York: Norton.

Langer, E. J. (1978). Rethinking the role of thought in social interaction. In J. H. Harvey, W. J. Ickes, & R. F. Kidd (Eds.), *New directions in attribution research* (Vol. 2). Hillsdale, NJ: Erlbaum.

Langer, E. J., & Abelson, R. P. (1974). A patient by any other name . . . : Clinician group differences in labeling bias. *Journal of Consulting and Clinical Psychology, 42,* 4–9.

McArthur, L. Z. (1981). What grabs you? The role of attention in impression formation and causal attribution. In E. T. Higgins, C. P. Herman, & M. P. Zanna (Eds.), *Social cognition: The Ontario Symposium* (Vol. 1). Hillsdale, NJ: Erlbaum.

Meehl, P. E. (1973). Why I do not attend case conferences. In P. Meehl, *Psychodiagnosis: Selected papers.* Minneapolis: University of Minneapolis Press.

Merton, R. K. (1957). *Social theory and social structure* (rev. ed.). New York: Free Press.

Metalsky, G. I., & Abramson, L. Y. (1981). Attributional styles: Toward a framework for conceptualization and assessment. In P. C. Kendall & S. E. Hollon (Eds.), *Assessment strategies for cognitive-behavioral interventions.* New York: Academic Press.

Miller, D. T., & Ross, M. (1975). Self-serving biases in the attribution of causality: Fact or fiction? *Psychological Bulletin, 82,* 213–215.

Mischel, W. (1968). *Personality and assessment.* New York: Wiley.

Monson, T. C., & Snyder, M. (1977). Actors, observers, and the attribution process: Toward a reconceptualization. *Journal of Experimental Social Psychology, 13,* 89–111.

Murray, H. A. (1938). *Explorations in personality.* New York: Oxford University Press.

______. (1962). *Explorations in personality.* New York: Wiley.

Newtson, D. (1973). Attribution and the unit of perception of ongoing behavior. *Journal of Personality and Social Psychology, 28,* 28–38.

Nisbett, R. E., & Wilson, T. D. (1977). Telling more than we can know: Verbal reports on mental processes. *Psychological Review, 84,* 231–259.

Orvis, B. R., Cunningham, J. D., & Kelley, H. H. (1975). A closer examination of causal inference: The roles of consensus, distinctiveness, and consistency information. *Journal of Personality and Social Psychology, 32,* 605–616.

Ostrom, T. M. (1981). Attribution theory: Whence and whither. In J. Harvey, W. Ickes, & R. Kidd (Eds.), *New directions in attribution research* (Vol. III). Hillsdale, NJ: Erlbaum.

Regan, D. R., & Totten, J. (1975). Empathy and attribution: Turning observers into actors. *Journal of Personality and Social Psychology, 32,* 850–856.

Renaud, H., & Estess, F. (1961). Life history interviews with one hundred normal American males: "Pathogenicity" of childhood. *American Journal of Orthopsychiatry, 31,* 796–802.

Rosenthal, R. (1966). *Experimenter effects in behavioral research.* New York: Appleton-Century-Crofts.

Rosenthal, R., & Jacobson, L. (1968). *Pygmalion in the classroom.* New York: Holt, Rinehart and Winston.

Ross, L. (1977). The intuitive psychologist and his shortcomings: Distortions in the attribution process. In L. Berkowitz (Ed.), *Advances in experimental social psychology* (Vol. 12). New York: Academic Press.

Ross, L., Bierbrauer, R., & Polly, S. (1974). Attribution of educational outcomes by professional and nonprofessional instructors. *Journal of Personality and Social Psychology, 29,* 609–618.

Scheff, T. J. (1966). *Being mentally ill: A sociological theory.* Chicago: Aldine.

Schopler, J., & Layton, B. (1972). Determinants of the self-attribution of having influenced another person. *Journal of Personality and Social Psychology, 22,* 326–332.

Schur, E. M. (1971). *Labeling deviant behavior.* New York: Harper & Row.

Shaver, K. G. (1970). Defensive attribution: Effects of severity and relevance on the responsibility assigned for an accident. *Journal of Personality and Social Psychology, 14,* 101–113.

Snyder, M. (1981). Seek, and ye shall find: Testing hypotheses about other people. In E. T. Higgins, C. P. Herman, & M. P. Zanna (Eds.), *Social cognition: The Ontario Symposium* (Vol. 1). Hillsdale, NJ: Erlbaum.

Starr, B. J., & Katkin, E. S. (1969). The clinician as an aberrant actuary: Illusory correlation and the incomplete sentence blank. *Journal of Abnormal Psychology, 74,* 670–675.

Storms, M. D. (1973). Videotape and the attribution process: Reversing actors' and observers' points of view. *Journal of Personality and Social Psychology, 27,* 165–175.

Surwit, R. S., & Jordan, J. S. (1987). Behavioral treatment of Raynaud's syndrome. In J. Hatch, J. G. Fisher, & J. D. Rugh (Eds.), *Biofeedback: Studies in clinical efficacy.* New York: Plenum.

Tetlock, P. E. (1980). Explaining teacher explanations of pupil performance: A self-presentation interpretation. *Social Psychology Quarterly, 43,* 283–290.

Turk, D. C., Meichenbaum, D. H., & Berman, W. H. (1979). Application of biofeedback for the regulation of pain: A critical review. *Psychological Bulletin, 86,* 1322–1338.

Walster, E. (1966). Assignment of responsibility for an accident. *Journal of Personality and Social Psychology, 3,* 73–79.

Weary, G. (1981). The role of cognitive, affective, and social factors in attributional biases. In J. H. Harvey (Ed.), *Cognition, social behavior, and the environment.* Hillsdale, NJ: Erlbaum.

Weary, G., & Arkin, R. M. (1981). Attributional self-presentation. In J. H. Harvey, W. Ickes, & R. F. Kidd (Eds.), *New directions in attribution research* (Vol. 3). Hillsdale, NJ: Erlbaum.

Weary Bradley, G. (1978). Self-serving biases in the attribution process: A reexamination of the fact or fiction question. *Journal of Personality and Social Psychology, 36,* 56–71.

Weiner, B. (1980). A cognitive (attribution)-emotion-action model of motivated behavior: An analysis of judgments of help-giving. *Journal of Personality and Social Psychology, 39,* 186–200.

Weiner, B., Graham, S., & Chandler, C. (1982). Pity, anger, and guilt: An attributional analysis. *Personality and Social Psychology Bulletin, 8,* 226–232.

Whitman, R. M., Kramer, M., & Baldridge, B. (1963). Which dream does the patient tell? *Archives of General Psychiatry, 8,* 277–282.

6 | Some Effects of Mood on Clinicians' Memory

Peter Salovey
Dennis C. Turk

THE effects of transient mood states on memory and judgment were first investigated by researchers in the early part of this century (reviewed by Rapaport, 1942). Following several decades during which the topic was viewed as tangential to the goals of a behavioristic science, researchers once again have returned to the study of mood states and their cognitive consequences (see recent reviews by Blaney, 1986; Isen, 1984; Mayer & Salovey, in press). Many of these investigators have conducted experiments in the service of some theory of memory and/or emotion, most commonly Bower's Network Theory of Affect (Bower, 1981, derived from Anderson & Bower, 1973; Collins & Loftus, 1975). The implications of this research for clinical work, however, have not been elaborated, perhaps due to caution about the stability of findings in this area (e.g., Bower & Mayer, 1985). Moreover, this body of research has been published in journals directed toward experimental rather than clinical psychologists and so findings with obvious clinical relevance are easily overlooked. In essence, this rapidly proliferating literature suggests that memory for people and events seems to be systematically affected by mood in several different ways, namely, in attentional focus, selective encoding, and retrieval of information. These mood effects on memory can and often do result in distortions that might bias judgment.

In this chapter, we will discuss the influence of affect on the memory, judgment, and behavior of clinicians. It should be pointed out, however, that this is not the way feelings states that evolve during therapy are discussed typically. Clinicians probably always experience feelings during the course of a therapy session. And, these feelings, at least according to some schools of psychotherapy, rather than serving as biasing influences on the course of therapy, are instead used as productive sources of information for the therapist. That is, the feelings aroused in the therapist during a therapeutic session are actively attended to and interpreted in the context of the relationship with the client. These feelings on the part of the clinician are usually thought of as part of the countertransference process, defined as the whole of the therapist's feelings and conscious and unconscious reactions to the patient (Heimann, 1950; see also Singer, this volume). Further, it is sometimes assumed that the feelings a client can arouse in a therapist are similar to the feelings that significant others in the client's environment might experience when dealing with this person. These feelings are then used as a tool in helping the therapist understand the client (Walrond-Skinner, 1986).

Most schools of psychotherapy, however, also emphasize the importance of gaining understanding of countertransference reactions and developing the maturity or skills necessary to distance oneself from the feelings generated by a therapy session (Kernberg, 1965). Psychodynamically oriented writers must have realized the potentially biasing impact of the therapist's mood state in recommending that clinicians learn to regulate such feelings. It is possible that these writers recognized that affect can influence thought in less than optimal ways for effective assessment and psychotherapy.

Consider the following scenario. Dr. Joseph Doakes, a psychotherapist in private practice, buys a Lotto ticket on the way to his office one morning. When the winning numbers are announced at 10:00 A.M., he discovers that he has won a prize. His mood, at this point, shifts in the positive direction. He now sees his first client, whom he finds it especially easy to attend to and learns about the client's successes during the past week. However, Dr. Doakes finds that he does not attend to or encode any information about possible client failures. Later in the session, Dr. Doakes recalls an incident from a past session giving evidence for the client's potential for further success. And, at the conclusion of the session, Dr. Doakes discovers that he can remember better something this client told him three weeks ago (the same day the good doctor found out his daughter did not need $5,000 worth of orthodontic work), but that he cannot remember much about last week's session (which was also the day he filed his income tax return).

Because of his positive mood state, initiated by events external to the therapy, Dr. Doakes exhibits several common effects that mood has on the processing of information. These include the tendency to (a) learn material better when it is congruent in tone with one's mood, (b) retrieve information from memory that is consistent in tone with one's mood, and (c) more easily remember material when one's mood state at the time of retrieval matches one's original mood state at the time the information was encoded. This chapter will deal with these kinds of influences of affect on memory, explore mood influences on judgment, decision making, and behavior, and then very briefly describe ways that clinicians can try to minimize any detrimental impact that these influences may have on their clinical activities (but see also Arnoult and Anderson, this volume). First, however, we will place the affect–cognition question in a broader theoretical context.

Overview of Affect Vis-à-vis Cognition

For the last decade, psychologists have debated the role played by affect relative to cognitive activities. For example, Zajonc (1980, 1984) and Lazarus (1982) have argued vociferously about the priority of affect versus cognition in determining responses to stimuli. Zajonc has claimed that affective responses can occur in the absence of higher order cognitive processes. He supports this view by citing studies showing that individuals exhibit affective responses to stimuli they have seen so briefly that they are unaware of having experienced them. Zajonc also uses findings from such "mere exposure" experiments (1980) to support his view that affective experience is distinct from cognition and that the two represent separate systems (a view shared by Izard, 1972, 1977; and Tomkins, 1962, 1963). Lazarus, whose view is more consistent with the approach of cognitive behaviorally oriented clinicians, disputes Zajonc's conclusions, proposing instead that affect arises out of a complex cognitive process requiring a series of appraisals (of stimuli) and judgments about them, although the individual need not be consciously aware of these appraisals.

Others (e.g., Bower, 1981; Clark & Isen, 1982) have attempted to integrate the workings of affect within information-processing paradigms without becoming entangled in the primacy of affect versus cognition debate. Bower, for example, believes that emotions and moods are central units (called "nodes") in the network of ideas (called "propositions") linked together by being associated in memory (see Figure 6–1 for an example). Still other researchers have discussed similar cognitively oriented views of the effects of affect on memory as well as on social behavior (e.g., Clark & Isen, 1982; Isen, 1984; Salovey & Rodin, 1985). These researchers argue that affective states increase the availability (i.e., ease of recall) of similarly toned thoughts, inferences, and judgments (see, in particular, Isen, Shalker, Clark, & Karp, 1978).

In Bower's Network Theory of Affect (Bower, 1981; Bower & Cohen, 1982) mood states activate relevant associations in memory, priming other material linked to them. This process facilitates learning and recall

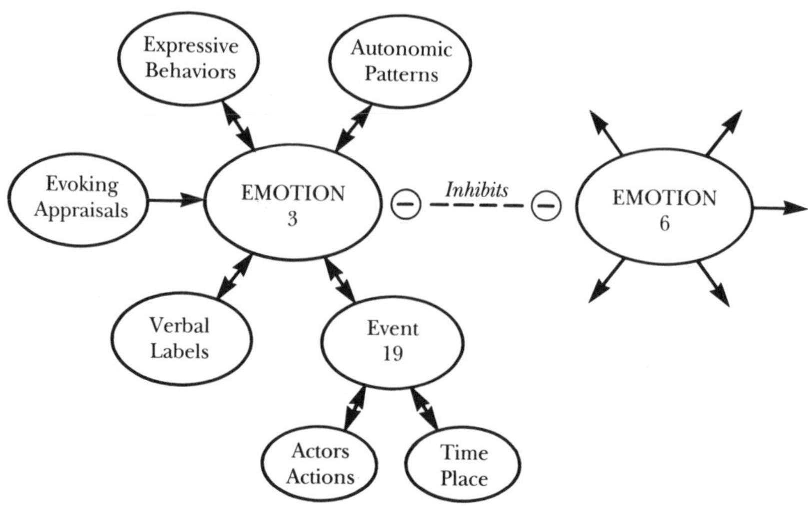

Figure 6–1. Fragment of a Memory Network Containing Emotion Nodes
Adapted from Bower, 1981.

of material that is consistent in emotional tone with the existing mood state (as Dr. Doakes discovered in the example described earlier). In the most comprehensive statement of this theory, Gilligan and Bower (1984) enumerate seven postulates: First, emotions are characterized as central units in memory, with many connections to related ideas, autonomic activity, muscular and expressive patterns, and events. Second, emotion-laden material is stored in the memory network in terms of subject–response–object idea units (e.g., Doakes wins lottery; Doakes feels happy). Third, thought emerges through the activation of these units within the network. Once one unit is stimulated in this way, material associated with it can also be primed, and, if raised above threshold, activated. Cognitive psychologists refer to this process as "spreading activation" (Collins & Loftus, 1975). Fourth, activation can be initiated by internal or external sources, including thought, physiological feedback, and environmental stimuli. Fifth, spreading activation is selective, reaching out primarily to associated memories and concepts. Sixth, associations among thoughts and ideas are formed during learning. When new material is learned, it is associated with whatever in memory is already active at the time. Seventh, "consciousness" consists of the network of associations activated at a given moment.

Research spawned by this theoretical tradition has identified several ways in which mood might affect memory. Each of these effects of mood on memory was illustrated in the Dr. Doakes example that opened this chapter. They will be defined more formally, however, here. The first will be called "encoding congruency" in this chapter, meaning that material congruent with one's current affective state is encoded into memory more readily. The second effect we will describe will be referred to as "recall congruency," the relative ease with which one can recall information from memory that is affectively consistent with one's current emotional state. A third common event is that material learned while in a particular affective state is better recalled when one is once again in that state, a phenomenon known as "state-dependent recall." Finally, there is a general tendency for material that is highly charged emotionally to be better learned and more easily recalled, the "mood intensity" effect.

Encoding Congruency

One can easily imagine the potentially biasing effects created by encoding congruency on the memory of clinicians. When a clinician's mood is made more positive temporarily because a client indicates that the therapy is going well, the clinician may be more likely to disregard and consequently not encode information presented by the client that might arouse negative affect. The clinician, later, may recall a falsely positive view of the outcome of this therapy case as a result of the encoding congruency effect.

In addition, clinicians' moods are affected by events outside the therapeutic hour. Like our Dr. Doakes, whose positive mood resulted from winning the lottery, therapists are more likely to encode information from clients that is consistent with their "extratherapeutic" mood states and to disregard mood-incongruent material.

In the laboratory, the encoding congruency effect has been found when subjects are induced to experience a particular mood and then read a story involving several characters. Later, once the mood has dissipated, subjects are better able to recall information about the character in the story whose affect is most like their own (Bower, Gilligan, & Monteiro, 1981). Bower et al. (1981) obtained their strongest effects using sad moods, but Nasby and Yando (1982) found that subjects were better able to recall positive information learned when they were happy than when they were sad or angry. The encoding congruency effect has been more difficult to observe using natural (rather than induced) changes in mood (e.g., Hasher, Rose, Zacks, Sanft, & Doren, 1985), but such studies have been criticized on methodological grounds (Mayer & Bower, 1985), because the naturally occurring mood states studied thus far have not been especially intense (e.g., investigators have compared normal individuals with Beck Depression Inventory Scores of 8 and above with individuals scoring below 8; a border-line clinical depression is usually not indicated by scores lower than 17, according to Burns, 1980).

Recall Congruency

The tendency to recall information that is consistent with one's mood state has been confirmed using a variety of laboratory mood-induction procedures—mood statements (e.g., Velten's, 1968), self-generated imagery, and hypnosis—and several different dependent measures (e.g., autobiographical memory content, retrieval speed). The problems for clinicians created by the mood-congruency effect are fairly obvious. In preparing for a session, clinicians may be more likely to recall and therefore inquire about issues consistent with their current moods. These questions could then elicit mood-congruent responses from clients (see Snyder & Thomsen, this volume). Certainly, information about a client's behavior during a prior session that is congruent with the clinician's current mood would be easier to recall than mood-incongruent information. And, in diagnostic work, clinicians may be more likely to recall the negative signs and symptoms associated with a particular category of pathology when they, themselves, are feeling bad. When the clinician is experiencing a particular mood state, information is likely to be recalled that confirms hypotheses generated when the clinician was in a similar affective state.

In general, the largest differences have been observed comparing the recall of positive material in positive and negative moods (Teasdale & Fogarty, 1979; Teasdale & Russell, 1983; Teasdale & Taylor, 1981; Teasdale, Taylor, & Fogarty, 1980). The most common pattern in these laboratory studies is that happy moods facilitate the recall of positive memories and inhibit the recall of negative memories, while sad moods inhibit the recall of positive memories but have no particular effect on negative memories (e.g., Natale & Hantas, 1982). However, individuals do seem slower to dismiss an *existing* unpleasant thought when sad than when happy (Sutherland, Newman, & Rachman, 1982), and actual clinical depressives are much quicker to retrieve negative as compared to positive memories than are nondepressives (Lloyd & Lishman, 1975; but see Clark & Teasdale, 1985).

State-dependent Recall

As in any state-dependent phenomenon (Eich, 1980; Eich, Weingartner, Stillman, & Gillin, 1975), mood, too, can serve as a contextually based discriminatory cue such that when learning and recall contexts match, memory is facilitated, and when the two contexts differ, memory is inhibited (just as certain behaviors carried out while intoxicated are difficult to recall until one is once again intoxicated).

The state-dependent recall effect for positive and negative moods has been demonstrated in carefully designed experiments involving the learning of a first list of information (when in a mood state), a second interfering list, and then a recall task while in the same or opposing mood as originally induced (Bower, Monteiro, & Gilligan, 1978; Schare, Lishman, & Spear, 1984). Moreover, there is even some evidence that the mood-state–dependent effect is observed in bipolar depressives as they shift between manic and depressive states (Weingartner, Miller, & Murphy, 1977). That is, material learned while manic is easier to recall in a subsequent manic episode and harder to recall during a depressive cycle. The recall of material learned while depressed is facilitated by a subsequent depressive state and inhibited by a subsequent manic episode.

The affective state of the therapist during a session is probably partially influenced by the client's affect, because therapists are taught and encouraged to empathize with their clients and because such empathy is a common human response. As a result, we would expect therapists to have an easier time recalling information from past sessions that matches the client's affective state in the current session than information in a different vein. For example, details about the client's childhood revealed during a tearful session some time before might not be followed up (because the details are not recalled) until the next tearful session. In addition, a therapist's own, independently generated mood state might influence processing; a death in his or her own family might cause information in sessions conducted immediately after to be suppressed until a later tragic event returns the therapist to the negative state once again.

Mood Intensity

Historically, it has been observed that affectively intense memories are remembered more accurately and over longer periods of time than affectively flat memories (Dutta & Kanungo, 1967, 1975; Holmes, 1970; Kanungo, 1968; Kanungo & Dutta, 1966; Robinson, 1980). For example, Dutta and Kanungo (1975) found that the perceived affective intensity of different memories is the best predictor of which are recalled.

The mood-intensity effect can be observed commonly in the therapeutic situation. Clients present therapists with a range of material, probably quickly exceeding the therapists' ability to process it all. So, therapists often use certain heuristics or rules-of-thumb to decide to which information they should carefully attend (cf. Turk & Salovey, 1985, 1986; Turk, Salovey, & Prentice, this volume), and one heuristic might be to listen carefully to material with a strong affective charge. But even if clinicians did not resort to this strategy in a conscious way, they might find that any material that arouses intense affect is, in fact, automatically better remembered. Once again, since clinicians tend to empathize with their clients, material that is affectively charged for the client is likely to create some congruent affect in the clinician, rendering it particularly memorable. For example, one of us (P.S.) can recall quite vividly a client who was particularly upset about the way she was treated by her husband. The ease with which this memory is recalled is partially a function of the intense affect that this woman evoked in her clinician—in this case, the affect was anger at her husband. Now, this might be a bias that serves the clinician well in most cases. After all, affectively charged material probably should be attended to quite carefully. However, it seems possible that clinicians might not encode adequately important but affectively flat material (affectively flat because the client has repressed attached emotion or because the emotion has been dealt with adequately) and, hence, easily forget some important detail.

Judgment and Decision Making

So far, we have been considering the impact of affect on memory. But therapists must do more than encode and recall information. They must use this information as the basis for making inferences and judgments about clients and about the processes of assessment and therapy. Hence, the influence of affect on memory has an indirect influence on inference and judgment. In the laboratory, however, the ways in which affect influences inference, judgment, and decision making has been examined quite directly. And these studies serve to inform us, in particular, about the effects of mood on the taking of risks.

Nearly every serious decision a clinician makes—to hospitalize a patient, to ask a particular question, to refer a client elsewhere—involves an assessment of risk. This appraisal process seems vulnerable to influence by a clinician's ongoing mood state. Although some researchers have found a linear relationship between mood and judgment such that happy subjects take more risks than affectively neutral subjects, who, in turn, take more risks than sad subjects (Deldin & Levin, 1986), the relationship between mood, judgment, and decision making is probably more complex than this. For example, Isen, Means, Patrick, and Nowicki (1982) reported that although happy individuals might be more likely to take risks than those who are neutral or sad, this effect of mood on risk taking holds for only rather mild risks. When risk is high, positive mood states may actually decrease risk taking. It seems that happy individuals do not want to risk ending their happy moods (Isen, 1985; Isen & Simmonds, 1978).

Isen et al. (1982) have identified the decision-making strategies used by individuals experiencing positive affect. Happy individuals are likely to reduce the complexity of the task and choose a simple decision-making strategy in order to engage in quick and simple kinds of cognitive processing (Isen & Daubman, 1984). Basically, Isen and her colleagues believe, positive affect "makes people tend to reduce the load on working memory" (p. 246). This reduction in memory load may occur because of the capacity required by the affect itself, or, perhaps, because—as noted above—individuals do not want to risk terminating their positive moods. When happy, people seem much more likely to use intuitive (and potentially error-prone) strategies as compared with more taxing, logical ones (Means, 1980, cited in Isen et al., 1982). They tend to "go with their gut." Moreover, these decision-making strategies seem to have behavioral consequences. At least for hypothetical decisions, happy individuals are ready to make risky decisions, i.e., bet on a "long shot" (Isen & Patrick, 1983), although the desire to maintain a pleasant mood seems to inhibit this kind of risk taking when the decisions are real. In that situation, happy subjects tend to prefer milder risks.

When individuals are made sad, perhaps by experiencing or hearing about a tragic event, their perception of the frequency of risks and of other undesirable events is increased, even if these are not related to the original tragic circumstances (Johnson & Tversky, 1983). Sad moods seem to cause a rather global shift in one's perceptions of the world, which is now seen as riskier and more dangerous than before. Johnson and Tversky (1983) asked subjects to read newspaper accounts of a fatal stabbing. Later, they were asked to estimate the frequency of a variety of grim occurrences such as natural disasters, fires, accidents, violent acts, technological disasters, and epidemics. Estimates of the frequency of all of these negative events rose after subjects read the initial story about the fatal stabbing. Thus, it appears that hearing about one negative event has a generalized effect on one's perceptions of danger. Negative affect seems to be a likely mediator of these effects, as subjects reported sadder moods after having read the initial story.

Overall, happy moods tend to simplify the decision-making process and result in greater risk taking, provided the potential losses are not too large. And sad moods tend to cause one to overestimate the risk involved in most aspects of life (a bias that should then result in more conservative decision-making strategies, but that conclusion has yet to be tested). For the clinician, either of these situations is not ideal. Clinicians in a more positive mood might persuade clients to be overly eager to try low-to-moderate risk solutions to problems when either a no-risk or, perhaps, a high-risk approach might have been more optimal. Further, clinicians experiencing a temporary negative mood may overpathologize, see substantial risks lurking behind every corner, or, at least, induce their clients into rather passive decision-making styles.

Mood and Attentional Focus

Recently, Salovey (1986; Salovey & Rodin, 1985) has suggested that mood causes a shift in the focus of one's attention to oneself. According to this hypothesis, when individuals have affective experiences, they become temporarily self-preoccupied. Their attention first turns away from external social cues and drifts inward, except when there is an explicit manipulation of salient external cues and a purposeful ambiguity of internal cues (e.g., Schachter & Singer, 1962). This process is thought to occur because it assists the individual in clarifying his or her emotional arousal evoked by (usually) unexpected stimuli. Individuals seem to focus attention on themselves during emotionally arousing experiences because emotion was originally a function of the relevance of the stimulus to the self (Snygg & Combs, 1949); highly self-relevant stimuli seem much more capable of eliciting emotional reactions than stimuli with less personal significance (Rogers, 1951; Salovey & Rodin, 1984). Moreover, self-focused attention serves to clarify and intensify emotional reactions (Scheier & Carver, 1977; Scheier, Carver, & Gibbons, 1981).

The implications of the hypothesis that intense moods lead to self-focused attention for clinical judgment and decision making are interesting. As has been emphasized, a clinician's mood might be determined empathically within the therapeutic session or extratherapeutically, that is, for reasons having nothing to do with a particular client. In either case, the arousal of any intense mood state might be accompanied by a tendency toward self-focused attention or introspection. The therapist may then have some difficulty attending to the nuances of the client's verbalizations and behavior. It seems possible that intense moods on the part of the therapist may thus interfere with optimal attention to the client.

The depression literature suggests other parallels between affect and self-focused attention which imply that therapists experiencing intense moods (and resultant self-focused attention) might show biases in cognitive processing and subsequent behavior that are quite similar to those of a depressed person. For example, as Smith and Greenberg (1981) and Pyszczynski and Greenberg (1985) note, depressives and self-focused nondepressives both show (a) increased self-evaluation tendencies, (b) intensified negative affect, (c) increased tendencies to make internal attributions for negative outcomes, (d) a marked accuracy in self-reports, and (e) increased tendencies to withdraw from tasks after failure.

Further, depressives tend to score higher than nondepressives on a variety of indices of self-awareness (Ingram & Smith, 1984; Smith & Greenberg, 1981; Smith, Ingram, & Roth, 1985) even though such self-focusing reveals all the more clearly, at least to the depressive, an array of self-deficiencies. Perhaps this was the phenomenon that prompted McGuire (1984) to write, "One does not have to be a depressive (though it helps) to realize that at times the self is all too much with us" (p. 73).

Mood and Motivation to Help

Let us consider two common mood states, joy and sorrow. And, let us assume that for the clinician these two states could originate from two different sources, the clinician's own experiences or the experiences of the client with whom the clinician empathizes. We will label moods created by the clinician's experiences as self-focused joy and self-focused sorrow. Moods deriving from the good fortunes or difficulties of the client could be called empathic joy or empathic sorrow. In a series of studies conducted at Stanford University, we were able to observe the effects of joy and sorrow (generated by the self or empathetically) on subjects' willingness to offer help. When individuals feel joyful, they tend to offer help to others when the joy is self-focused, but they tend to withhold help when the joy is empathically generated (Rosenhan, Salovey, & Hargis, 1981).

On the other hand, when sadness is self-focused, helping is not very likely, but empathic sorrow motivates one to help others (Thompson, Cowan, & Rosenhan, 1980). These mood-induced changes in helpfulness probably reflect changes in one's beliefs about one's resources relative to others and one's expectations about one's abilities to carry out helping activities (Rosenhan, Karylowski, Salovey, & Hargis, 1981). In fact, recent evidence (Salovey, 1986) suggests that self-generated happiness seems to promote helping by making thoughts about charity more available to the helper as compared with less altruistically oriented thoughts about helping such as reciprocity (i.e., tit-for-tat). These thoughts seem superimposed on a more general tendency for positive mood to increase individuals' perceived "helping self-efficacy" (Salovey, 1986). It seems that happy people see themselves as much more capable of carrying out a variety of helping acts.

The implications for clinical work are that, paradoxically, clinicians might have great difficulty offering help to clients following successes in the client's life or, more obviously, following failures in the therapist's external activities. It appears that help would be much more forthcoming following some pleasant event in the therapist's private life or when the client is experiencing misery with which the therapist can empathize.

Moods have consequences for clinically relevant behaviors other than helping as well. Positive moods make people more willing to initiate conversations with others (Batson, Coke, Chard, Smith, & Taliaferro, 1979), and happy individuals express greater liking for people whom they have just met (Gouaux, 1971; Griffitt, 1970; Veitch & Griffitt, 1976). In general, it seems that individuals in happy moods perceive themselves as more capable of coping with the world and are more generous with their own resources (Isen, 1970). Further, happy individuals act to maximize their happiness and minimize the chances that their good moods could be replaced by any kind of distress (Forest, Clark, Mills, & Isen, 1979; Isen & Patrick, 1983; Isen & Simmonds, 1978).

Avoiding the Biasing Consequences of Mood States

Let us assume that, for the most part, mood states themselves are rather unavoidable, nor would we, in fact, want to avoid them. The question then becomes, given I, as a clinician, may be experiencing some mood state, how can I keep it from unduly influencing the way that I interact with a particular client? In this sense, one can reduce bias by engaging in any of a number of "debiasing" strategies that we have described in more detail elsewhere (Turk & Salovey, 1986; see also Arnoult & Anderson, this volume).

In particular, the clinician is probably well served by always attempting to generate competing causal hypotheses for understanding any clinical observation (Anderson, 1982; Einhorn & Hogarth, 1982), and including as one competing hypothesis that the clinical observation might be partially determined by the clinician's affective state. Once alternative hypotheses have been generated, questions can be formulated that falsify one hypothesis while confirming a second one (Einhorn & Hogarth, 1982), and erroneous inferences can be easily replaced with better alternatives.

Additionally, clinicians may want to undergo the "bias inoculation" procedure that we have described (Turk & Salovey, 1986), whereby they are provided with actual experiences and can then observe how their moods affect their memories, "inoculating" them against ignoring these factors in more important clinical contexts. For example, clinicians may want to participate in mood induction procedures and then literally observe the kinds of autobiographical memories that are most likely to occur to them. Further, clinicians might find it useful to question themselves (i.e., self-interrogate) about their moods at the start of each therapy session. They may even want to record their mood state in their process notes so that mood-generated biases can later be discovered and accounted for.

Summary

Research concerning the effects of mood on thought, judgment, and behavior has been carried out for quite some time now. However, the implications of this work for clinical judgment generally have not been made explicit. It seems clear, however, that clinicians, along with lay people, are susceptible to biases emanating from the tendency to learn and recall information that is consistent with one's ongoing mood state. And, as clinicians, it is important for us to be aware of these potential biases and to consider ways of reducing their impact. As we have done on other occasions (e.g., Turk & Salovey, 1985), it seems appropriate to conclude with Meehl's (1954) warning that "We of all people, ought to be highly suspicious of ourselves . . . [and] have no right to assume that entering the clinic has resulted in some miraculous mutation and made us singularly free from ordinary errors" (p. 27–28)—errors, in this case, deriving from the ebb and flow of commonly experienced mood states.

References

Anderson, C. A. (1982). Inoculation and counterexplanation: Debiasing techniques in the perseverance of social theories. *Social Cognition, 1,* 126–139.

Anderson, J. R.. & Bower, G. H. (1973). *Human associative memory.* Washington, DC: Winston & Sons.

Batson, C. D., Coke, J. S., Chard, F., Smith, D., & Taliaferro, A. (1979). Generality of the "glow of goodwill": Effects of mood on helping and information acquisition. *Social Psychology Quarterly, 42,* 176–179.

Blaney, P. H. (1986). Affect and memory: A review. *Psychological Bulletin, 99,* 229–246.

Bower, G. H. (1981). Mood and memory. *American Psychologist, 36,* 129–148.

Bower, G. H., & Cohen, P. R. (1982). Emotional influences in memory and thinking: Data and theory. In M. S. Clark & S. T. Fiske (Eds.), *Affect and cognition: The 17th Annual Carnegie Symposium on Cognition.* Hillsdale, NJ: Erlbaum.

Bower, G. H., Gilligan, S. G., & Monteiro, K. P. (1981). Selectivity of learning caused by affective states. *Journal of Experimental Psychology: General, 110,* 451–473.

Bower, G. H., & Mayer, J. D. (1985). Failure to replicate mood-dependent retrieval. *Bulletin of the Psychonomic Society, 23,* 39–42.

Bower, G. H., Monteiro, K. P., & Gilligan, S. G. (1978). Emotional mood as a context of learning and recall. *Journal of Verbal Learning and Verbal Behavior, 17,* 573–585.

Burns, D. D. (1980). *Feeling good: The new mood therapy.* New York: Signet.

Clark, D. M., & Teasdale, J. D. (1985). Constraints on the effects of mood on memory. *Journal of Personality and Social Psychology, 48,* 1595–1608.

Clark, M. S., & Isen, A. M. (1982). Toward understanding the relationship between feeling states and social behavior. In A. Hastorf & A. Isen (Eds.), *Cognitive social psychology.* New York: Elsevier.

Collins, A. M., & Loftus, E. F. (1975). A spreading-activation theory of semantic processing. *Psychological Review, 82,* 407–428.

Deldin, P. J., & Levin, I. P. (1986). The effect of mood induction in a risky decision-making task. *Bulletin of the Psychonomic Society, 24,* 4–6.

Dutta, S., & Kanungo, R. N. (1967). Retention of affective material: A further verification of the intensity hypothesis. *Journal of Personality and Social Psychology, 5,* 476–481.

———. (1975). *Affect and memory: A reformulation.* Oxford, England: Pergamon.

Eich, J. E. (1980). The cue-dependent nature of state-dependent retrieval. *Memory and Cognition, 8,* 157–173.

Eich, J. E., Weingartner, H., Stillman, R. C., & Gillin, J. C. (1975). State-dependent accessibility of retrieval cues in the retention of a categorized list. *Journal of Verbal Learning and Verbal Behavior, 14,* 408–417.

Einhorn, H. J., & Hogarth, R. M. (1982). *A theory of diagnostic inference:* I. *Imagination and the psychophysics of evidence.* Unpublished manuscript, University of Chicago.

Forest, D., Clark, M. S., Mills, J., & Isen, A. M. (1979). Helping as a function of feeling state and nature of the helping behavior. *Motivation and Emotion, 3,* 161–169.

Gerrig, R. J., & Bower, G. H. (1982). Emotional influences on word recognition. *Bulletin of the Psychonomic Society, 19,* 197–200.

Gilligan, S. G., & Bower, G. H. (1984). Cognitive consequences of emotional arousal. In C. Izard, J. Kagen, & R. Zajonc (Eds.), *Emotions, cognition, and behavior.* New York: Cambridge University Press.

Gouaux, C. (1971). Induced affective states and interpersonal attraction. *Journal of Personality and Social Psychology, 20,* 37–43.

Griffitt, W. B. (1970). Environmental effects of interpersonal affective behavior: Ambient effective temperature and attraction. *Journal of Personality and Social Psychology, 15,* 240–244.

Hasher, L., Rose, K. C., Zacks, R. T., Sanft, H., & Doren, B. (1985). Mood, recall, and selectivity effects in normal college students. *Journal of Experimental Psychology: General, 114,* 104–118.

Heimann, P. (1950). On counter transference. *International Journal of Psychoanalysis, 31,* 81–84.

Holmes, D. S. (1970). Differential change in affective intensity and the forgetting of unpleasant personal experiences. *Journal of Personality and Social Psychology, 15,* 234–239.

Ingram, R. E., & Smith, T. W. (1984). Depression and internal versus external focus of attention. *Cognitive Therapy and Research, 8,* 139–152.

Isen, A. M. (1970). Success, failure, attention and reactions to others: The warm glow of success. *Journal of Personality and Social Psychology, 15,* 294–301.

———. (1984). Toward understanding the role of affect in cognition. In R. S. Wyer & T. K. Srull (Eds.), *Handbook of social cognition* (Vol. 3). Hillsdale, NJ: Erlbaum.

———. (1985). Asymmetry of happiness and sadness in effects on memory in normal college students: Comments on Hasher, Rose, Zacks, Sanft, and Doren. *Journal of Experimental Psychology: General, 114,* 388–391.

Isen, A. M., & Daubman, K. A. (1984). The influence of affect on categorization. *Journal of Personality and Social Psychology, 97,* 1206–1217.

Isen, A. M., & Patrick, R. (1983). The effect of positive feelings on risk taking: When the chips are down. *Organizational Behavior and Human Performance, 31,* 194–202.

Isen, A. M., Means, B., Patrick, R., & Nowicki, G. P. (1982). Positive affect and decision making. In M. S. Clark & S. T. Fiske (Eds.), *Affect and cognition: The 17th Annual Carnegie Symposium on Cognition.* Hillsdale, NJ: Erlbaum.

Isen, A. M., Shalker, T. E., Clark, M., & Karp, L. (1978). Affect, accessibility of material in memory, and behavior: A cognitive loop? *Journal of Personality and Social Psychology, 36,* 385–393.

Isen, A. M., & Simmonds, S. F. (1978). The effect of feeling good on a helping task that is incompatible with good mood. *Social Psychology, 41,* 345–349.

Izard, C. E. (1972). *The face of emotion.* New York: Appleton-Century-Crofts.

______. (1977). *Human emotions.* New York: Plenum.

Johnson, E. J. & Tversky, A. (1983). Affect, generalization, and the perception of risk. *Journal of Personality and Social Psychology, 45,* 20–31.

Kanungo, R. N., (1968). Retention of affective material: Role of extroversion and intensity of affect. *Journal of Personality and Social Psychology, 8,* 63–68.

Kanungo, R. N. & Dutta, S. (1966). Retention of affective material: Frame of reference or intensity. *Journal of Personality and Social Psychology, 4,* 27–35.

Kernberg, O. (1965). Notes on countertransference. *Journal of the American Psychoanalytic Association, 13,* 38–56.

Lazarus, R. S. (1982). Thoughts on the relation between emotion and cognition. *American Psychologist, 37,* 1019–1024.

Lloyd, G. G., & Lishman, W. A. (1975). Effect of depression on the speed of recall of pleasant and unpleasant experiences. *Psychological Medicine, 5,* 173–180.

Mayer, J. D. (1986). How mood influences cognition. In N. E. Sharkey (Ed.), *Advances in cognitive science 1.* Chichester, England: Ellis Horwood.

Mayer, J. D., & Bower, G. H. (1985). Naturally occurring mood and learning: Commentary on Hasher et al. *Journal of Experimental Psychology: General, 114,* 396–403.

Mayer, J. D., & Bremer, D. (1985). Assessing mood with affect-sensitive tasks. *Journal of Personality Assessment, 49,* 95–99.

Mayer, J. D., & Salovey, P. (in press). Personality moderates mood's effect on cognition. In J. Forgas & K. Fiedler (Eds.), *Affect, cognition, and social behavior.* Toronto: Hogrefe.

Mayer, J. D., & Volanth, A. J. (1985). Cognitive involvement in the emotional response system. *Motivation and Emotion, 9,* 261–275.

McGuire, W. J. (1984). Search for the self: Going beyond self-esteem and the reactive self. In R. A. Zucker, J. Aronoff, & A. I. Rabin (Eds.), *Personality and the prediction of behavior.* New York: Academic Press.

Meehl, P. E. (1954). *Clinical versus statistical prediction.* Minneapolis: University of Minnesota Press.

Nasby, W., & Yando, R. (1982). Selective encoding and retrieval of affectively valent information: Two cognitive consequences of children's mood states. *Journal of Personality and Social Psychology, 43,* 1244–1253.

Natale, M., & Hantas, M. (1982). Effect of temporary mood states on selective memory about the self. *Journal of Personality and Social Psychology, 42,* 927–934.

Pyszczynski, T., & Greenberg, J. (1985). Depression and preference for self-focusing stimuli after success and failure. *Journal of Personality and Social Psychology, 49,* 1066–1075.

Rapaport, D. (1942). *Emotions and memory.* Baltimore: Williams & Wilkins.

Robinson, J. A. (1980). Affect and retrieval of personal memories. *Motivation and Emotion, 4,* 149–176.

Rogers, C. B. (1951). *Client-centered therapy.* Boston: Houghton Mifflin.

Rosenhan, D. L., Karylowski, J., Salovey, P., & Hargis, K. (1981). Affect and altruism. In J. P. Rushton & R. M. Sorrentino (Eds.), *Altruism and helping behavior.* Hillsdale, NJ: Erlbaum.

Rosenhan, D. L., Salovey, P., & Hargis, K. (1981). The joys of helping: Focus of attention mediates the impact of positive affect on altruism. *Journal of Personality and Social Psychology, 40,* 899–905.

Salovey, P. (1986). *The effects of mood and focus of attention on self-relevant thoughts and helping intention.* Dissertation submitted to the Department of Psychology, Yale University, December 1986.

Salovey, P., & Rodin, J. (1984). Some antecedents and consequences of social-comparison jealousy. *Journal of Personality and Social Psychology, 47,* 780–792.

———. (1985). Cognitions about the self: Connecting feeling states to social behavior. In P. Shaver (Ed.), *Self, situations, and social behavior: Review of personality and social psychology,* (Volume 6). Beverly Hills, CA: Sage.

Schachter, S., & Singer, J. E. (1962). Cognitive, social and physiological determinants of emotional state. *Psychological Review, 62,* 379–399.

Schare, M. L., Lishman, S. A., & Spear, N. E. (1984). The effects of mood variation on state-dependent retention. *Cognitive Therapy and Research, 8,* 387–408.

Scheier, M. F., & Carver, C. S. (1977). Self-focused attention and the experience of emotion: Attraction, repulsion, elation, and depression. *Journal of Personality and Social Psychology, 35,* 625–636.

Scheier, M. F., Carver, C. S., & Gibbons, F. X. (1981). Self-focused attention and reactions to fear. *Journal of Research in Personality, 15,* 687–699.

Smith, T. W., & Greenberg, J. (1981). Depression and self-focused attention. *Motivation and Emotion, 5,* 323–331.

Smith, T. W., Ingram, R. E., & Roth, D. L. (1985). Self-focused attention and depression: Self-evaluation, affect, and life stress. *Motivation and Emotion, 9,* 381–389.

Snygg, D., & Combs, A. W. (1949). *Individual behavior.* New York: Harper.

Sutherland, G., Newman, B., & Rachman, S. (1982). Experimental investigations of the relations between mood and intrusive, unwanted cognitions. *British Journal of Medical Psychology, 55,* 127–138.

Teasdale, J. D., & Fogarty, S. J. (1979). Differential effects of induced mood on retrieval of pleasant and unpleasant events from episodic memory. *Journal of Abnormal Psychology, 88,* 248–257.

Teasdale, J. D., & Russell, M. C. (1983). Differential effects of induced mood on the recall of positive, negative, and neutral words. *British Journal of Clinical Psychology, 22,* 163–171.

Teasdale, J. D., & Taylor, R. T. (1981). Induced mood and accessibility of memories: An effect of mood state or of induction procedure. *British Journal of Clinical Psychology, 20,* 39–48.

Teasdale, J. D., Taylor, R., & Fogarty, S. J. (1980). Effects of induced elation-depression on the accessibility of memories of happy and unhappy experiences. *Behavior, Research, and Therapy. 18,* 339–346.

Tomkins, S. S. (1962). *Affect, imagery, and consciousness.* (Vol. 1: *The positive affects.*) New York: Springer.

______. (1963). *Affect, imagery, and consciousness.* (Vol. 2: *The negative affects.*) New York: Springer.

Thompson, W. C., Cowan, C. L., & Rosenhan, D. L. (1980). Focus of attention mediates the impact of negative affect on altruism. *Journal of Personality and Social Psychology, 38,* 291–300.

Turk, D. C., & Salovey, P. (1985). Cognitive structures, cognitive processes, and cognitive-behavior modification: II. Judgments and inferences of the clinician. *Cognitive Therapy and Research, 9,* 19–33.

______. (1986). Clinical information processing: Bias inoculation. In R. Ingram (Ed.), *Information processing approaches to psychopathology and clinical psychology.* Orlando, FL: Academic.

Veitch, R., & Griffitt, W. (1976). Good news—bad news: Affective and interpersonal effects. *Journal of Applied Social Psychology, 6,* 69–75.

Velten, E. A. (1968). A laboratory task for induction of mood states. *Behavior Research and Therapy, 6,* 473–482.

Walrond-Skinner, S. (1986). *A dictionary of psychotherapy.* London: Routledge & Kegan Paul.

Weingartner, H., Miller, H., & Murphy, D. L. (1977). Mood-state dependent retrieval of verbal associations. *Journal of Abnormal Psychology, 86,* 276–284.

Zajonc, R. B. (1980). Feeling and thinking: Preferences need no inferences. *American Psychologist, 35,* 151–175.

______. (1984). On the primacy of affect. *American Psychologist, 39,* 117–123.

7 Interactions Between Therapists and Clients: Hypothesis Testing and Behavioral Confirmation

Mark Snyder
Cynthia J. Thomsen

IT has been estimated that over 400 types of psychotherapy are available to those seeking assistance with psychological problems (Karasu, 1985, cited by Kazdin, 1986). This vast array of therapeutic orientations on the market suggests that no one form of psychotherapy has emerged as clearly superior to the others. Yet, these therapies do differ in numerous ways, not only in terms of their preferred methods of treatment, but also in terms of their underlying theoretical conceptualizations of psychopathology. As Kazdin (1986) has observed, "The techniques . . . are considered to reflect different, although not necessarily diametrically opposed, conceptual views about the nature of the dysfunction, the focus of treatment, and the processes and/or techniques required to produce therapeutic change" (p. 95).

In addition, although most theories of psychopathology agree that the presence of certain conditions and the occurrence of particular events potentiate the development of psychopathology, current points of view differ greatly in terms of the *specific* conditions and events thought to be "psychogenic." Yet, despite their myriad differences, and although the popularity of various schools of psychotherapy has waxed and waned over the years, by and large these theories of psychopathology, and the therapies based upon them, continue to endure.

In part, the coexistence of many and diverse forms of therapy reflects a lack of clear empirical support for the ascendancy of any one over the others. Although a great deal of effort has been expended in assessing the validity of various orientations, the results have generally been mixed, sometimes favoring one type of therapy and sometimes another. In fact, Smith, Glass, and Miller (1980), in a meta-analysis of 475 studies, found no systematic differences in success rates among different therapies, despite dramatic differences in philosophy and procedure (cf. American Psychiatric Commission on Psychotherapies, 1982; Kazdin & Wilson, 1978; Luborsky, Singer, & Luborsky, 1975; Miller & Berman, 1983; Shapiro & Shapiro, 1982; Smith & Glass, 1977). However, recently, some clinical researchers have obtained evidence for the effectiveness of particular treatments for specific disorders (e.g., the combination of antidepressant medications and cognitive therapy for treating depression; see Rush, 1982; Sacco & Beck, 1985).

Sources of Belief in Therapeutic Orientations

In the absence of conclusive evidence supporting the definite superiority of any one approach, what might lead a particular therapist to persist in adhering to a theoretical and therapeutic orientation? Presumably, therapists must be receiving some support for the validity and efficacy of their own particular "brand" of therapy if they continue to practice it. We suggest that there are at least three main sources from which a therapist might garner such support.

First, a therapist's peers and colleagues may support his orientation. Graduate training programs often selectively inculcate their students with a particular theoretical and therapeutic position (see Houts, 1984), and the social support of advisers, supervisors, and peers may firmly establish confidence in the particular perspective that is normative in any program. Such factors may continue to operate long after graduate training is completed, helping to sustain and perpetuate a therapist's theoretical identity.

Second, some support for a therapist's preferred orientation may be derived from published information about that form of therapy. Indeed, it is probably possible to find evidence that appears to support virtually any form of therapy. For example, Kazdin (1983) has suggested that a researcher's investment in a particular approach often affects the way research is conducted, with the result that confirmatory conclusions become more likely. In fact, meta-analyses of psychotherapy outcome research have consistently obtained positive correlations between outcome effect, size, and measurement reactivity to demand artifacts (e.g., Miller & Berman, 1983; Shapiro & Shapiro, 1982; Smith et al., 1980; cf. Basham, 1986).

In addition, when evaluating contradictory empirical reports, therapists may be likely to conclude that research supporting their own position is more reliable and better conducted; at the same time, research with incompatible conclusions may be perceived as irrelevant or unconvincing. For example, Mahoney (1977) presented journal reviewers with manuscripts that described identical experiments, the manuscripts differing only in whether the results confirmed or disconfirmed the reviewers' theoretical orientations. When the results supported their beliefs, reviewers evaluated the methodology positively and recommended acceptance of the manuscript, with perhaps some minor revisions. When the results contradicted their views, however, reviewers criticized the methodology and suggested substantial revisions or outright rejection of the manuscript. Little wonder, then, that "the same studies often are simultaneously praised and criticized on substantive and/or methodological grounds, and are cited in support of different conclusions" (Kazdin, 1986, p. 95; cf. Glass, McGaw, & Smith, 1981).

Third, clinical experience may constitute a particularly powerful and highly persuasive source of evidence that bolsters therapists' beliefs in the validity of their own approaches. For a variety of reasons, the impact of personal clinical experience may outweigh research-based empirical evidence, even though the former may be based on much more limited numbers of cases. Research on attitude–behavior relations suggests that attitudes formed through direct experience are more strongly linked to subsequent behavior than attitudes formed through indirect experience (e.g., Fazio & Zanna, 1981; Manstead, Proffitt, & Smart, 1983; Smith & Swinyard, 1983). Moreover, concrete, vivid, case-history information has a greater influence on social judgments than more pallid, abstract, statistical information (e.g., Anderson, 1983; Nisbett & Ross, 1980; Taylor & Thompson, 1982). Thus, because personal experience with clinical cases is likely to be a more direct, more vivid, and more concrete source of information than scientific reports and statistical summaries of empirical research, we would expect that therapists weigh their personal clinical experience quite heavily in evaluating the accuracy of particular theories of psychopathology and particular approaches to therapy. In accord with this line of reasoning, Barlow (1981) has concluded that "clinical research has little or no influence on clinical practice" (p. 147).

The Consequences of Belief in Therapeutic Orientations

Of what consequence is it that practitioners may be firm believers in the validity of their particular therapeutic and theoretical orientations? We would not for a moment suggest that therapists should not practice what they believe in or that they should practice what they do not believe in. However, we do suggest that therapists' beliefs may exert powerful influences, often unintended and unforeseen, on interactions between therapists and their clients. A considerable body of research evidence demonstrates that social beliefs often function as self-fulfilling prophecies. Based upon their beliefs about how other people will behave, individuals often treat others in ways that cause them to actually behave in ways that confirm these beliefs (for one recent review, see Snyder, 1984). Do such "behavioral confirmation" processes occur in the context of interactions between therapists and clients? That is, do therapists induce their clients to behave in ways that support and confirm the beliefs that therapists bring to bear on the therapeutic situation? Do clients, in the course of their interactions with therapists, come to behave in accord with their therapists' particular theoretical and therapeutic orientations? Before addressing these and related questions about therapist–client interactions (which are the central concerns of this chapter), let us define more fully the behavioral confirmation process.

Behavioral Confirmation in Social Interaction

Behavioral confirmation refers to a process in which one individual's preconceived *beliefs* and prior *expectations* about another person channel their interactions in such ways that these initial beliefs (even when they are based on erroneous stereotypes or hypotheses of dubious validity) come to be *confirmed* by the other person's *behavior*. Behavioral confirmation has been demonstrated in a wide variety of laboratory and nonlaboratory contexts and for a wide range of beliefs and expectations, including stereotypes about the personalities of those with attractive or unattractive physical appearances (Andersen & Bem, 1981; Snyder, Tanke, & Berscheid, 1977), conceptions of sex and gender roles (Skrypnek & Snyder, 1982; von Baeyer, Sherk, & Zanna, 1981; Zanna & Pack, 1975), expectations of racial differences (Word, Zanna, & Cooper, 1974), arbitrary designations of differences between individuals in abilities and performance competencies (King, 1971; Rosenthal & Jacobson, 1968), and anticipations of the likely personalities of other people (e.g., Snyder & Swann, 1978; Swann & Guiliano, in press).

In one investigation of behavioral confirmation in social interaction, Snyder et al. (1977) examined the effects on interactions between pairs of college-age men and women of the commonly held stereotype that physically attractive people possess more socially appealing personalities than the physically unattractive. Before participating in a "getting acquainted" telephone conversation with a female partner, each man was randomly assigned a snapshot (ostensibly of his partner) that portrayed a woman who was either physically attractive or physically unattractive. Men who believed their partners to be attractive expected them to be more poised and socially adept, and consequently treated them with much more warmth and friendliness than men who believed their partners to be unattractive. And, as a result of the men's behavior, the women behaved in a manner that provided behavioral confirmation of the men's initial beliefs about them. Those women thought to be attractive (regardless of their actual physical attractiveness) reciprocated the overtures of the men and actually came to behave in a friendly and sociable manner. In sharp contrast, women who were believed by their partners to be physically unattractive adopted cool and aloof postures during the conversation.

Psychotherapists, no doubt, hold many of the same sorts of beliefs and expectations (e.g., stereotypes about sex, race, attractiveness) investigated in studies of behavioral confirmation in social interaction. Perhaps, then, interactions between therapists and clients may contain the possibility of behavioral confirmation outcomes. Try as they may to set such beliefs aside, therapists' stereotypes about the sex, race, appearance, and social class of their clients have self-fulfilling consequences on their dealings with them. Indeed, such factors often do influence clinical judgments (e.g., Barocas & Vance, 1974; Brown, 1970; Cash, Kehr, Polyson, & Freeman, 1977; Scharf & Bishop, 1979). The influences of these stereotyped preconceptions on clinical judgments are likely to be the first steps in the behavioral confirmation process in psychotherapy (cf. Turk & Salovey, 1986).

In addition, and of particular relevance for our current concerns, clinicians bring to therapy a host of beliefs dictated by the particular theoretical and therapeutic orientations to which they adhere. The beliefs provide additional opportunities for the occurrence of behavioral confirmation within psychotherapy. Different therapeutic orientations are associated with different characteristic views of the nature, causes, and treatment of particular disorders (e.g., Kazdin, 1986). The beliefs may provide therapists with numerous expectations about their clients' behavior that may, in the course of therapy, come to be supported through behavioral confirmation. As a result of such behavioral confirmation processes, for instance, Freudians may induce their patients to speak of their troubles in Freudian terms and the clients of Rogerians may come to talk of their problems in terms appropriate to the Rogerian point of view. (This point is further developed in the chapter by Arnoult and Anderson in this volume.)

Hypothesis Testing in Social Interaction

Behavioral confirmation, the research literature tells us, may be initiated also by beliefs held in the form of tentative *hypotheses* (open to question and subject to test) about other people. That is, when people attempt to use their interactions as opportunities to *test* the accuracy of their beliefs and intuitions about other people, they may operate in ways that lead the targets of their hypotheses to behave as if the hypotheses under scrutiny were valid, even when they are not. In an initial demonstration of this phenomenon, Snyder and Swann (1978, Experiment 1) asked college students to test the hypothesis that a target person was either an extrovert or an introvert. To test the hypothesis, participants selected questions to ask the target person. Students working with the propositions that the target was extroverted chose to ask questions that preferentially solicited evidence of extroverted behavior (e.g., "What would you do if you wanted to liven things up at a party?"); those testing the introvert hypothesis chose favored questions that probed for instances of introversion (e.g., "What factors make it hard for you to really open up to people?").

In this and related demonstrations of hypothesis-testing processes in social interaction (for a review, see Snyder and Gangestad, 1981), people systematically chose to solicit evidence whose presence would tend to confirm the very hypotheses under scrutiny. This "confirmatory hypothesis testing" phenomenon seems to occur even when the expected accuracy of the hypothesis is low (Snyder & Swann, 1978, Experiment 3), incentives are offered for accuracy (Snyder & Swann, 1978, Experiment 4), the initial hypothesis contains information about disconfirming as well as confirming attributes (Snyder & Campbell, 1980), the hypothesis testers formulate the questions themselves rather than choosing them from a prepared list (Swann & Guiliano, in press), and for traits other than introversion and extroversion (e.g., Swann & Guiliano, in press). To be sure, this line of research has drawn the attention of critics (e.g., Trope & Bassok, 1982); for a detailed listing of these criticisms and relevant and persuasive empirical answers to them, see Swann and Guiliano (in press).

It appears, then, that the use of such confirmatory hypothesis-testing strategies is a rather widespread phenomenon. Moreover, these strategies influence not only the ways that people *gather* evidence, but also the *outcome* of attempts to test hypotheses. The end product of hypothesis-testing activities is often behavioral confirmation, with the target of the hypothesis coming to behave in accord with the hypothesis under scrutiny. When Snyder and Swann (1978) gave people the opportunity to assess their hypotheses directly (by actually interviewing the targets of their research), the hypothesis testers concluded that their propositions had been supported. More significantly, ratings of the targets' behavior by outside observers corroborated the hypothesis testers' conclusions. These observers verified that the targets had in fact come to behave in a manner consistent with the hypotheses being tested, even though these hypotheses had been assigned on a fully random basis, and hence had no necessary validity.

Interactions Between Therapists and Clients

This program of research on hypothesis testing is of considerable potential relevance to the therapeutic context. In many ways, and at many stages, interactions between therapists and clients constitute hypothesis-testing situations. When initially diagnosing a client, the therapist explicitly constructs hypotheses about which diagnostic categories are appropriate for the client's problems and sets out to assess their validity. For example, the therapist might have an initial hunch that a particular patient merits a diagnosis of paranoid schizophrenia. He might therefore direct his questions toward determining the presence of relevant symptomatology such as hostility, suspiciousness, and hypervigilance, while not probing so diligently for evidence of symptomatology relevant to other diagnoses. Will such hypothesis-testing activities make it more likely that this patient will display signs that provide behavioral confirmation for the hypothesized diagnosis?

Once an initial diagnosis has been settled upon, the therapist often seeks to illuminate the causal origins of the disorder. During this stage of therapy, clinicians' theoretical beliefs about the etiology of the particular disorder in question provide them with hypotheses about events and conditions predisposing to pathology that are likely to be found in the patient's background. The clinician may then proceed to test these hypotheses by asking questions to determine the presence of such pathogenic factors. If the therapist believes that paranoid schizophrenics often come from families in which the mother behaved in a cold and hostile manner toward the child, she may preferentially query the patient about instances in which the mother's behavior fitted this profile, to the possible neglect of probing for instances in which the mother contradicted the profile. Will such hypothesis-testing activities induce patients to reveal instances of past experience that confirm the hypothetical explanation of their current condition?

Even the treatment phase of therapy may incorporate a substantial hypothesis-testing component, as therapists continually monitor the effectiveness of their interventions in improving the patient's condition. In effect, the therapist at this stage is testing the hypothesis that a specific form of treatment is particularly efficacious for treating the client's disorder. Thus, for instance, believers in the cognitive-behavioral approach to therapy may regard their dealings with clients as opportunities to validate the therapeutic effectiveness of their preferred approach. Will such hypothesis-testing activities lead therapists to have particular success with their preferred modes of treatment, not because of any necessary superior efficacy on its part but because acting on their beliefs in its efficacy produces behavioral confirmation for their faith in it?

At each of these stages, then, as therapists proceed to test their hypotheses, they may preferentially search for, preferentially solicit, and preferentially elicit information that is relevant to and consistent with their beliefs and expectations. And, as a result of the therapist's confirmatory strategies, the responses of clients may be constrained in such a way that they ultimately come to confirm the therapist's initial beliefs through their behavior, consequently providing evidence for the validity and utility of the therapist's preferred theoretical perspective and therapeutic orientation.

In this chapter, we propose to examine some of the processes and outcomes of interactions between therapists and clients. Specifically, in the following sections, we will consider the manner in which hypothesis testing and behavioral confirmation may influence the therapeutic endeavor as the clinician pursues three major therapeutic goals: (1) *diagnosis,* or defining the nature of the client's problem; (2) *explanation,* or elucidating the causal origins of the client's problem; and (3) *treatment,* or applying interventions designed to ameliorate or eliminate the problem.

Diagnosis: Defining the Client's Problem

To locate a particular client within his or her system of beliefs about psychopathology, a therapist must first form a *working hypothesis* about the nature of the client's problem and then proceed to test that hypothesis. The importance of this initial diagnosis should not be underestimated. Intake judgments determine the allocation of counseling and clinical resources (Bordin, 1968; Callis, 1965; Pellegrine, 1971; Sharp & Marra, 1971) and "form the basis for making predictions about the behavior of the client, the length of treatment, and the type of counseling that will be most appropriate" (Bishop & Richards, 1984, p. 398).

Considering the importance of the initial diagnosis, it may be somewhat surprising to discover that substantial research has documented the tendency of mental health professionals, regardless of their level of experience or theoretical orientation, to form clinical impressions of patients *very* quickly (Gauron & Dickinson, 1969; Meehl, 1960; O'Leary, Speltz, Donovan, & Walker, 1979; Oskamp, 1965; Sandifer, Hordern, & Green, 1970). In fact, Gauron and Dickinson (1969) discovered that therapists often form their initial diagnostic impressions within the first 30 to 60 *seconds* of observing the patient! Although other estimates have been somewhat higher (for example, Sandifer, Hordern, and Green, 1970, concluded that "the first three minutes of observation have a significant, and sometimes apparently decisive, impact upon the final diagnostic decision," p. 968), clinicians generally do seem to arrive at an initial diagnosis very rapidly.

Sources of Diagnostic Hypotheses

How can therapists assess their clients' disorders so quickly? The rapidity of diagnosis may stem from several sources of information available very early, if not immediately, in contacts between therapists and clients. Thus, in the initial stages of clinical interactions, clients frequently state their own beliefs about what is causing their problems (Bandura, 1969; Mischel, 1977; Strupp & Luborsky, 1962). By providing therapists with presenting problems, clients are in effect providing them with hypotheses about the nature of their disorders, hypotheses that therapists then may proceed to test. For example, if a client enters therapy claiming that he or she has been feeling depressed, the therapist may begin with the working hypothesis that the client is indeed depressed.

A slightly different situation occurs when clients enter therapy less voluntarily, perhaps because they have been referred by the legal system (courts or parole boards) or by a family member (in the case of minors). Under these circumstances, clients are likely to be less cooperative in informing therapists about the reasons for their presence in therapy. However, it is likely that information about the nature of the client's problem will have been offered by the referring agent, thus providing therapists with initial working hypotheses that may guide and channel attempts to gather evidence relevant to diagnostic processes.

Moreover, when clients have received previous treatment, therapists normally have access to their records. Prior diagnoses may provide another source of information about the likely nature of clients' current disorders. In fact, the opinions of a therapist's colleagues may substantially influence his diagnosis. Temerlin (1968) examined the effect of overhearing a colleague's diagnostic opinion about a "patient" on therapists' subsequent diagnoses. After hearing a high-prestige colleague remark that the patient was "a very interesting man because he looked neurotic but was actually quite psychotic" (Temerlin, 1968, p. 349), psychiatrists, clinical psychologists, and graduate students in clinical psychology listened to a tape-recorded interview with what was actually a "normal, healthy man" (Temerlin, 1968, p. 349). Psychiatrists proved to be most influenced by the colleague's diagnostic comment: 60 percent of them judged the patient to be psychotic, and none judged him to be mentally healthy; the remaining 40 percent diagnosed the patient to be neurotic or to have a character disorder. Clinical psychologists and graduate students in clinical psychology were less influenced by the suggested diagnosis (with 28 percent and 11 percent respectively diagnosing the patient as psychotic). However, "control" judges (matched with the psychiatrists and psychologists for professional identity but given no diagnostic suggestions) in *no* instance arrived at a diagnosis of psychosis (Temerlin, 1968; cf. Langer & Abelson, 1974).

Testing Diagnostic Hypotheses

The working hypotheses that therapists form and test may reflect (in addition to the influences of the client's presenting problem, referral source, and previous therapeutic experience) systematic differences among therapists in the diagnostic categories they can and do use. To a large extent, these differences may be determined by the "cognitive accessibility" of particular diagnostic classifications, or the ease with which different diagnostic categories come to mind. Categories that have been employed recently and/or frequently show enhanced cognitive accessibility and have increased probability of being employed in subsequent categorization and judgment (see Higgins & King, 1981, for a review); in addition, people differ in the extent to which particular categories are *chronically* accessible (Higgins, King, & Mavin, 1982). Since specific types of clinical practices (e.g., community mental health centers, Veteran's Administration hospitals, psychiatric wards) tend to be characterized by clients suffering from particular forms of psychopathology, it is likely that therapists are selectively exposed to particular types of disorders within their practices. And if, in their own clinical practices, therapists are repeatedly exposed to a particular disorder (say, paranoid schizophrenia), that diagnostic category may show a relatively permanent increase in accessibility. As a result, the therapist may be more likely to categorize ambiguous cases in terms of that disorder rather than employing other, equally plausible, classifications (tending, for example, to diagnose cases that present a mixed pattern of symptoms, only some of which are characteristic of paranoid schizophrenia, as paranoid schizophrenic). Furthermore, since theoretical orientations differ in the extent to which they emphasize particular forms of pathology, clinicians with different theoretical perspectives may systematically differ in the types of diagnostic categories that are chronically most accessible to them. Hence, they may differ in terms of the diagnostic categories they characteristically employ, with, for example, psychoanalysts and behavioral therapists reaching quite different diagnoses based upon the same constellation of symptoms and behavior.

In fact, there is evidence that therapists do differ in the frequency with which they employ particular diagnostic classifications. These differences among therapists are detectable even when their clients come from the same population and have been randomly assigned to therapists, presumably eliminating the possibility of actual differences in the composition of different case loads (e.g., Borreson, 1965). Moreover, research has demonstrated differences among therapists in their tendency to diagnose significant pathology (Ash, 1949), and therapists' preferences for particular types of problems can and do influence intake judgments (Eells & Guppy, 1963). Finally, there is some evidence that therapists with different therapeutic orientations differ in their initial clinical judgments (Bishop & Richards, 1984; Houts, 1984).

Thus, the fact that therapists arrive at working diagnoses so quickly becomes easier to understand when one realizes that they are often provided with working hypotheses by the client's presenting problem, by other referral sources, by the client's therapeutic history, or by their own particularly accessible diagnostic categories. If therapists accept these working hypotheses as ones to be evaluated by further diagnostic activities, the hypotheses may guide them in the types of symptoms they perceive to be relevant to the case. As a result, therapists may choose to inquire selectively about these symptoms, neglecting to ask about other potentially relevant symptomatology. A client, by responding (quite understandably) only to those questions which are asked, may report only symptoms that are indeed concordant with the therapist's initial expectations. Other symptomatology, simply because it has not been explored by the therapist, may not come to light so readily.

For example, a therapist with the working hypothesis that a client suffers from depression may probe for evidence of potentially relevant symptoms and causes of depression and not for symptoms and causes of some other potentially applicable diagnostic category, say, anxiety. The client, in response, may attempt to report symptoms relevant to the therapist's line of questioning, ignoring other symptoms that the therapist does not seem interested in. Perhaps the client will respond affirmatively to queries about changes in sleeping and eating habits, but neglect to report the occurrence of anxiety attacks because he or she has not been questioned about them. Thus, the therapist, right from the start, may be more likely to find evidence supportive of the working hypothesis rather than another diagnostic category, if only because the working hypothesis is the sole hypothesis under consideration.

Furthermore, as a result of differences in the readiness with which therapists employ particular diagnostic classifications, two therapists may arrive at two quite different diagnoses (say, schizophrenia and bipolar affective disorder) after observing the same client. Particularly if the client is not a clear-cut case and possesses some symptoms characteristic of each disorder, therapists may categorize the client in terms of the potentially applicable categories most cognitively accessible for them. What would be the effect of the different diagnostic classifications employed by the two therapists? Research on hypothesis testing and behavioral confirmation suggests that, in this situation, the client's reported symptoms might differ a great deal depending on the therapist conducting the interview. The initial diagnostic hypothesis may channel each therapist's line of questioning so that the client responds only with symptoms relevant to the hypothesis, in effect providing behavioral confirmation for the therapist's initial diagnostic hypothesis.

If interviewed by a therapist whose working hypothesis is schizophrenia, the client may be questioned primarily about attributes associated with schizophrenia. However, the therapist whose working hypothesis is bipolar affective disorder might probe preferentially for symptoms typically associated with manic depression. To the extent that the client's symptomatology is actually a mixed pattern, both diagnosticians will find evidence confirming their own working hypothesis even though, had each tested the other's working hypothesis, he or she would have concluded that it too was the correct diagnostic classification. Thus, particularly in instances where, according to the DSM-III, two different disorders are characterized by similar constellations of symptoms, the categorical option that is most cognitively accessible may guide the clinician's selection of an initial diagnostic hypothesis. And this hypothesis, in turn, may direct the future course of the therapist–client interaction in such a way that it ultimately comes to be confirmed.

Explanation: Identifying Causal Origins of the Problem

A stage in therapy conceptually distinct from (although temporally overlapping with) diagnosis involves attempts to explain the origins and development of the client's problems. Although therapists with different theoretical perspectives may vary in the emphasis they place on this therapeutic goal (with, for example, behaviorists focusing more on current maintaining factors than on historical causal factors), all therapists at some level seek to understand how and why the disorder developed by attempting to identify the conditions that have caused and now maintain it. To do so, they may rely on their beliefs about factors that predispose people to psychopathology. Therapists, in addition to having beliefs about the particular symptoms associated with various forms of pathology, typically have beliefs about the factors and conditions that are implicated in the development of specific disorders. Clinicians with differing theoretical and therapeutic perspectives may differ greatly in their formulations of the particular causes implicated in the origins of particular disorders. Thus, for example, Freudians may see phobias as the result of displaced anxiety caused by disturbed psychosexual development; at the same time, behaviorists may view phobias as the products of conditioning or avoidance learning.

Testing Hypotheses About Origins of the Problem

In effect, after reaching a diagnosis, therapists' beliefs about the causal origins of particular forms of psychopathology may provide expectations about conditions and events likely to be present in the backgrounds of clients with specific disorders. These beliefs and expectations then may function as *hypotheses* about the sorts of background factors that the client is likely to have experienced. These hypotheses, in turn, may channel subsequent therapeutic interactions in such a way that they come to be confirmed by the client's behavior.

If, for example, a practitioner adheres to the theory that the development of paranoia is due to a person's inability to deal with homosexual tendencies (a theory emanating from Freud), a client diagnosed as paranoid may be queried about close relationships with members of the same sex or about conflicts with members of the other sex, but not about positive heterosexual experiences or about other factors that might be relevant and present in the client's background. With such a confirmatory hypothesis-testing strategy, therapists may elicit evidence consistent with their hypotheses about the associations between a particular disorder and specific causal factors. In the current example, the client, even if entirely free of homosexual conflicts, is likely to have had some negative heterosexual experiences (who among us has not?) as well as some close same-sex relationships (once again, who has not?) and, if probed selectively about these experiences, will be particularly likely to describe them. Thus, in this example, as a result of the manner in which the hypothesis has been tested, behavioral confirmation may be obtained for the therapist's initial hypothesis about the causal origins of the client's problem as well as for the global theory of paranoia that generated the hypothesis in the first place.

In a fashion not unlike this example, other theories postulating linkages between current disorders and particular historical factors may determine which questions are asked of clients, constraining the possible range of answers so that clients ultimately may confirm a therapist's initial theories of psychopathology. In fact, there is evidence that therapists do employ confirmatory hypothesis-testing strategies. Wilson Dallas and Baron (1985), in a replication of Snyder and Swann's (1978) initial demonstration, asked therapists to interview college students in order to test hypotheses about them. As did the college student interviewers in Snyder and Swann's experiment, therapists chose to ask questions of the target person that preferentially solicited confirmatory evidence for their hypotheses. Therapists evaluating the hypothesis that the student was an introvert chose to ask questions that probed for evidence of introversion; those testing the hypothesis that the target was extroverted asked questions that selectively solicited instances of extroversion.

The college students in the Wilson Dallas and Baron experiment, in response to this directive line of questioning, confirmed the therapists' hypotheses during the interview. Students for whom the introverted hypothesis was being assessed behaved in an introverted manner during the interview; those subjected to the extroverted hypothesis presented themselves in an extroverted manner. Interestingly, although independent judges' ratings indicated that the students had behaved in a manner congruent with the therapists' hypotheses, the therapists' own ratings did not reflect this fact. Either the therapists were unresponsive to the students' actual behavior or they were unwilling or unable to report their reactions to the students.

Backgrounds for Behavioral Confirmation

But, the reader may be asking: How do confirmatory hypothesis-testing processes lead to behavioral confirmation consequences? Do these processes somehow invent, create, or manufacture events and conditions in the client's background that were not there to begin with? That is, even if therapists do provide clients with strong cues pointing toward appropriate or approved topics, encouraging them to provide evidence of background events that confirm therapists' etiological beliefs, behavioral confirmation can occur only to the extent that clients do have some "pathogenic" events in their backgrounds. After all, it is rather unlikely that clients, even highly compliant ones, would completely fabricate confirmatory evidence merely to please their therapists. Rather, it seems more likely that behavioral confirmation of clinicians' theories about the causal origins of psychopathology may occur only when clients actually have experienced events of a pathogenic nature.

In the spirit of this argument, Renaud and Estess (1961) have provided evidence that a wide variety of circumstances thought to be pathogenic may be discovered even in the backgrounds of people suffering no psychological difficulties, let alone in the backgrounds of those who do suffer psychological problems. They conducted life-history interviews with 100 men who had been chosen precisely because their adult lives gave no indication whatsoever of "problems." These men had no histories of mental or psychological conflict and complained of no problems of personal, social, marital, or occupational adjustment. Furthermore, according to all objective indices, these men were functioning at a normal, or even superior, level in all major life domains. They possessed excellent health, had exhibited superior educational and occupational accomplishment, and had effective relationships with authority figures, peers, spouses, and children.

Interviews conducted with these men, similar in scope to clinical intake interviews and covering all major areas of life, yielded rather striking information. Quite simply, the life histories of these "ordinary" people were laden with the kinds of "traumatic events" and "pathogenic factors" that are usually encountered in the histories of psychiatric patients whose functioning is presumably impaired by their symptoms. More specifically, Renaud and Estess (1961) found that the life histories of these "normal" men were rife with

> overt parental discord as seen in divorce or separation; covert parental discord as manifested in lengthy periods of withdrawal; seclusiveness or lack of mutuality; excessively rigid or overindulgent patterns of discipline, or both; resolution of oedipal anxieties through overidentification with one parent to the exclusion of the other; unresolved sibling rivalries; repressive and unrealistic approaches to sexual information and sexual practices; frequent maternal physical complaints of a type recognized today as related to tension and conflict. (p. 795)

The life histories abounded, in short, with background factors "*at least* as severe" (p. 795, their italics) as those that practitioners in clinical and therapeutic settings typically point to in accounting for the development of psychological disorders. In fact, Renaud and Estess quite candidly admitted that, had these men come to them complaining of "colitis, ulcers, phobias, work inhibitions, incapacitating shyness, etc." (p. 795), they would have had no trouble finding evidence of the sorts of background problems associated with these conditions.

Renaud and Estess's study dramatically demonstrates that apparently "normal" people may have experienced many of the "traumatic" or "pathogenic" background factors thought to predispose one to the development of psychopathology. Of course, the presence of these factors in the backgrounds of normals is unlikely to be discovered, since they are seldom interviewed by clinicians. Nevertheless, the backgrounds of these people (and presumably those of many who do find their way into therapy) may be rich sources of evidence in support and confirmation of any of a wide variety of theories about the origins and development of psychopathology—should these people ever become the targets of therapeutic attempts to test hypotheses. That is, the evidence may be there all along, ready and waiting for a hypothesis to guide the search for it and a confirmatory hypothesis-testing strategy to ferret it out.

Our suggestions about hypothesis-testing processes and behavioral confirmation outcomes have their counterparts in the writings of others concerned with diagnostic and explanatory activities. For example, Gauron and Dickinson (1969) have observed:

> What typically occurred was that once the doctor had reached a preliminary conclusion, he temporarily at least discarded other possibilities and approached the case from the point of view of validating his initial impression. He was then not attuned to data suggesting other possibilities that he was not considering. . . . In the very process of reducing

> his own 'booming, buzzing confusion' about the case by imposing some guiding principles about what might be going on, the psychiatrist preset himself to look for those things that would support his conclusion. In the very act of reaching a diagnostic decision so rapidly and efficiently, he placed himself in the situation of taking a position he felt he must defend until some strikingly better alternative came along. (p. 203)

Treatment: Intervening to Ameliorate the Problem

In what ways might the treatment phase of therapy afford opportunities for hypothesis testing and behavioral confirmation? During the treatment phase, as therapists implement interventions designed to alleviate their clients' problems, there are two major types of expectations that might exert self-fulfilling influences on the therapeutic interaction. First, therapists typically have expectations about their clients' prognosis, that is, about the likelihood that they will benefit from treatment and exhibit improvement as a result of it. Second, therapists may have expectations about the ways in which clients will respond to particular therapeutic interventions. These expectations in effect provide therapists with hypotheses about the processes and outcomes of therapy. As therapists proceed to test these hypotheses, might their behavior toward clients reflect these expectations? Might clients, in return, come to display behaviors that confirm their therapists' initial beliefs?

Testing Hypotheses About Prognosis

Prognostic judgments, like diagnostic ones, are typically formed quite early in the therapeutic process (e.g., Gauron & Dickinson, 1969). In part, assessments of a client's likely prognosis may depend upon the therapist's beliefs about the prognosis typically associated with the diagnosed disorder. Thus, for example, if the treatment literature indicates that depression is fairly amenable to therapeutic intervention and that psychopathy is not, therapists may have more optimistic expectations for clients diagnosed as depressed than for those diagnosed as psychopathic. These expectations then may influence the course of therapeutic interactions so that clients ultimately confirm these expectations, with (in our example) depressed clients showing greater and faster improvement than psychopathic ones.

To the extent that prognostic forecasts derive from objective evidence of real differences among disorders, behavioral confirmation may play only a minor role (if any) in therapy outcomes. However, other, more subjective judgments influence therapists' prognostic expectations about their clients. A great deal of evidence indicates that therapists exhibit a general tendency to form initial impressions of clients very quickly, classifying them as either "good patients" or "bad patients" (Arnhoff, 1954; Houts & Galante, 1985; Mehlman, 1952; Pasamanick, Dinitz, & Lefton, 1959; Schmidt & Fonda, 1956; Soskin, 1954; Strupp, 1958). These initial affective reactions are associated with therapists' prognostic expectations (e.g., Barocas & Vance, 1974; Brown, 1970). Thus, a therapist who has an initially positive reaction to a client is likely to be more optimistic about the client's prognosis than one who formed a negative first impression of that same client.

What are the effects of these differential expectations? Positive therapist impressions and their associated prognostic expectations often are the precursors of successful treatment outcomes (Bishop, Sharf, & Adkins, 1975; Brown, 1970; Goldstein, 1960; Mills & Abeles, 1965; Rosenzweig & Harford, 1972; Shader, Kellam, & Durell, 1967; Sharf & Bishop, 1979; Stoler, 1963). Also, clients' post-treatment ratings of their own degree of improvement are to some extent predictable from their therapists' initial affective reactions and their prognostic judgments (Saltzman, Luetgert, Roth, Creaser, & Howard, 1976; Sharf & Bishop, 1979). Similarly, therapists' final assessments of client improvement are significantly related to their initial affective impressions of clients and to their early prognostic expectations (Brown, 1970; Saltzman et al., 1976). Even the number of therapeutic sessions that the clients ultimately attend is to some extent predictable from therapists' early affective impressions (Bishop, Sharf, & Adkins, 1975; Brown, 1970).

What might account for this strong and consistent pattern of findings? One explanation is behavioral confirmation processes. To the extent that therapists like particular clients and expect them to improve, they may treat them in a more positive manner, with the eventual result that clients come to confirm therapists' expectations. Those expected to exhibit rapid improvement may do so; those not expected to respond so well may not. There is, of course, an alternative explanation for relations between therapists' expectations and therapeutic outcomes. Therapists simply may be extraordinarily accurate at predicting which clients will be most responsive to treatment. Rather than being an actual cause of therapeutic outcomes, liking and prognostic judgments merely may reflect therapists' accurate assessments of their clients' likelihood of improvement. However, there is evidence against this interpretation. Therapists often form very different first impressions of the same client, even when they have been exposed to an identical sample of that client's behavior (e.g., by watching exactly the same videotape of the client; Houts & Galante, 1985; Strupp, 1958), demonstrating that therapists' impressions are not based solely upon objective attributes of the client.

Furthermore, these initial evaluative impressions of the client tend to persist. For example, Houts and Galante (1985) found that regardless of the information therapists later learned about a client's improvement, those who had formed an initially positive impression formed subsequent impressions that were uniformly more positive than those whose initial expressions were negative. Studies of ongoing therapeutic interactions have similarly found that therapists' impressions of clients stabilize quite quickly. For example, Meehl (1960) found that therapists' impressions formed by the fourth clinical interaction were not significantly different from those at the 24th contact.

The stability of therapist impressions may reflect the fact that clients do not change much over the course of therapy. However, this explanation loses plausibility when one considers that recent meta-analyses have indicated that people in psychotherapy *do* exhibit improvement relative to nontherapeutic controls (e.g., Shapiro & Shapiro, 1982; Smith & Glass, 1977). Instead, the evidence indicates that stability of therapists' impressions may be, to a great degree, due to the influence of these early assessments on subsequent interpretations and evaluations of the client's behavior (e.g., Houts & Galante, 1985).

But, do therapists' evaluative impressions actually affect their *behavior* toward clients in the course of therapy? Although we know of no experimental investigations that have directly examined this question, there is evidence that is highly suggestive of the influence of therapist impressions on their later behavior. Strupp (1958) found that therapists who had initially formed either positive or negative impressions of a client (after watching the identical videotape) differed greatly in the manner of treatment planned for the client. Those who had positive initial reactions prescribed more tolerant treatment plans; those with negative initial impressions dictated more rigid and moralistic regimens. We may speculate that recipients of rigid and moralistic treatments might respond negatively, thereby confirming the therapists' initially negative expectations. Those favored with more tolerant treatment plans might respond with greater improvement, thus providing support for their therapists' initially positive expectations.

Testing Hypotheses About Effectiveness of Interventions

During the treatment phase, therapists also may formulate and test hypotheses about the efficacy of particular therapeutic interventions for treating their clients' specific disorders. And, since different schools of thought specify different sorts of interventions, therapists of differing orientations may hold divergent expectations about the therapeutic techniques likely to prove most efficacious. However, because practitioners typically employ the techniques prescribed by their theoretical and therapeutic orientations, they most likely will be engaging primarily in those activities they hypothesize, expect, and assume to be most successful and effective. Even therapists who don't subscribe uniformly to one particular therapeutic orientation (and who instead consider themselves "eclectics" who pick and choose among therapies) may nevertheless, in treating any specific client, be operating with a therapeutic technique chosen precisely because they have positive expectations about its effectiveness for that client's specific problem.

How might these hypotheses and expectations be translated into practice? Therapists might, by means of their verbal and nonverbal behavior, communicate their expectations about the types of behavioral changes they expect to occur. As a result, to the extent that clients are motivated to cooperate with their therapists (and perhaps to justify their investment of time, effort, and money in therapy; cf. Cooper, 1980), clients may selectively display—or selectively present to the therapist—behaviors consistent with their therapists' expectations.

Do therapists' expectations influence therapeutic outcomes? Although there is little in the way of direct evidence, there is much in the way of suggestive evidence. Several studies have documented the tendency for clients to become increasing similar to their therapists and to display increasing congruence with their therapists' theoretical orientation over the course of therapy. For example, Rosenthal (1955) found that patients who showed greater-than-average improvement in therapy (based on self-reported improvement and on ratings by naive interviewers) also shifted their moral values in the direction of greater congruence with their therapists (cf. Welkowitz, Cohen, & Ortmeyer, 1967). Although this research was not designed to assess the mechanisms by which clients' values come to parallel more closely those of their therapists, we can speculate that those who shifted their values were responding to their therapists' implicit expectations and thus confirming these expectations with their behavior.

Similarly, clients tend to report improvement in terms appropriate to their therapists' orientation (Murray, 1956; Rogers & Dymond, 1954). Thus, clients of Rogerian therapists may speak of their improvements in terms of approaching self-actualization, and patients of Freudian analysts may describe improvements that involve working through long-repressed psychological conflicts. Even dreams may come to reflect therapists' expectations. Whitman, Kramer, and Baldridge (1963) monitored dreams for 13–16 nights by awakening sleepers and asking them to report their dreams. Surprisingly, they found that, in examining the dreams reported to therapists, "Major changes or deletions occurred 3 times more frequently than did the complete forgetting of an awakening" (p. 278). Moreover, an analysis of these omissions and distortions revealed that references to certain topics (construed by the researchers as threatening ones) were regularly deleted or modified. Perhaps, the participants in this study selectively reported their dreams so as to eliminate "inappropriate" material and to make them conform more closely to their therapists' expectations.

If such findings do reflect the operation of behavioral confirmation processes, how are therapists' expectations conveyed to clients? One likely mechanism involves reward and punishment. Therapists may convey approval or disapproval of clients either through explicit rewards and punishments or through more indirect nonverbal messages. For example, it is known that therapists high in "hostility anxiety" are likely to ignore or avoid topics with overtly hostile content; as a result, clients tend to change the expressed object of their hostility or to abandon topics with hostile content altogether (Bandura, Lipsher, & Miller, 1960).

That therapists reinforce clients for talking about their problems in an approved manner and extinguish nonapproved content may help explain why clients come to speak of their difficulties in terms appropriate to their therapists' orientations. Therapists of diverging theoretical orientations may elicit different types of changes in their clients, changes that confirm the type of improvement predicted by their orientation. In fact, Kopta, Newman, McGovern, and Sandrock (1986) found that therapists with differing theoretical orientations (psychodynamic, cognitive-behavioral, family systems, and eclectic) differed substantially in the types of information on which they focused in verbal interactions with clients. A particularly revealing illustration of this point is provided by an analysis of Carl Rogers's therapeutic interactions. One of the fundamental tenets of Rogers's therapy is the provision of unconditional positive regard to the client. However, an analysis of Rogers's own interactions with clients revealed that, far from being unconditional, his regard (or at least his reinforcement) was apparently contingent upon the content of his clients' verbalizations. In effect, Rogers reinforced "approved" material and extinguished "nonapproved" material through subtly communicated cues (Truax & Carkhuff, 1967; cf. Murray & Jacobson, 1971).

Taken together, these considerations (of therapists' expectations about their clients' therapeutic prognoses and their beliefs about the effectiveness of interventions prescribed by their therapeutic orientations) point to possible self-fulfilling outcomes in the treatment phase of therapist–client interactions. Therapists may find that their clients spend as little or as long in therapy as they expect them to, that their clients improve or fail to improve just as they expect them to, that their clients say and do the things that they expect them to say and do in therapy, and that therapeutic techniques work as effectively or ineffectively as they expect them to—all because of the self-fulfilling impact of acting upon their beliefs, expectations, assumptions, and hypotheses about their clients and about their preferred modes of therapy.

Applicability to Clinical Contexts

In this chapter, we have sought to analyze the role of hypothesis testing and behavioral confirmation in the processes and outcomes of psychotherapy. Specifically, we have attempted to apply the results of experiments on hypothesis testing and behavioral confirmation to interactions between therapists and their clients. In addition, we have described several lines of research in the clinical domain that have yielded results congruent with our thesis that behavioral confirmation may occur in therapeutic contexts. We are aware that few of these studies were explicitly designed to address the question of whether therapy may lead to behavioral confirmation outcomes, and hence conclusions based upon this research must be tentative. Furthermore, in some cases, plausible alternative explanations could be generated to account for the findings obtained in particular studies. Nonetheless, we believe that when viewed as a whole, the results of clinical investigations, as well as studies of behavioral confirmation, converge on a highly plausible account of the possible role of hypothesis testing and behavioral confirmation in therapist–client interactions.

In our efforts to apply the results of experiments on behavioral confirmation to the clinical domain, we have focused, in turn, on the diagnosis, explanation, and treatment phases of the therapeutic situation. We recognize that some caution must be exercised when generalizing from experiments conducted primarily in the psychological laboratory, typically with college students as participants. However, we should point out that there have been demonstrations of behavioral confirmation in nonlaboratory contexts and with participants other than college students.

In an investigation that stimulated a long line of research, Rosenthal and Jacobson (1968) informed elementary school teachers that some of their students were "late bloomers," thus leading them to believe that these children had a great deal of unrealized potential. Although the children had been selected randomly, by the end of the year they showed noticeable intellectual gains, presumably because the teachers treated the supposed "late bloomers" in ways that helped their performance to improve. Similarly, King (1971) informed a welding instructor that some of his trainees had unusually high aptitude. Chosen at random, and knowing nothing of their designation as high aptitude workers, these men nonetheless showed superior achievement throughout the welding course. To the extent that the psychotherapeutic treatment situation represents an educational and/or a training situation, then, the same behavioral confirmation outcomes that occur between teachers and students and between instructors and trainees may occur between therapists and clients. Indeed, as we have seen, there is at least one demonstration of the formulation of confirmatory hypothesis-testing strategies (a known precursor of behavioral confirmation) among professional therapists (Wilson Dallas & Baron, 1985).

Perhaps, it might be argued, the clinical situation is immunized against behavioral confirmation by the fact that there is so much at stake. Therapists and clients, to the extent that they perceive therapy as consequential, may be highly motivated to avoid dealing with each other in ways that generate behavioral confirmation. Such motivations notwithstanding, there actually are reasons to believe that the psychotherapeutic situation is one especially well suited to the occurrence of behavioral confirmation processes.

First, the motivation that may appear to protect against behavioral confirmation actually may contribute to its occurrence. Typically, both therapist and client are highly motivated to discover the nature and source of the problem as well as to treat it. In seeking to understand the client's problem, the therapist explicitly formulates and tests hypotheses, and the client (at least the motivated one) attempts to cooperate in providing answers the therapist will find relevant and useful. In addition, the therapist engages in therapeutic activities designed to ameliorate or eliminate the client's problems. The client who genuinely wishes to solve his or her problem may accept these influence attempts as legitimate and may become highly compliant with the therapist's wishes and expectations.

Second, therapeutic interactions are situations in which typically there is a large differential between client and therapist in their relative power and expertise. Such situations of differential power and professional expertise are known to be particularly likely arenas for the occurrence of self-fulfilling prophecies (e.g., Rosenthal, 1976). Moreover, since therapists are clearly in a "one-up" position, clients often are highly motivated to earn their therapists' approval (e.g., Schwartz, Friedlander, & Tedeschi, 1986). In this regard, it is worth noting that people who are high in need for approval are most likely to provide behavioral confirmation for the expectations of others (e.g., Laszlo & Rosenthal, 1970; Smith & Flenning, 1971; Todd, 1975; cf. Harris & Rosenthal, 1976). Thus, to the extent that the therapeutic situation arouses the need for approval (or attracts people high in need for approval as clients), it may be a context in which clients are especially likely to confirm therapists' beliefs, expectations, and hypotheses.

Third, the very subject matter of therapy may provide additional opportunities for behavioral confirmation. The topics under discussion in therapy are often highly subjective and, therefore, unverifiable. This is particularly true of topics such as dreams and emotions. But even in the case of past events and behaviors, there is a great deal of latitude for clients to present themselves in ways congruent with therapists' expectations. We do not mean to imply here that clients are necessarily deceitful, deliberately falsifying their past histories, dreams, or subjective states when recounting them to the therapist (although, to be sure, this can occur). Rather, we are suggesting that clients, even with the best of intentions (perhaps, because of their good intentions) may inadvertently select which events to report and how to report them, particularly when drawing on memories of events that transpired quite some time ago. Such a data base may provide an abundant harvest of evidence to confirm therapists' expectations and hypotheses about their clients' histories.

For these reasons, interactions between therapists and clients may be particularly conducive to behavioral confirmation processes. Needless to say, we do not mean to argue that therapists' beliefs, expectations, and hypotheses will always (or even usually) induce clients to behave in ways that appear to confirm those preconceptions. We do, however, mean to argue that, within the range of variability of interpersonal situations, therapist–client interactions are ones with structural and motivational features that, more so than other social interactions that lack these features, may set the stage for self-fulfilling outcomes. It must remain, we should point out, for researchers to document the actual frequency with which confirmatory hypothesis testing and behavioral confirmation occur in clinical and therapeutic contexts.

Concluding Remarks

Let us be emphatic: it is not our intent to derogate the psychotherapeutic enterprise or its practitioners. The value of psychotherapy has been well established (e.g., Smith, Glass, & Miller, 1980). Rather, our purpose has been to explore and attempt to illuminate some of the dynamics of interactions between therapists and clients. Needless to say, examples of possible negative effects of the phenomena and processes we have discussed are easy to generate, including the perpetuation of erroneous diagnoses, diminished prospects for recovery of clients mistakenly labeled with poor prognostic expectations, spurious confirmation, and perpetuation of invalid theories of psychopathology, and so on. As such, suggestions for ways to minimize some of these negative effects of hypothesis testing and behavioral confirmation are beginning to appear in the literature (see Arkes, 1981; Arnoult & Anderson, this volume; Fischhoff, 1982).

Nevertheless, we expect as well that *positive* therapeutic outcomes may result from those same phenomena and processes of hypothesis testing and behavioral confirmation. To the extent that therapists believe in the efficacy of their therapeutic interventions, those interventions may be more effective than they otherwise would be, simply by virtue of the self-fulfilling effects of therapists' faith in them. Similarly, if therapists hold prognostic expectations that are particularly (perhaps even overly) optomistic, clients might improve more rapidly than they otherwise would have. The frequency of such salutary consequences of behavioral confirmation in therapist–client interactions (as well as those of their negative counterparts) remains to be assessed in relevant empirical investigations.

In closing, let us return to our point of departure. We began by noting that therapy has been something of a growth industry, with a large and increasing number of different forms of psychotherapy on the market. In the early 1960s, the number of different types of psychotherapy was estimated at 60 (Garfield, 1982), by the mid-1970s more than 250 techniques had been delineated (Herink, 1980), and current estimates range as high as 400 (Karasu, 1985, cited in Kazdin, 1986). Thus, the proliferation of therapeutic techniques continues. Having analyzed the possible role of hypothesis testing and behavioral confirmation in therapist–client interactions, we are now in a position to offer some perspective on this state of affairs.

The persistence and coexistence of these many and diverse forms of psychotherapy may, in part, reflect the operation of behavioral confirmation processes. Practitioners of differing persuasions, acting on their confident belief in the prescriptions for therapy provided by their particular schools of thought, may behave toward clients in ways that elicit behavioral confirmation for the theoretical and therapeutic orientations they adhere to. In like fashion, and welcome or not, the blossoming of even more brands of therapy may be ensured by the self-fulfilling consequences of hypothesis-testing processes and behavioral confirmation outcomes in interactions between therapists and clients.

Acknowledgments

We are grateful to Beatrice Ellis for her helpful suggestions and for her comments on an earlier version of this manuscript.

References

American Psychiatric Commission on Psychotherapies. (1982). *Psychotherapy research: Methodological and efficacy issues.* Washington, DC.

Andersen, S., & Bem, S. L. (1981). Sex typing and androgyny in dyadic interaction. *Journal of Personality and Social Psychology, 41,* 74–86.

Anderson, C. A. (1983). Abstract and concrete data in the perseverance of social theories: When weak data lead to unshakable beliefs. *Journal of Experimental Social Psychology, 19,* 93–108.

Arkes, H. R. (1981). Impediments to accurate clinical judgment and possible ways to minimize their impact. *Journal of Consulting and Clinical Psychology, 49,* 323–330.

Arnoff, F. N. (1954). Some factors influencing the unreliability of clinical judgments. *Journal of Clinical Psychology, 10,* 272–275.

Ash, P. (1949). The reliability of psychiatric diagnoses. *Journal of Abnormal and Social Psychology, 44,* 272–277.

Bandura, A. (1969). *Principles of behavior modification.* New York: Holt, Rinehart & Winston.

Bandura, A., Lipsher, D. H., & Miller, P. E. (1960). Psychotherapists' approach-avoidant reactions to patients' expressions of hostility. *Journal of Consulting Psychology, 24,* 1–8.

Barlow, D. H. (1981). On the relation of clinical research to clinical practice: Current issues, new directions. *Journal of Consulting and Clinical Psychology, 49,* 147–155.

Barocas, R., & Vance, F. L. (1974). Physical appearance and personal adjustment counseling. *Journal of Counseling Psychology, 21,* 96–100.

Basham, R. B. (1986). Scientific and practical advantages of comparative design in psychotherapy outcome research. *Journal of Consulting and Clinical Psychology, 54,* 88–94.

Bishop, J. B., & Richards, T. F. (1984). Counselor theoretical orientation as related to intake judgments. *Journal of Counseling Psychology, 31,* 398–401.

Bishop, J. B., Sharf, R. S., & Adkins, D. M. (1975). Counselor intake judgments, client characteristics, and number of sessions at a university counseling center. *Journal of Counseling Psychology, 23,* 557–559.

Bordin, E. S. (1968). *Psychological counseling* (2nd ed.). New York: Appleton-Century-Crofts.

Borreson, A. M. (1965). Counselor influence on diagnostic classification of client problems. *Journal of Counseling Psychology, 12,* 252–258.

Brown, R. D. (1970). Experienced and inexperienced counselors' first impressions of clients and case outcomes: Are first impressions lasting? *Journal of Counseling Psychology, 17,* 550–558.

Callis, R. (1965). Diagnostic classification as a research tool. *Journal of Counseling Psychology, 12,* 238–243.

Cash, T. F., Kehr, J., Polyson, J., & Freeman, V. (1977). The role of physical attractiveness in peer attribution of psychological disturbances. *Journal of Consulting and Clinical Psychology, 45,* 987–993.

Cooper, J. (1980). Reducing fears and increasing assertiveness: The role of dissonance reduction. *Journal of Experimental Social Psychology, 16,* 199–213.

Eells, K., & Guppy, W. (1963). Counselor's valuations of and preferences for different types of counseling problems. *Journal of Counseling Psychology, 10,* 146–155.

Fazio, R. H., & Zanna, M. P. (1981). Direct experience and attitude-behavior consistency. In L. Berkowitz (Ed.), *Advances in experimental social psychology* (Vol. 14). New York: Academic Press.

Fischhoff, B. (1982). Debiasing. In D. Kahneman, P. Slovic, & A. Tversky (Eds.), *Judgment under uncertainty: Heuristics and biases.* New York: Cambridge University Press.

Garfield, S. L. (1982). Eclecticism and integration in psychotherapy. *Behavior Therapy, 13,* 610–623.

Gauron, E. F., & Dickinson, J. K. (1969). The influence of seeing the patient first on diagnostic decision-making in psychiatry. *American Journal of Psychiatry, 126,* 199–205.

Glass, G. V., McGaw, B., & Smith, M. L. (1981). *Meta-analysis in social research.* Beverly Hills, CA: Sage.

Goldstein, A. P. (1960). Therapist and client expectation of personality change in psychotherapy. *Journal of Counseling Psychology, 7,* 180–184.

Harris, M. J., & Rosenthal, R. (1986). Counselor and client personality as determinants of counselor expectancy effects. *Journal of Personality and Social Psychology, 50,* 362–369.

Herink, R. (1980). *The psychotherapy handbook.* New York: New American Library.

Higgins, E. T., & King, G. A. (1981). Accessibility of social constructs: Information-processing consequences of individual and contextual variability. In N. Cantor & J. F. Kihlstrom (Eds.), *Personality, cognition, and social interaction.* Hillsdale, NJ: Erlbaum.

Higgins, E. T., King, G. A., & Mavin, G. H. (1982). Individual construct accessibility and subjective impressions and recall. *Journal of Personality and Social Psychology, 43,* 35–47.

Houts, A. C. (1984). Effects of clinician theoretical orientation and patient explanatory bias on initial clinical judgments. *Professional Psychology: Research and Practice, 15,* 284–293.

Houts, A. C., & Galante, M. (1985). The impact of evaluative disposition and subsequent information on clinical impressions. *Journal of Social and Clinical Psychology, 3,* 201–212.

Kazdin, A. E. (1983). Treatment research: The investigation and evaluation of psychotherapy. In M. Hersen, A. E. Kazdin, & A. S. Bellack (Eds.), *The clinical psychology handbook.* New York: Pergamon Press.

———. (1986). Comparative outcome studies of psychotherapy: Methodological issues and strategies. *Journal of Consulting and Clinical Psychology, 54,* 95–105.

Kazdin, A. E., & Wilson, G. T. (1978). *Evaluation of behavior therapy: Issues, evidence, and research strategies.* Cambridge, MA: Ballinger.

King, A. S. (1971). Self-fulfilling prophecies in training the hard-core: Supervisors' expectations and the underpriviledged workers' performance. *Social Science Quarterly, 52,* 369–378.

Kopta, S. M., Newman, F. L., McGovern, M. P., & Sandrock, D. (1986). Psychotherapeutic orientations: A comparison of conceptualizations, interventions, and treatment plan costs. *Journal of Consulting and Clinical Psychology, 54,* 369–374.

Langer, E. J., & Abelson R. P. (1974). A patient by any other name . . . : Clinician group difference in labeling bias. *Journal of Consulting and Clinical Psychology, 42,* 4–9.

Laszlo, J. P., & Rosenthal, R. (1970). Subject dogmatism, experimenter status, and experimenter expectancy effects. *Personality, 1,* 11–23.

Luborsky, L., Singer, B., & Luborsky, L. (1975). Comparative studies of psychotherapy: Is it true that "everyone has won and all must have prizes"? *Archives of General Psychiatry, 32,* 995–1008.

Mahoney, M. (1977). Publication prejudices: An experimental study of confirmatory bias in the peer review system. *Cognitive Therapy and Research, 1,* 161–175.

Manstead, A. S. R., Proffitt, C., & Smart, J. L. (1983). Predicting and understanding mothers' infant-feeding intentions and behavior: Testing the theory of reasoned action. *Journal of Personality and Social Psychology, 44,* 657–671.

Meehl, P. E. (1960). The cognitive activity of the clinician. *American Psychologist, 15,* 19–27.

Mehlman, B. (1952). The reliability of psychiatric diagnoses. *Journal of Abnormal and Social Psychology, 47,* 577–578.

Miller, R. C., & Berman, J. S. (1983). The efficacy of cognitive behavior therapies: A quantitative review of the research evidence. *Psychological Bulletin, 94,* 39–53.

Mills, D. H., & Abeles, N. (1965). Counselor needs for affiliation and nurturance as related to liking for clients and counseling process. *Journal of Counseling Psychology, 12,* 353–358.

Mischel, W. (1977). On the future of personality measurement. *American Psychologist, 32,* 246–254.

Murray, E. J. (1956). The content-analysis method of studying psychotherapy. *Psychological Monographs, 70* (13, Whole No. 420).

Murray, E. J., & Jacobson, L. I. (1971). The nature of learning in traditional and behavioral psychotherapy. In A. E. Bergin & S. L. Garfield (Eds.), *Handbook of psychotherapy and behavior change: An empirical analysis.* New York: Wiley.

Nisbett, R., & Ross, L. (1980). *Human inference: Strategies and shortcomings of social judgment.* Englewood Cliffs, NJ: Prentice-Hall.

O'Leary, M. R., Speltz, M. L., Donovan, D. M., & Walker, R. D. (1979). Implicit preadmission screening criteria in an alcoholism treatment program. *American Journal of Psychiatry, 136,* 1190–1193.

Oskamp, S. (1965). Overconfidence in case-study judgments. *Journal of Consulting Psychology, 29,* 261–265.

Pasamanick, B., Dinitz, S., & Lefton, M. (1959). Psychiatric orientation and its relation to diagnosis and treatment in a mental hospital. *American Journal of Psychiatry, 116,* 127–132.

Pellegrine, R. J. (1971). Repression-sensitization and perceived severity of presenting problem of four hundred and forty-four counseling center clients. *Journal of Counseling Psychology, 18,* 333–336.

Renaud, H., & Estess, F. (1961). Life history interviews with one hundred normal American males: "Pathogenicity" of childhood. *American Journal of Orthopsychiatry, 31,* 786–802.

Rogers, C. R., & Dymond, R. (1954). *Psychotherapy and personality change.* Chicago: University of Chicago Press.

Rosenthal, D. (1955). Changes in some moral values following psychotherapy. *Journal of Consulting Psychology, 19,* 431–436.

Rosenthal, R. (1976). *Experimenter effects in behavior research* (Enlarged ed.). New York: Irvington.

Rosenthal, R., & Jacobson, L. (1968). *Pygmalion in the classroom.* New York: Holt, Rinehart & Winston.

Rosenzweig, S. P., & Harford, T. (1972). Correlates of therapists' initial impressions of patients in a psychiatric day center. *Psychotherapy: Research, Theory, and Practice, 9,* 126–129.

Rush, A. J. (Ed.). (1982). *Short-term psychotherapies for depression.* New York: Guilford Press.

Sacco, W. P., & Beck, A. T. (1985). Cognitive therapy for depression. In E. Beckham & W. R. Leber (Eds.), *Handbook of depression: Treatment, assessment and research.* Homewood, IL: Dorsey Press.

Saltzman, C., Luetgert, M. J., Roth, C. H., Creaser, J., & Howard, L. (1976). Formation of a therapeutic relationship: Experiences during the initial phase of psychotherapy as predictors of treatment duration and outcome. *Journal of Consulting and Clinical Psychology, 44,* 546–555.

Sandifer, M. G., Hordern, A., & Green, L. M. (1970). The psychiatric interview: The impact of the first three minutes. *American Journal of Psychiatry, 126,* 968–973.

Schmidt, H. O., & Fonda, C. P. (1956). The reliability of psychiatric diagnosis. *Journal of Abnormal and Social Psychology, 52,* 262–267.

Schwartz, G. S., Friedlander, M. L., & Tedeschi, J. T. (1986). Effects of clients' attributional explanations and reasons for seeking help on counselors' impressions. *Journal of Counseling Psychology, 33,* 90–93.

Shader, R. I., Kellam, S. G., & Durell, J. (1967). Social field events during the first week of hospitalization as predictors of treatment outcome for psychotic patients. *Journal of Nervous and Mental Disease, 145,* 142–153.

Shapiro, D. A., & Shapiro, D. (1982). Meta-analysis of comparative therapy outcome studies: A replication and refinement. *Psychological Bulletin, 92,* 581–604.

Sharf, R. R., & Bishop, J. B. (1979). Counselors' feelings toward clients as related to intake judgments and outcome variables. *Journal of Counseling Psychology, 26,* 267–269.

Sharp, W. H., & Marra, H. A. (1971). Factors related to classification of client problem, number of counseling sessions, and trends of client problems. *Journal of Counseling Psychology, 18,* 117–122.

Skrypnek, B. J., & Snyder, M. (1982). On the self-perpetuating nature of stereotypes about women and men. *Journal of Experimental Social Psychology, 18,* 277–291.

Smith, M. L., & Glass, G. V. (1977). Meta-analysis of psychotherapy outcome studies. *American Psychologist, 32,* 752–760.

Smith, M. L., Glass, G. V., & Miller, T. I. (1980). *The benefits of psychotherapy.* Baltimore: Johns Hopkins University Press.

Smith, R. E., & Flenning, F. (1971). Need for approval and susceptibility to unintended social influence. *Journal of Consulting and Clinical Psychology, 36,* 383–385.

Smith, R. E., & Swinyard, W. R. (1983). Attitude-behavior consistency: The impact of product trial versus advertising. *Journal of Marketing Research, 20,* 257–267.

Snyder, M. (1984). When belief creates reality. In L. Berkowitz (Ed.), *Advances in experimental social psychology* (Vol. 16). New York: Academic Press.

Snyder, M., & Campbell, B. H. (1980). Testing hypotheses about other people: The role of the hypothesis. *Personality and Social Psychology Bulletin, 6,* 421–426.

Snyder, M., & Gangestad, S. (1981). Hypothesis-testing processes. In J. H.

Harvey, W. Ickes, & R. F. Kidd (Eds.), *New directions in attribution research* (Vol. 3). Hillsdale, NJ: Erlbaum.

Snyder, M., & Swann, W. B., Jr. (1978). Hypothesis-testing processes in social interaction. *Journal of Personality and Social Psychology, 36,* 1202–1212.

Snyder, M., Tanke, E. D., & Berscheid, E. (1977). Social perception and interpersonal behavior: On the self-fulfilling nature of social stereotypes. *Journal of Personality and Social Psychology, 35,* 656–666.

Soskin, W. F. (1954). Frames of reference in personality assessment. *Journal of Clinical Psychology, 10,* 107–114.

Stoler, N. (1963). Client likability as a variable in the study of psychotherapy. *Journal of Consulting Psychology, 27,* 168–175.

Strupp, H. H. (1958). The psychotherapist's contribution to the treatment process. *Behavior Science, 3,* 34–67.

Strupp, H. H., & Luborsky, L. (1962). *Research in psychotherapy.* (Vol. 2). Washington, DC: American Psychological Association.

Swann, W. B., Jr., & Guiliano, T. (in press). Confirmatory search strategies in social interaction: How, when, why and with what consequences? *Journal of Social and Clinical Psychology.*

Taylor, S. E., & Thompson, S. C. (1982). Stalking the elusive "vividness" effect. *Psychological Review, 89,* 155–181.

Temerlin, M. K. (1968). Suggestion effects in psychiatric diagnosis. *Journal of Nervous and Mental Disease, 147,* 349–353.

Todd, J. (1975). Social evaluation orientation, task orientation, and deliberate cuing in experimenter expectancy effects. *British Journal of Social and Clinical Psychology, 14,* 27–31.

Trope, Y., & Bassok, M. (1982). Confirmatory and diagnosing strategies in social information gathering. *Journal of Personality and Social Psychology, 43,* 22–34.

Truax, C. B., & Carkhuff, R. R. (1967). *Toward effective counseling and psychotherapy.* Chicago: Aldine.

Turk, D. C. & Salovey, P. (1986). Clinical information processing: Bias inoculation. In R. E. Ingram (Ed.), *Information processing approaches to clinical psychology.* Orlando, FL: Academic Press.

von Baeyer, C. L., Sherk, D. L., & Zanna, M. P. (1981). Impression management in the job interview: When the female applicant meets the male (chauvinist) interviewer. *Personality and Social Psychology Bulletin, 7,* 45–52.

Welkowitz, J., Cohen, J., & Ortmeyer, D. (1967). Value system similarity: Investigation of patient-therapist dyads. *Journal of Consulting Psychology, 31,* 48–55.

Whitman, R. M., Kramer, M., & Baldridge, B. (1963). Which dream does the patient tell? *Archives of General Psychiatry, 8,* 277–282.

Wilson Dallas, M. E., & Baron, R. S. (1985). Do psychotherapists use a confirmatory strategy during interviewing? *Journal of Social and Clinical Psychology, 3,* 106–122.

Word, C. O., Zanna, M. P., & Cooper, J. (1974). The nonverbal mediation of self-fulfilling prophecies in interracial interaction. *Journal of Experimental Social Psychology, 10,* 109–120.

Zanna, M. P., & Pack, S. J. (1975). On the self-fulfilling nature of apparent sex differences in behavior. *Journal of Experimental Social Psychology, 11,* 584–591.

PART III — A New Look at Clinical Theory

Rationalism, Constructivism, and the Transference

8 Rationalism and Constructivisim in Clinical Judgment

Michael J. Mahoney

THE important complexities of clinical judgment have captured professional interest in psychology and psychiatry for much of the 20th century. Whatever else they may disagree about, therapists of diverse theoretical orientations concur that important judgments are involved in psychological services. The appropriate nature and focus of those judgments has captured less consistency of opinion, however, and the literature on clinical judgment ranges far and wide in its analyses (Arkes, 1981; Goldberg, 1968; Meehl, 1954, 1973; Wiggins, 1981; Wiggins & Hoffman, 1968). The classic contributions of the 1950s and 1960s came close to equating "clinical judgment" with "diagnostic validity," and Meehl's (1954, 1973) classic works in the area have been among the most frequently misinterpreted (Faust, in press).

The traditional association of "clinical judgment" and "psychodiagnosis" is not surprising given the emphases of the earliest and most influential works in the field (Chapman & Chapman, 1967, 1969; Goldberg, 1968; Meehl, 1954, 1973; Wiggins, 1981; Wiggins & Hoffman, 1968). Although they have come under increasingly critical scrutiny over recent years, clinical assessment and diagnostics remain at the heart of mainstream psychological services (Korchin & Schuldberg, 1981; Wade & Baker, 1977). This state of affairs has been both applauded and lamented by assessment proponents and critics (Meehl, 1978).

This chapter draws on material published in M. J. Mahoney (in press), *Human Change Processes: Notes on the Facilitation of Personal Change* (New York: Basic Books), and is printed by permission.

As I see it, *clinical judgment covers an infinite array of layered movements in perception, action, feeling, and thought.* The counselor's judgmental processes go much further and deeper than his or her diagnostic interpretations. They include—among many other things—tacit models of (a) human nature, (b) the "real" world, (c) the nature of change, (d) the nature of effective counseling, and (e) each client's idiosyncratic psychological needs. Session by session, the therapist attempts to facilitate knowledge via the procedural "language" (techniques) of one or more of the almost 300 psychotherapies currently acknowledged (Herink, 1980; Mahoney, in press). In so doing, the service provider necessarily makes countless decisions that are predominantly tacit. These decisions, in turn, constrain future decision options so that a selective stochastic process becomes self-perpetuating. First impressions are stubborn, and tacit assumptions seldom permit the experience of their own disconfirmation (Snyder & Thomsen, this volume).

It would be misleading, however, to suggest that the psychological processes involved in clinical judgment are categorically different from those observed universally in the moment-to-moment negotiations of everyday life. As recently demonstrated in epistemology, all acts of knowing—and, indeed, all sensation, feeling, and action—entail some form of judgment or valenced contrast (Guidano, 1987; Mahoney, 1985, in press; Weimer, in press, a, b; see also Elstein, this volume). The implicit difference between "clinical" and "nonclinical" judgment, then, lies primarily in there being very different connotations and expectations associated with the former. Clinical judgment invites special attention because it addresses the complex undertaking of one person attempting to understand ("know") and help another. Whether as psychometrician or counselor, the specialist will—for better and for worse—influence those whom he assesses and counsels. One would hope that the selection and training of such professionals would assure that their assessments and advice are qualitatively superior to that of their untrained peers. The data on this point are less than reassuring, however, and they suggest the need for a much closer scrutiny of human judgment, professional and otherwise (Bradley, 1981; Cohen, 1981; Einhorn & Hogarth, 1978; Faust, 1982, 1984, in press; Kahneman, Slovic, & Tversky, 1982; Kahneman & Tversky, 1973; Mahoney, 1976, 1977; Mahoney & DeMonbreun, 1977; Nisbett & Ross, 1980; Tversky & Kahneman, 1971, 1974; Weimer, 1979).

Through my own admittedly limited lenses of knowing, I see the cognitive and developmental (process/systems) sciences as offering many valuable models for the study of human judgment and knowing. Research on the limitations and processes of human knowing has already demonstrated the promise of these approaches. Rather than reiterate or extend some of these analyses of human knowing processes (clinical and otherwise), I will instead concentrate my remarks on the two major frameworks from which such processes have been conceptualized. Briefly, I will outline the difference between rationalistic and realistic metatheories of knowledge and what have come to be called "constructivistic" and developmental metatheories.

Revolution and Evolution in Cognitive Metatheories

While psychology and the social sciences were struggling with the merits and implications of the "cognitive revolution" in the 1970s (Dember, 1974; DeMey, 1982; Dennett, 1978, 1984; Fodor, 1981; Gardner, 1985; Mahoney, 1974; Palermo, 1971), substantial developments were already underway within the cognitive perspectives that these disciplines were endorsing. Despite agreement on the overall merits of acknowledging and studying human cognition, cognitive specialists have begun to diverge in their preferred conceptualizations of cognitive processes. Although it may be oversimplifying the matter, one way of viewing these divergences is in terms of their endorsement or rejection of traditional *realism* and *rationalism.*

Realism and Rationalism

The fundamental differences among current cognitive perspectives are focused on basic assumptions about (a) *ontology* (the nature of reality), (b) *epistemology* (theories of knowledge and knowing), and (c) *theories of causation.* In its most extreme and naive forms, *realism presumes a singular, stable, external reality that is accurately revealed by one's senses.* This assumption is both ontological and epistemological in nature because of its dual assertions about the nature of reality and the implicit role of sense data in coming to know such a reality.

Rationalism presumes that thought is superior to sense and most powerful in determining experience. One way of thinking about both realism and rationalism is to invoke the metaphor of edges or boundaries. Traditionally, realism has drawn a sharp boundary between that which is internal or external, changing or unchanging, and clear or ambiguous. As to processes in knowing, realism has endorsed a conservative "felt/sensed" epistemology. In the extreme, this has come to be called the doctrine of immaculate perception (Mahoney, 1974). Rationalism, for its part, also draws a boundary. In rationalism, the primary distinction is between thought and experience, mind and body. Implicit in traditional rationalism is the belief that thought is the most powerful domain of human activity. The idea that mental representation is more powerful than circumstances has appealed to practitioners and clients alike for many centuries.

Constructivism and Motor Metatheories

The most powerful challenges to realism and rationalism have emanated from both historical and contemporary sources. *Constructivisim asserts that humans actively create and construe their personal and social realities.* Contemporary proponents of constructivism question whether reality is fundamentally external and stable and whether human thought is meaningfully separable from human feeling and action (Guidano, 1984, 1987; Hayek, 1952, 1978, 1982; Joyce Moniz, 1985; Mahoney, 1985, in press; Mancuso & Adams-Webber, 1982; Neimeyer, 1985; Varela, 1979; Watzlawick, 1984; Weimer, 1977, 1982).

A fundamental aspect of modern constructivism has been its endorsement of what Weimer (1977) has termed *motor metatheories* of mind. These are theories that portray the human mind as proactive (as well as reactive) in nature. The important contrast here is between this active "inside-out" portrayal of cognition and the more passive "outside-in" perspective offered by *sensory metatheories.* The latter, which have until recently dominated information-processing approaches, portray the brain as a collector of information via the senses, and the information collected is presumed to reside in the external world:

> Common to these positions is an implicit notion that cognition is to be understood "from the outside inward," that it is a matter of the structuring of sensory information by intrinsically sensory systems, and that the products of cognition must somehow subsequently be married (in a peculiar sort of shotgun wedding) to action. (Weimer, 1977, p. 270)

Where sensory metatheories highlight the role of feedback mechanisms in learning and adaptation, motor metatheories emphatically add *feedforward mechanisms* that actively constrain and influence moment-to-moment experience patterns. For the constructivist, then, the hallowed distinction between input and output must be challenged:

> What the motor metatheory asserts is that there is no sharp separation between sensory and motor components of the nervous system which can be made on functional grounds and that the mental or cognitive realm is intrinsically motoric, like all the nervous system. The mind is intrinsically a motor system, and the sensory order by which we are acquainted with external objects as well as ourselves . . . is a product of what are, correctly interpreted, constructive motor skills. (Weimer, 1977, p. 272)

These challenging reconstructions have not been popular in some traditional quarters, to be sure, in that much of modern psychology remains fascinated with linear models of causality and simple, "technified" strategies of intervention (Mahoney, 1986a).

Starting with the questionable premise that human experience can be neatly divided into cognitive, behavioral, and affective components, contemporary psychological theories have offered models of causation that rank these components hierarchically (or sequentially). For the behaviorists, behavior is the prime mover in adjustment; for the cognitive psychologists, the first force is cognition. Likewise, affective theorists emphasize emotional processes as the primary crucibles for psychological development. Later in this chapter, I will demonstrate how adherence to these different perspectives will influence clinical practice.

The Developmental and Systems Movements

Constructivism and motor metatheories represented revolutions (or at least "evolutions") within the cognitive movement itself. It is important to note, however, that the generic cognitive revolution that has permeated late 20th-century psychology has not been the only trend of importance. Several thematic changes in our ways of conceptualizing human experience have emerged and accelerated over the last few decades. Most pertinent to the present discussion are what might be called the *developmental movement* and the *systems movement.* The former refers not only to the growth of interest in human psychological development across the lifespan, but also to the increasing interest in fundamental *processes* of change.

The systems movement has also become increasingly visible over the last few decades. Although its origins can be traced to general systems theory and other manifestations of the cognitive revolution (Gardner, 1985), it is also clear that both systems thinking and an emphasis on general processes pervade the overall study of complex phenomena (Bateson, 1972, 1979; Cook, 1980, Hayek, 1964, 1978; Land, 1973; Laszlo, 1983; Pattee, 1973; Weimer, 1982, in press,a,b). Conceptual emphasis has shifted away from reductionism and unilinear determinism and toward an acknowledgment of complex systems, reciprocal interdependence, and codevelopment over time.

Two illustrations of these trends are relevant to the present discussion. *Evolutionary epistemology* involves the study of knowing systems and their development over time. Although its historical origins are diverse, psychological interest in evolutionary epistemology is relatively recent (Campbell, 1974; 1975; Jantsch, 1980, 1981; Mahoney, in press; Reynolds, 1981). Along with increasing ratios of brain to body and neocortex to lower brain, our neurological and systemic evolution suggest punctuated "quantum leaps" in our development (Dobzhansky, 1962; Gould,

1977, 1980; Jerison, 1973, 1976; Land, 1973; Mahoney, in press; Passingham, 1982; Washburn & Moore, 1980; Wilson, 1980).

The heterarchical (quasi-horizontal) organization of the brain may help account for the "mystery" of *desynchrony* in human experience (Rachman, 1980), in which various measures of cognitive, behavioral, affective, and physiological change are minimally correlated. It also suggests significant possibilities for refining our understanding of such phenomena as *relapse, regression,* and *resistance* (Mahoney, 1985, in press; Marlatt & Gordon, 1985; Wachtel, 1982). Briefly stated, the human brain is not organized to afford "centralized (executive) control," but wisely reflects a "decentralized (coalitional) control" organization that forces subsystems and subprocesses to continuously compete for momentary "ascendancy." Earlier patterns of adaptation, for example, are never totally "eliminated" but can be potentially "overridden" by more viable patterns. During episodes of acute or chronic stress, fatigue, or disorder, older habitual patterns may again appear. Indeed, the earliest and most fundamental ordering processes in the nervous system appear to "resist" (protect against) too much or too rapid change, so that oscillations of progression and regression are not surprising and, as we will see, have important implications for the process of counseling (Mahoney, 1985, in press). Moreover, recent work in evolutionary epistemology dovetails nicely with constructivism and motor metatheories of cognition in emphasizing that *viability* is much more important than *validity* in mental representations of self and world.

Autopoiesis refers to self-development in complex, open systems. Nobel Prize winner Ilya Prigogine showed that the tendency of mass and energy to seek a totally balanced, static equilibrium is observed only in *closed* systems (e.g., the universe), but does not apply in *open, developing systems* (as in living organisms, nascent galaxies, etc.). As Prigogine and his colleagues have empirically and theoretically demonstrated (Prigogine, 1980; Prigogine & Stengers, 1984), self-organizing systems demonstrate a powerful *negentropic* (ordering) capacity that transforms their own basic structure when the system's dynamic equilibrium is sufficiently challenged by "perturbations" (a reformulation of Newton's Second Law of Thermodynamics). Disorder and disequilibrium are "natural" phenomena that play an integral role in a system's transformation toward a more viable, higher-order organization (Brent, 1978; Dell, 1982; Jantsch, 1980; 1981; Maturana, 1975; Maturana & Varela, 1980; Varela, 1979; Zeleny, 1980).

This principle of structural and functional transformation is called "*order through fluctuation*" and acknowledges the basic oscillatory nature of virtually all developmental processes (Mahoney, 1985, in press). In human systems, moment-to-moment experience is integrated and assimilated via first- and second-order cognitive processes (Bateson, 1972, 1979). First-order processes involve the *assimilation* of current experience into existing structures that constrain the nature and range of phenomenological content (Piaget, 1970, 1981). *Accommodation,* which reflects a proactive change in knowing structures (also known as *schemas,* or *schemata;* see chapter by Turk, Salovey, and Prentice, and appendix, this volume), occurs when extant assimilative structures are unable to resolve and equilibrate current environmental perturbations. When an experience does not "fit" with expectations and memory structures, the latter must be modified or vindicated. Regressive development involves an entrenchment in prior knowing structures, while progressive development involves a transformational shift to higher-order contexts or *metacognition* (Flavell, 1979; Guidano & Liotti, 1983; Lakatos, 1970; Mahoney, 1985).

Social Learning and Attachment Theories

Albert Bandura's social learning theory represents another trend in conceptualizing and facilitating human psychological development. According to many observers, it was Bandura's (1969) book *Principles of Behavior Modification* that inspired an accelerating trend toward studying central (versus peripheral) processes in human adjustment (Mahoney & Arnkoff, 1978). His emphases on *vicarious learning processes, self-regulation, cognitive representation,* and *causal reciprocity* helped inaugurate the cognitive revolutions in both behavior therapy and psychology at large. Likewise, his theory of *self-efficacy* has emphasized the central importance of beliefs about personal ability and the complexity of causal influences in human performance (Bandura, 1977).

The interdependence of social relationships and personal belief–behavior systems has also been emphasized by John Bowlby (1969, 1973, 1979, 1980, 1985). Bowlby's *attachment theory* asserts that personal meaning systems are generated, maintained, and transformed in the context of emotional attachments. The most formative of attachment relationships, according to Bowlby, are those that develop (or fail to develop) in early life, although emotional attachments and detachments continue to influence and reflect well-being throughout the lifespan. Bowlby's work and the developmental sciences in general have come to play an increasingly visible role in recent cognitive theories and therapies (Guidano, 1984, 1987; Guidano & Liotti, 1983, 1985; Mahoney, 1980, 1981, in press). In fact, developmental and constructivist issues form the primary dimensions that appear to differentiate the "old" and "new" looks in cognitive psychotherapies (Mahoney, in press).

The Cognitive Sciences and Clinical Judgment

The emergent themes reviewed in the last section—constructivism, motor metatheories, developmental and systems approaches, and the social contexts of self—reflect what may well be the first major differentiation within the cognitive revolution. Strictly rationalist theorists—personified by Albert Ellis and orthodox rational–emotive therapy—argue for the causal supremacy of *beliefs* about self and world. Counselors who have adopted a rationalist metatheory of helping tend to emphasize "reality contact," "realistic thinking," and "rationality" as the preferred paths toward individual psychological development. For the extreme rationalist, disorder and irrationality are synonymous. The developmentalists and constructivists, on the other hand, challenge traditional concepts of reality, knowing, and rationality, as well as of disorder, disease, and development (Guidano, 1984, 1987; Hayek, 1952, 1982; Joyce Moniz, 1985; Mahoney, in press; Watzlawick, 1984; Weimer, 1977, 1979, 1982).

Philosophical Differences

In brief, the major distinctions between rationalist and developmental perspectives can be highlighted as follows (see Table 8–1). *Ontologically,* modern rationalists tend to be realists. They believe (a) in a singular, stable, and external reality whose understanding constitutes (b) the primary task and capacity of the "higher" mental processes. The developmentalists, by way of contrast, endorse relativistic and multiple approaches to reality. In their opinion, reality is not singular, stable, or neatly external. It is, instead, complex, dynamic, and both individual and collective. Rationalists tend to portray the brain as a curator of information gleaned from sense data that reliably reflect an external order. Developmentalists and constructivists, on the other hand, tend to portray the brain as an active sculptor of experience, proactively "projecting" its "expectations" onto each next milli-moment of development.

Epistemologically, rationalists defend a curious marriage of sense data and quasi-pure intellect. For the rabid rationalist, knowledge and knowing are sure categories. Knowledge is authorized or justified by various information sources: sense experience, empirical data, logic, science, expert authority, revelation, etc. Inferences and judgments are deemed rational (and therefore right) when they conform to current standards for *epistemic warrant* (Weimer, 1979).

For the developmentalists, however, *knowing is a complex process that involves active explorations toward ordering (understanding) and controlling valenced experiences.* Knowledge is physical (behavioral), emotional, and

TABLE 8–1
Philosophical Differences Between Rationalist and Developmental Cognitive Theories

Issue/Area	*Rationalist View*	*Developmental View*
1. *Ontology* (the nature of reality)	*Realism*—reality is singular, stable, and external.	*Relativism*—realities are individual and collective constructions of order in experience.
2. *Epistemology* (theories of knowing)	*Rationalism*—knowledge is authorized as valid by logic or reason; reality is revealed via the senses.	*Constructivism*—knowing is behavioral and emotional as well as cognitive; the validity of knowledge is less important than its viability; sensation is proactive.
3. *Theories of causation*	*Associationism*—learning and change are linear chains of discrete causes and effects.	*Structural differentiation*—learning and development involve refinements and transformations of mental representations.

representational. Knowing and learning do not entail absolute levels of objectivity and certainty. Put in other terms, we do not survive and develop because our mental representations of self–world relationships are progressively more valid, but because they are more viable. The difference is of enormous epistemic importance. Validity presumes that knowledge is correct, true, accurate, and enduring. Thus, a genuinely "valid" finding or phenomenon is considered "real." The foundational concept in ontological validity is *correspondence;* rationalists and realists tend to presume a potentially perfect (absolute) correspondence between mental representations and the "external" world. "Reality contact" and "rational living" are portrayed as essential themes of personal development (Weimer, 1979).

The constructivists and developmentalists, however, challenge these notions and propose that individual processes must first be viable (in the literal evolutionary sense) if the individual is to survive. *Viability,* when applied to knowing processes, refers to such qualities as flexibility, generativity, complexity, and resilience. As cross-cultural and anthropological research have shown, technically inaccurate beliefs may still afford adaptive behavior patterns, and generously warranted beliefs may nevertheless engender maladaptive consequences. From developmental and constructivistic perspectives, all knowledge and knowing are inherently participatory (Varela, 1979).

Not surprisingly, these differences between the perspectives are reflected in their epistemological preferences. With some exceptions, rationalists and realists in psychology tend to be *logical positivists, operationists,* and *justificationists.* The constructivists and developmentalists, however, are more often *"critical rationalists," "ethno-phenomenologists,"* and vocal *nonjustificationists* (Laudan, 1977; Mahoney, 1976; Weimer, 1979). These differences are spelled out more extensively elsewhere, and their assumptions and differential implications are worthy of reflection. For the moment, it is important to note only that orthodox rationalists believe in authorized (guaranteed) knowledge and a stable reality that it can approximate. The constructive developmentalists, on the other hand, believe that all knowing organisms are embodied, self-developing "theories" of relationships. Acting, feeling, and knowing are inseparable expressions of adaptation and development. From this perspective, "knowing" (scientific and otherwise) is seldom technically logical, but always pervasively psychological.

At the level of *causal analysis,* the fundamental difference between traditional realists-rationalists and constructive developmentalists has to do with mechanisms of change and causal processes. Traditionally, realists and rationalists have leaned heavily toward *associationism* and *functionalism.* From these perspectives, learning involves the contiguous or contingent chaining of discrete events in the fashion first described by Aristotle. Such learning by association is said to apply not only at the stimulus–response (input–output) realm but also between specific nerves and synapses within the nervous system. Constructive developmentalists are quick to point out, however, that associationism and what is called "billiard-ball determinism" have recently been shown to be critically flawed at both conceptual and empirical levels (Bandura, 1969; Bever, Fodor, & Garrett, 1968; Brewer, 1974; Dulany, 1968; Mahoney, 1984a). In place of associationism and conditioning as the primary mechanisms of change, constructive developmentalists invoke the *structural differentiation* proposed by the likes of Hayek (1952), Piaget (1970), Werner (1948), and Wundt (1912). From this cosmological perspective, learning and change involve structural transformations in knowing. The latter entail the differentiation of previous mental representations toward more complex, higher order cognitive classifications and organizations.

Before addressing some of the theoretical differences that reflect on these philosophical issues, two technicalities merit mention. First, constructive developmental perspectives are not "irrational," "antirational," or "arational" in nature. Such dichotomous thinking is unfortunately less rare than one might hope. Constructivism is admittedly "radical" in its assertions:

> Radical constructivism, thus, is *radical* because it breaks with convention and develops a theory of knowledge in which knowledge does not reflect an "objective" ontological reality, but exclusively an ordering and organization of a world constituted by our experience. The radical constructivist has relinquished "metaphysical realism" once and for all and finds himself in full agreement with Piaget, who says, "Intelligence organizes the world by organizing itself." (von Glaserfeld, 1984, p. 24)

But what is radical about constructivism is not a rejection of rationalism so much as a transformation of what it may mean to be and act rationally (Weimer, in press,a,b). The tradition of rationalism and its valuation of knowledge has never been so widely adopted. What is at issue is the meanings and processes associated with the kinds of knowing we consider adaptive, viable, and valuable.

The second technicality has to do with different uses of the term "constructivism." Throughout this chapter, I have been using constructivism in what might be called the psychological sense to denote perspectives that portray the mind as active, interactive, and representationally generative. This is essentially the same usage employed by other psychological constructivists (Guidano, 1984, 1987; Joyce Moniz, 1985; Kelly, 1955; Neimeyer, 1985; von Glaserfeld, 1984; Watzlawick, 1984).

There is another, very different meaning associated with constructivism, however. In what might be called the "philosophical sense," constructivism refers to rationalistic interventionism. In this sense, it refers to rationalized attempts to impose order and control in complex, open systems. Hayek (1952, 1978) and Weimer (1977, 1982, in press,a,b)—who are psychological constructivists—are opposed to philosophical constructivism. Their argument, with which I concur (Mahoney, in press), is that regulatory interventions in complex, open systems tend to produce many unexpected and far-ranging results that are generally less viable than those emerging out of the natural "catallaxy" (open exchange dynamics). The practical implications of their view highlight the warrant for caution in systemic interventions and the wisdom of respecting individual differences and freedom in development.

Theoretical Differences

When there are basic philosophical differences, there will necessarily be differences in theoretical conceptualization. This is clearly the case with the rationalist–developmental distinction here emphasized. As is briefly outlined in Table 8–2, some very fundamental theoretical differences

Table 8–2
Theoretical Differences Between Rationalist and Developmental Cognitive Theories

Concept/Issue	*Rationalist View*	*Developmental View*
1. Basic functions of human nervous system	To *control* and direct action and feeling via *valid mental representations.*	To *order* and organize experience via *viable mental representations.*
2. Nature of representation	Representations are accurate *copies* that *correspond* to the "real" world.	Representations are predominantly *tacit constructions* of order that *constrain* but do not specify plans of action.
3. Body–brain relationship	*Cerebral primacy:* the brain leads and the body follows.	*Somatopsychic unity:* body and brain are inseparable and interdependent.
4. Cognition–behavior–affect relationship	*Rational supremacy:* "higher" intellectual processes can and should direct feelings and actions.	*Holism:* thought, feeling, and action are structurally and functionally inseparable.
5. Nature of emotionality	*Emotions as problems:* negative and intense affect is to be controlled or eliminated.	*Emotions as primitive, powerful knowing processes:* disorder and affective intensity are natural elements of development.

help identify these two metatheories. To begin with, their views on the *basic functions of the nervous system* diverge considerably. Rationalists tend to view the brain and nervous system as recipients and repositories of information imparted logically and sensorially. A healthy and functional nervous system is one that renders accurate (valid) mental representations of reality, and—of equal importance—translates those representations into effective controls on action and feeling. For the developmentalists, however, the primary task and talent of the nervous system is the idiosyncratic construction of ordered experience. From this perspective, mental representations are not to be judged by their validity (which is technically unknowable) or their power to control, but by their capacity to afford adaptation and development.

The two perspectives also view representation quite differently.

Orthodox rationalists tend to view *cognitive representation* in terms of correspondence and storage. "Good" representations are those that involve accurate, explicit, and extensive "copies" of the external world. These copies are said to be encoded and stored in memory for access when expedient. In some early expressions of cognitive psychology, the copies were compared to "templates" that afforded a higher order "match-to-sample" classification (Neisser, 1967, 1976). Constructive developmentalists, by way of contrast, reject the idea of such explicit models or templates in the mind and suggest instead that abstract or tacit *schemata,* or schemas, are the norm in cognitive representation (cf. Goldfried & Robins, 1983). Constructivism suggests that these schemata are not explicit "blueprints" for action that reflect valid estimations of reality. Rather, they are tacit scaffoldings for experience that constrain but do not specify particulars (Hayek, 1978; Mahoney, in press).

The theoretical differences that may be most central to the distinction in question have to do with *body–brain relationships* and the *relationships among thought, feeling, and action.* Rationalists tend to believe in cerebral primacy and rational supremacy. *Cerebral primacy* refers to the belief that the brain is the primary or leading edge in human development. This is such a pervasive assumption in Western science that it is seldom acknowledged and appraised. A recent discovery in evolutionary anthropology illustrates the point. Until very recently, the dominant view in evolutionary theory was that encephalization preceded bipedalism (Gould, 1977, 1980). The sudden evolutionary leap among primates from quadruped to biped—with its transformational consequences for manual differentiation and brain structure—was thought to have been caused by a sudden increase in brain size. With the recent discovery of a small-brained *Homo erectus* ("Lucy"), however, it became clear that brain development did not precede body development (Mahoney, in press). The two were (and are) inseparable. Somewhere in that realization lies a simultaneous acknowledgement of the brain sciences *and* the integral role of behavior in neural development.

Rational supremacy refers to what may well be the cardinal assumption in classical rationalism—namely, that the "higher" intellectual processes should dominate functionally over the more primitive dimensions of action and feeling. This is the essence of the stoic philosophies of Epictetus and Marcus Aurelius that begot the "positive thinking," "mind cure," and "rational" therapies of the late 19th and 20th centuries. "As you think, so shall you act and feel" is their explicit motto, and their message is clear. In this sense, it is the rationalistic cognitivists who occupy the cognitive apex of a thought-feeling-action triangle. The developmentalists, on the other hand, head for the center of the triangle and propose that these three categories—thought, feeling, and action—are a conceptual legacy with questionable partitions. Modern anatomical, physiological, and functional analyses suggest that traditional distinctions between sensory and motor processes, for example, are untenable, and that the quest for a "prime mover" in the triumvirate is misplaced (Mahoney, 1984b, in press; Weimer, 1977). From a developmental perspective, cognition, behavior, and affect represent interdependent expressions of holistic and systemic processes. To the extent that their conceptual differentiation is useful, they are each very important aspects of an individual's attempts to adapt and develop.

The *nature of emotionality* is the last issue on which I will comment here. In essence, rationalists have traditionally viewed emotions as epiphenomena and/or problems. Negative and intense emotions have been particularly denigrated, with the practical corollary that they should be controlled or eliminated. The evolution of our current concepts of feeling could easily consume a few volumes, and this would not include the history of attempts to control our own feelings. The abridged conclusion of such a survey would, I believe, suggest that we are now in the throes of an intensive evolutionary struggle involving the conflict between head and heart. Intense and chronic negative affects are common among seekers of psychological services. Emotional disorders and psychopathology are veritable synonyms in modern psychology. For a variety of reasons, intensely negative emotions have come to be defined as psychological problems. From the rationalist perspective, all intense emotions (regardless of valence) have a disorganizing effect on behavior.

Developmentalists generally acknowledge this disorganizing effect, but they hasten to add that disorganization represents a developmental phase that precedes reorganization. From a developmental perspective, feelings are primitive and powerful knowing processes that underly their neocortical offspring (MacLean, 1973; Mahoney, in press). They represent an evolutionary leap subsequent to reptilian reflexivity and prior to higher primate reflection. Buoyed by recent work in chemistry, physics, and biology on the role of disorder and disequilibrium in systems development, several developmental theorists have begun to suggest a more positive and progressive conceptualization of affective intensity (Brent, 1978, 1984; Dell, 1982; Guidano, 1987; Mahoney, in press). In these renditions, emotional intensity reflects a significant deviation from affective equilibrium, often (though not always) associated with an identifiable stressor. When current coping skills are inadequate to resolve this disequilibrium, the individual (as a system of systems) becomes distressed, disorganized, and—in medical models—"dis-eased." Oscillations (waves) of order and disorder ensue, and emotional intensity may increase. In *regressive* development, this pattern of disorder continues indefinitely due to the individual's inability to break out of self-perpetuating cycles. In *progressive* development, however, the disorder and disequilibrium intensify and higher order knowing structures emerge. These cognitive transformations allow a dynamic equilibrium to be reestablished and maintained until they, in turn, meet demands that initiate another phase of disorder.

Practical Differences

Needless to say, these philosophical and theoretical differences beget still further differences in professional practice. The most salient of these are outlined in Table 8–3. When it comes down to *intervention emphases,* for example, rationalists tend to focus on current problems and their control while developmentalists focus on developmental history and current developmental processes. Likewise, there are important differences in the tacit and explicit goals of the two forms of therapy. Rationalists tend to be teleological, deriving the "direction" of preferred development and its facilitation from the designation of explicit short- and long-term goals (which usually involve the control or elimination of current "symptomatology"). Developmentalists, on the other hand, tend to emphasize "teleonomic" direction (literally, direction without a goal), which acknowledges and affirms the fundamental wisdom of self-organizing processes in systems development.

In the *conceptualization of problems,* rationalists are likely to equate problems with negative affect and symptoms, both of which reflect psychological deficits or dysfunctions that need to be redressed, regulated, or eradicated. This view can be contrasted with the developmental rendition of problems as discrepancies between demands on the organism and current adaptive capacities. From a developmental perspective, problems are expressions of disorder. Acute episodes of disorder reflect sudden and/or substantial shifts in ambient demands, while chronic disorders represent habitually ineffective (but self-perpetuating) cycles of crisis. When conceptualized in this way, problems become powerful opportunities for learning and current contents (instances) of higher order patterns and processes (Mahoney, in press).

Among rationalists, the most common conceptualization of affect portrays intense and negative emotions as expressions of irrational and unrealistic beliefs. "As you think, so shall you feel" is the foundational assumption. Unpleasant affect (dysphoria, or distress) is conceptualized as the result of "*wrong* thinking," and the latter is equated with invalid, distorted, and "unrealistic" thinking. This approach can be differentiated from the developmental view, which conceptualizes affect as a primitive and powerful form of knowing (Guidano, 1987; Mahoney, in press). Feelings somehow integrate past, present, and anticipated expe-

TABLE 8–3
Practical Differences Between Rationalist and Developmental Cognitive Therapies

Issue/Theme	*Rationalist View*	*Developmental View*
1. Intervention emphases	a. Ahistorical b. Problem-focused c. Control-focused d. Teleological	a. Historical b. Process-focused c. Development-focused d. Teleonomic
2. Conceptualization of problems	Problems are deficits, dysfunctions, or their emotional correlates; they should be redressed, controlled, or eliminated.	Problems are current and recurrent discrepancies between challenges and capacities; they reflect limits in current capacities and should not be mistaken for their abstract ordering processes.
3. Conceptualization of affect	Affect, especially intense and negative, *is* the problem; irrational and unrealistic cognitions are its cause.	Affect expresses a primitive and powerful form of knowing; emotional experience, expression, and exploration should be encouraged.
4. Resistance	Resistance reflects (a) lack of motivation, (b) ambivalence, or (c) motivated avoidance. Resistance is an impediment to therapeutic change and must be "overcome."	Resistance reflects natural self-protective processes that guard systemic integrity and resist rapid or substantial "core" change. Resistance should be worked *with* rather than *against.*
5. Insight	Insight into irrational and unrealistic beliefs is necessary and (almost) sufficient for therapeutic change.	Insight may help to transform personal meanings and scaffold change, but emotional and behavioral enactments are also very important.
6. Therapeutic relationship	The therapeutic relationship entails technical instruction and guidance.	The therapeutic relationship entails a safe, caring, and intense context in and from which the client can explore and develop relationships with self and world.
7. Relapse and regression	These phenomena reflect failures in maintenance and generalization that should be avoided and minimized.	These phenomena reflect limits in current capacity and/or cycles (or spirals) in psychological development; they involve important opportunities for learning.

riences, and—much more consistently than their neocortical counterparts—they covary with pituitary, endocrine, and lymphatic activities. It is not surprising, therefore, that developmental cognitive therapists tend to encourage emotional experience, expression, and exploration.

Practical approaches to *resistance* constitute yet another difference between these two metatheories. For orthodox rationalists, resistance represents motivational deficit, ambivalence, or avoidance. As such, it is the antithesis of change and should be minimized or avoided wherever possible and "overcome" when necessary. Simply put, resistance is either laziness or irrational fear (Ellis, 1985; Wachtel, 1982). From a developmental perspective, however, resistance reflects natural and healthy self-protective processes that guard against changing too much, too quickly. In this view, resistance to core structural change is fundamentally adaptive and should therefore be worked "with" rather than "against" (Bugental & Bugental, 1984; Mahoney, in press). Reluctance to change (and its complementarity—reluctance to stop changing) reflects order- and integrity-protecting processes of a fundamental nature. Respect for these processes is more likely to facilitate progressive psychological development than denial or attempted domination of them.

Insight represents a complex topic in human change processes. On some levels, it is clear that beliefs and "awareness" may facilitate or impede learning and performance (Bandura, 1969; Brewer, 1974; Mahoney, 1974; Spielberger & DeNike, 1966). The primary goal of the "insight therapies" is to produce awareness, with the assumption that insight can dramatically accelerate or improve adaptive changes. In classical psychoanalysis, insight was fostered by explicitly instructing the client to attend to their thoughts, dreams, feelings, and behaviors. This same basic prescription is used in rational–emotive therapy and cognitive–behavior therapy. A major difference, however, is that these rationalist cognitive approaches encourage the client to translate their self-talk and behavior into action and to actively "restructure" them.

Developmentalists also tend to encourage self-exploration and insight, and they employ experiential exercises to help integrate the relevant cognitive, behavioral, and affective processes. From a developmental perspective, however, insight is a subtype of a family of processes that might be called *metacognitive* (Flavell, 1979; Guidano, 1987; Mahoney, 1985, in press). In the holistic interpretation of metacognition, it is a higher order level of knowing that appears to involve perceptual, conceptual, and experiential components. In essence, metacognition refers to knowing about knowing, but there are many fascinating subtleties to its import. For example, developmentalists do not view "awareness" and "consciousness" in the same manner, and they caution against attributing too much power to explicit awareness. There are times when attention to and awareness of one's self may actually interfere with performance (Borkovec & O'Brien, 1977; Hayek, 1978; Jerome, 1980; Nideffer, 1976; Polanyi, 1958, 1966).

Rationalist and developmental approaches also differ in their conceptualizations of the therapeutic relationship. For the former, a professional helping relationship is one that entails the service, that is, the delivery, of technical instruction and guidance. What is imparted in effective rational therapy is knowledge and information, along with skills in their use. When such knowledge and information can be imparted via audiovisual and mechanical means, the relative unimportance of the human relationship in counseling becomes apparent (see Singer, this volume).

Developmental therapies view the helping relationship as a critically important and unique social exchange which, when it "works," helps to establish a safe and supportive context. It is in and from this context that the client can explore and develop relationships with self and world (Bowlby, 1973; Guidano, 1987; Guidano & Liotti, 1983, 1985; Mahoney, in press). This view is consistent with humanistic approaches in this (and several other) regards, and it herein aligns itself with psychoanalytic and neo-analytic thought on the therapeutic relationship (and its ongoing processes). For Freud and many others, intense emotional relationships constitute the crucibles in which psychological patterns are forged and altered. Whether it is one's relationship with a parent, sibling, friend, lover, therapist, or child, such emotionally charged attachments bear powerfully on one's experience and development. There are differences, to be sure, in how developmental and psychoanalytic writers have portrayed and pursued the helping relationship, but their mutual endorsement of its importance is worth noting.

Finally, there are differences between rationalist and developmental approaches to relapse, recidivism, and regression. For the classical rationalist, these phenomena reflect failures in generalization and maintenance, which, in turn, suggest insufficient or inconsistent use of the knowledge and information imparted during therapy. A psychological "setback" signifies a probable deficit in the client's motivation or learning. Hence, such setbacks or relapses should be avoided if at all possible. From the developmental view, setbacks and the recurrence of prior (and less viable) psychological patterns are natural and virtually inevitable aspects of psychological development (Mahoney, in press; Marlatt & Gordon, 1985). Thus viewed, such phenomena represent nonlinear regressions and cycles in epistemic differentiation. A temporary relapse or regression to lower levels of functioning may reflect a quasi-catabolic process whose significance can be appreciated only when viewed in relation to its anabolic counterparts (e.g., "leaps forward"). Among other interesting implications, the developmental view of relapse and regression suggests very different emphases in counseling.

Concluding Remarks

This chapter began with a brief acknowledgment of the complexities involved in clinical judgment. The most important decisions in psychological counseling, in my opinion, are not those confined to traditional assessments and diagnostic classification. Although these activities cannot be separated from the overall endeavor of professional psychological services, they play a less formative role in actual psychotherapy than many other tacit judgments about human nature, the nature of change, and principles of effective helping. These tacit judgments, in turn, reflect basic assumptions about ontology (the nature of reality), epistemology (the nature of knowing), and the nature of causation and change.

The bulk of this chapter has focused on philosophical, theoretical, and practical differences between the two major approaches to human knowing, learning, and psychological development. I have characterized realism as a tradition that presumes a singular, stable, and external order. In classical empiricism, this reality is reliably and validly revealed via sense data. Rationalism additionally asserts that thought is superior to the senses and that the human mind transforms sensory messages into accurate mental models that correspond to the real world. Constructivism proposes, on the other hand, that humans actively create order in their experience and literally construct the realities to which they react. Adding developmental and systems perspectives, constructivism endorses a process-oriented, epigenetic model of psychological differentiation.

From all of this it is hopefully apparent that the cognitive, systems, and developmental sciences have much to offer the field of clinical judgment. Moreover, the metatheories that differentiate approaches within these sciences have significantly different implications for conceptualizing clinical judgment processes. Cognitive perspectives that reflect a realist–rationalist tradition, for example, may be more likely to emphasize a single, stable diagnosis and an approach to therapy that focuses on reality contact and what the counselor and culture consider rational adaptation. Ahistorical and nondevelopmental approaches may likewise focus on current environmental circumstances and contingencies rather than on longstanding and early-established patterns of experiencing self and world. Perspectives that presume relatively simple causal mechanisms are less likely to look at multiplicity, complexity, and reciprocity among causal influences, and they may also tend to "locate" problems predominantly "in" clients rather than examining the system of systems that may be involved (including families, friends, co-workers, and local and planetary society).

I have elsewhere argued that constructivism and the developmental and systems approaches present formidable challenges to many traditional views in psychology (Mahoney, 1986b). From the presentation in this chapter it should also be apparent that I consider these perspectives much more viable and promising than their current alternatives. I believe that constructivist approaches to assessment, for example, are more valuable than realist or rationalist assessments. To date, constructivist assessment has been dominated by Kelly's personal construct theory and has yielded some fascinating portrayals of human psychological organization (Mancuso & Adams-Webber, 1982; Neimeyer, 1985). One of the major differences between constructivist and rationalist assessment, as I see it, has to do with how assessment is approached and how an individual's responses are interpreted. In the rationalist tradition, clients are asked standardized questions for which the responses are usually constrained (by multiple choices, degrees of agreement, etc.). A client's responses are then compared to actuarial norms for "identified" populations, and the client is classified according to his correspondence with such norms. In a constructivist assessment—perhaps best illustrated by Kelly's (1955) "rep grid" approach—the client's responses are generally less constrained and the client (rather than the therapist or test expert) generates the constructs most expressive of his or her psychological make-up. Besides attending to the contents and constructs invoked by a client, the constructivist as psychometrician is also more likely to attend to the processes and judgments inherent in the client's responses. Theoretically at least, such an approach should lead to the therapist having a better sense of the client's private "assumptive world," expressed in terms and concepts emanating from that world.

The clinical judgments that pervade ongoing counseling, referrals, and terminations are also influenced by the metatheories that the therapist consciously or unconsciously endorses. A case example may help illustrate this point. At a recent conference, I was a member of a panel of clinicians who were asked to outline a treatment plan for a young woman who had sought therapy for depression and loneliness. She was 26 years old, unemployed, and had been living with her parents since dropping out of college after one semester. She complained about not having friends and was particularly interested in meeting a "boy" and "falling in love." She was an only child and reported a history of shyness and apparent parental overprotection from an early age.

One panel member who identified himself as "an orthodox behavior therapist" recommended that the young woman be given social skills training and guided through a desensitization hierarchy directed at dating and sexual intimacy. Another "psychodynamic" therapist said that she felt the client had not resolved some issues concerning sexual maturity, and that treatment should focus on her unresolved conflicts about leaving home and particularly on her relations with her father. I found myself in more agreement with the psychodynamic therapist than the behaviorist, although my emphases and concerns were focused differently. Given that the client's developmental history reflected a paucity of friendships, no siblings, and no prior romances, I felt that social skills training and a hierarchy aimed at sexual intimacy were premature. The family dynamics and the client's apparently anxious attachment to her parents were also of concern to me. I, too, recommended intensive therapy but with an emphasis on encouraging the client to explore her beliefs, feelings, and daily behaviors regarding her relationship with herself, with her parents, and with the world at large. Teaching the young woman socialization skills and encouraging her to explore the world outside her home could be introduced as later elements in counseling, I thought, but they should be preceded by first establishing therapy as a safe and caring context from which to operate and by more thoroughly addressing her expectations about relationships and intimacy. The ultimate question regarding our differing clinical appraisals, however, is not which of our conjectural analyses was "right" (valid) but which was more likely to be viable and helpful for the client.

Although I have only been able to touch upon highlights in my discussion of trends and differentiating issues, my remarks have hopefully offered some scaffoldings for understanding traditional and more recent expressions of the growing interface between cognitive and clinical sciences. More extensive commentaries and a presentation of a cognitive developmental approach are offered elsewhere (Mahoney, in press). It will be interesting to review these traditions and trends after the cognitive movement has undergone another decade of development and differentiation.

I shall, therefore, close with a reiteration of my fundamental sense that the cognitive and developmental sciences have much to offer the psychological theorist and therapist. Whether rationalist or constructivist in flavor, those perspectives that acknowledge and explore the complexities of human experience—and particularly the "inner," private, and personal aspects of that experience—clearly promise a more adequate understanding than those that deny or denigrate these dimensions. The cognitive revolution and its sequelae constitute major phenomena in late 20th-century psychology (DeMey, 1982; Fodor, 1981; Gardner, 1985). The importance of their direction should not be lost in our reflections on their differentiations.

References

Arkes, H. E. (1981). Impediments to accurate clinical judgment and possible ways to minimize their impact. *Journal of Consulting and Clinical Psychology, 49,* 323–330.

Arkowitz, H., & Messer. H. (Eds.) (1984). *Psychoanalytic and behavior therapy: Is integration possible?* New York: Plenum.

Bandura, A. (1969). *Principles of behavior modification.* New York: Holt, Rinehart & Winston.

———. (1976). Social learning perpsectives on behavior change. In A. Burton (Ed.), *What makes behavior change possible?* New York: Brunner/Mazel.

———. (1977). Self-efficacy: Toward a unifying theory of behavioral change. *Psychological Review, 94,* 191–215.

———. (1978). The self-system in reciprocal determinism. *American Psychologist, 33,* 344–358.

———. (1985). Model of causality in social learning theory. In M. J. Mahoney & A. Freeman (Eds.), *Cognition and psychotherapy.* New York: Plenum.

———. (1986). *Social foundations of thought and action: A social cognitive theory.* Englewood Cliffs, NJ: Prentice-Hall.

Bateson, G. (1972). *Steps to an ecology of mind.* New York: Ballantine.

———. (1979). *Mind and nature: A necessary unity.* New York: Bantam.

Bever, T. G., Fodor, J. A., & Garrett, M. (1968). A formal limit of associationism. In T. R. Dixon & D. L. Horton (Eds.), *Verbal behavior and general behavior theory.* Englewood Cliffs, NJ: Prentice-Hall.

Borkovec, T. D., & O'Brien, G. T. (1977). Relation of autonomic perception and its manipulation to the maintenance and reduction of fear. *Journal of Abnormal Psychology, 86,* 163–171.

Bowlby, J. (1969). *Attachment and loss.* Vol. I: *Attachment.* New York: Basic Books.

———. (1973). *Attachment and loss.* Vol. II: *Separation: Anxiety and anger.* New York: Basic Books.

———. (1979). *The making and breaking of affectional bonds.* London: Tavistock.

———. (1980). *Attachment and loss.* Vol. III: *Loss: Sadness and depression.* London: Hogarth Press.

———. (1985). The role of childhood experience in cognitive disturbance. In M. J. Mahoney & A. Freeman (Eds.), *Cognition and psychotherapy.* New York: Plenum.

Bradley, J. V. (1981). Overconfidence in ignorant experts. *Bulletin of the Psychonomic Society, 17,* 82–84.

Brent, S. B. (1978). Prigogine's model for self-organization in nonequilibrium systems: Its relevance for developmental psychology. *Human Development, 21,* 374–387.

Brewer, W. F. (1974). There is no convincing evidence for operant or classical conditioning in adult humans. In W. B. Weimer & D. S. Palermo (Eds.), *Cognition and the symbolic processes* (Vol. 1). Hillsdale, NJ: Erlbaum.

Bugental, J. F. T., & Bugental, E. K. (1984). A fate worse than death: The fear of changing. *Psychotherapy, 21,* 543–549.

Campbell, D. T. (1974). Evolutionary epistemology. In P. A. Schlipp (Ed.), *The philosophy of Karl Popper,* Vol. 14, I & II. LaSalle, IL: Open Court Publishing.

———. (1975). On the conflicts between biological and social evolution and between psychology and moral tradition. *American Psychologist, 30,* 1103–1126.

Chapman, L. J., & Chapman, J. P. (1967). Genesis of popular but erroneous psychodiagnostic observations. *Journal of Abnormal Psychology, 72,* 193–204.

______. (1969). Illusory correlation as an obstacle to the use of valid psychodiagnostic signs. *Journal of Abnormal Psychology, 74,* 271–280.

Cohen, L. J. (1981). Can human irrationality be experimentally demonstrated? *The Behavioral and Brain Sciences, 4,* 317–331.

Cook, N. D. (1980). *Stability and flexibility: An analysis of natural systems.* New York: Pergamon.

Dell, P.F. (1982). Beyond homeostasis: Toward a concept of coherence. *Family Process, 21,* 21–41.

Dember, W. N. (1974). Motivation and the cognitive revolution. *American Psychologist, 29,* 161–168.

DeMey, M. (1982). *The cognitive paradigm.* Boston: D. Reidel.

Dennett, D. C. (1978). *Brainstorms: Philosophical essays on mind and psychology.* Cambridge, MA: MIT Press.

______. (1984). *Elbow room: The varieties of free will worth wanting.* Cambridge, MA: MIT Press.

Dobzhansky, T. (1962). *Mankind evolving: The evolution of the human species.* New Haven: Yale University Press.

Dulany, D. E. (1968). Awareness, rules, and propositional control: A confrontation with S-R behavior theory. In T. R. Dixon & D. L. Horton (Eds.), *Verbal behavior and general behavior therapy.* Englewood Cliffs, NJ: Prentice-Hall.

Einhorn, H. J., & Hogarth, R. M. (1978). Confidence in judgment: Persistence of the illusion of validity. *Psychological Review, 85,* 395–416.

Ellis, A. (1985). *Overcoming resistance: Rational-emotive therapy with difficult clients.* New York: Springer.

Faust, D. (1982). A needed component in prescriptions for science: Empirical knowledge of human cognitive limitations. *Knowledge, 3,* 555–570.

______. (1984). *The limits of scientific judgment.* Minneapolis: University of Minnesota Press.

______. (in press). Research on human judgment and its meaning for clinical practice and research. *Professional Psychology.*

Flavell, J. H. (1979). Metacognition and cognitive monitoring: A new area of cognitive-developmental inquiry. *American Psychologist, 34,* 906–911.

Fodor, J. A. (1981). *Representations: Philosophical essays on the foundations of cognitive science.* Cambridge, MA: MIT Press.

Gardner, H. (1985). *The mind's new science: A history of the cognitive revolution.* New York: Basic Books.

Goldberg, L. R. (1968). Simple models or simple processes? Some research on clinical judgments. *American Psychologist, 23,* 25–33.

Goldfried, M. R. (Ed.) (1982). *Converging themes in psychotherapy.* New York: Springer.

Goldfried, M. R., & Robins, C. (1983). Self-schemas, cognitive bias, and the processing of learning experiences. In P. C. Kendall (Ed.), *Advances in cognitive-behavioral research and therapy* (Vol. 2). New York: Academic Press.

Gould, S. J. (1977). *Ever since Darwin: Reflections in natural history.* New York: Norton.

______. (1980). *The panda's thumb: More reflections in natural history.* New York: Norton.

Guidano, V. F. (1984). A constructivist outline of cognitive processes. In M. A.

Reda & M. J. Mahoney (Eds.), *Cognitive psychotherapies: Recent developments in theory, research, and practice.* Cambridge, MA: Ballinger.

———. (1987). *Complexity of the self.* New York: Guilford.

Guidano, V. F., & Liotti, G. (1983). *Cognitive processes and emotional disorders.* New York: Guilford.

———. (1985). A constructivistic foundation for cognitive therapy. In M. J. Mahoney & A. Freeman (Eds.), *Cognition and psychotherapy.* New York: Plenum.

Hayek, F. A. (1952). *The sensory order.* Chicago: University of Chicago Press.

———. (1964). The theory of complex phenomena. In M. Bunge (Ed.), *The critical approach to science and philosophy: Essays in honor of K. R. Popper.* New York: Free Press.

———. (1978). *New studies in philosophy, politics, economics, and the history of ideas.* Chicago: University of Chicago Press.

———. (1982). The Sensory Order after 25 years. In W. B. Weimer & D. S. Palermo (Eds.), *Cognition and the symbolic processes* (Vol. 2). Hillsdale, NJ: Erlbaum.

Herink, R. (1980). *The psychotherapy handbook.* New York: New American Library.

Howard, K. L., & Orlinsky, D. E. (1972). Psychotherapeutic process. *Annual Review of Psychology, 23,* 615–668.

Jantsch, E. (1980). *The self-organizing universe: Scientific and human implications of the emerging paradigm of evolution.* New York: Pergamon.

Jantsch, E. (Ed.). (1981). *The evolutionary vision: Toward a unifying paradigm of physical, biological, and sociocultural evolution.* Boulder, CO: Westview Press.

Jerison, H. (1973). *Evolution of the brain and intelligence.* New York: Wiley.

———. (1976). Paleoneurology and the evolution of mind. *Scientific American, 234,* 90–101.

Jerome, J. (1980). *The sweet spot in time.* New York: Summit.

Joyce Moniz, L. (1985). Epistemological therapy and constructivism. In M. J. Mahoney & A. Freeman (Eds.), *Cognition and psychotherapy.* New York: Plenum.

Kahneman, D., Slovic, P., & Tversky, A. (Eds.). (1982). *Judgment under uncertainty: Heuristics and biases.* New York: Cambridge University Press.

Kahneman, D., & Tversky, A. (1973). On the psychology of prediction. *Psychological Review, 80,* 237–251.

Kelly, G. A. (1955). *The psychology of personal constructs.* New York: Norton.

Korchin, S. J., & Schuldberg, D. (1981). The future of clinical assessment. *American Psychologist, 36,* 1147–1159.

Lakatos, I. (1970). Falsification and the methodology of scientific research programmes. In I. Lakatos & A. Musgrave (Eds.), *Criticism and the growth of knowledge.* Cambridge, MA: Cambridge University Press.

Land, G. T. L. (1973). *Grow or die: The unifying principle of transformation.* New York: Dell.

Laudan, L. (1977). *Progress and its problems: Towards a theory of scientific growth.* Berkeley: University of California Press.

Laszlo, E. (1983). *Systems science and world order: Selected studies.* New York: Pergamon.

MacLean, P. D. (1973). *A triune concept of brain and behavior.* Toronto: University of Toronto Press.

Mahoney, M. J. (1974). *Cognition and behavior modification.* Cambridge, MA: Ballinger.

______. (1976). *Scientist as subject: The psychological imperative.* Cambridge, MA: Ballinger.

______. (1977). Publication prejudices: An experimental study of confirmatory bias in the peer review system. *Cognitive Therapy and Research, 1,* 161–175.

______. (1979). Cognitive and non-cognitive views in behavior modification. In P. O. Sjoden, S. Bates, & W. S. Dockens (Eds.), *Trends in behavior therapy.* New York: Plenum.

______. (1980). Psychotherapy and the structure of personal revolutions. In M. J. Mahoney (Ed.), *Psychotherapy process: Current issues and future directions.* New York: Plenum.

______. (1981). La importancia de los procesos evolutivos para la psicoterapia. *Analysis y modification de conducta, 7,* 155–170.

______. (1984a). Psychoanalysis and behaviorism: The yin and yang of determinism. In H. Arkowitz & S. Messer (Eds.), *Psychoanalytic and behavior therapy: Is integration possible?* New York: Plenum.

______. (1984b). Integrating cognition, affect, and action: A comment. *Cognitive Therapy and Research, 8,* 585–589.

______. (1985). Psychotherapy and human change processes. In M. J. Mahoney & A. Freeman (Eds.), *Cognition and psychotherapy.* New York: Plenum.

______. (1986a). The tyranny of technique. *Counseling and Values, 30,* 169–174.

______. (1986b). *Participatory epistemology: The implications of psychology of science.* Paper presented at the First National Conference on Psychology of Science, Memphis State University, April, 1986.

______. (in press). *Human change processes: Notes on the facilitation of personal development.* New York: Basic Books.

Mahoney, M. J., & Arnkoff, D. (1978). Cognitive and self-control therapies. In S. Garfield & A. Bergin (Eds.), *Handbook of psychotherapy and behavior change.* New York: Wiley.

Mahoney, M. J., & DeMonbreun, B. G. (1977). Psychology of the scientist: An analysis of problem-solving bias. *Cognitive Therapy and Research, 1,* 229–238.

Mancuso, J. C., & Adams-Webber, J. R. (Eds.) (1982). *The construing person.* New York: Praeger.

Marlatt, G. A., & Gordon, J. R. (Eds.). (1985). *Relapse prevention: Maintenance strategies in the treatment of addictive behaviors.* New York: Guilford.

Maturana, H. R. (1975). The organization of the living: A theory of the living organization. *International Journal of Man-Machine Studies, 7,* 313–332.

Maturana, H. R., & Varela, F. G. (1980). *Autopoiesis and cognition: The realization of the living.* Boston: Reidel.

Meehl, P. E. (1954). *Clinical versus statistical prediction: A theoretical analysis and a review of the evidence.* Minneapolis: University of Minnesota Press.

______. (1973). *Psychodiagnosis: Selected papers.* Minneapolis: University of Minnesota Press.

______. (1978). Theoretical risks and tabular asterisks: Sir Karl, Sir Ronald, and the slow progress of soft psychology. *Journal of Consulting and Clinical Psychology, 46,* 806–834.

Neimeyer, R. A. (1985). Personal constructs in clinical practice. In P. C. Kendall (Ed.), *Advances in cognitive-behavioral research and therapy* (Vol. 2). New York: Academic Press.

Neisser, U. (1967). *Cognitive psychology.* Englewood Cliffs, NJ: Prentice-Hall.

———. (1976). *Cognition and reality.* San Francisco: Freeman.

Nelson, K. E., & Nelson, K. (1978). Cognitive pendulums and their linguistic realization. In K. E. Nelson (Ed)., *Children's language* (Vol. I). New York: Gardner Press.

Nideffer, R. M. (1976). *The inner athlete.* New York: Crowell.

Nisbett, R. E., & Ross, L. (1980). *Human inference: Strategies and shortcomings of social judgment.* Englewood Cliffs, NJ: Prentice-Hall.

Passingham, R. (1982). *The human primate.* San Francisco: Freeman.

Palermo, D. S. (1971). Is a scientific revolution taking place in psychology? *Science Studies, 1,* 135–155.

Pattee, H. H. (Ed.). (1973). *Hierarchy theory: The challenge of complex systems.* New York: George Braziller.

Piaget, J. (1970). *Psychology and epistemology: Towards a theory of knowledge.* New York: Viking.

———. (1981). *Intelligence and affectivity: Their relationship during child development.* Palo Alto, CA: Annual Reviews.

Polanyi, M. (1958). *Personal knowledge: Towards a post-critical philosophy.* Chicago: University of Chicago Press.

———. (1966). *The tacit dimension.* New York: Doubleday.

Prigogine, I. (1980). *From being to becoming: Time and complexity in the physical sciences.* San Francisco: Freeman.

Prigogine, I., & Stengers, I. (1984). *Order out of chaos: Man's new dialogue with nature.* New York: Bantam.

Prochaska, J. O. (1984). *Systems of psychotherapy: A transtheoretical analysis.* Homewood, IL: Dorsey Press.

Rachman, S. J. (1980) Emotional processing. *Behaviour Research and Therapy, 18,* 51–60.

Reynolds, P. C. (1981). *On the evolution of human behavior: The argument from animal to man.* Berkeley: University of California Press.

Rice, L. N., & Greenberg, L. S. (1984). *Patterns of change.* New York: Guilford.

Spielberger, C. D., & DeNike, L. D. (1966). Descriptive behaviorism versus cognitive theory in verbal operant conditioning. *Psychological Review, 73,* 306–326.

Tversky, A., & Kahneman, D. (1971). Belief in the law of small numbers. *Psychological Bulletin, 76,* 105–110.

———. (1974). Judgment under uncertainty: Heuristics and biases. *Science, 183,* 1124–1131.

Varela, F. J. (1979). *Principles of biological autonomy.* New York: Elsevier North Holland.

von Glaserfeld, E. (1984). An introduction to radical constructivism. In P. Watzlawick (Ed.), *The invented reality: Contributions to constructivism.* New York: Norton.

Wachtel, P. L. (Ed.). (1982). *Resistance: Psychodynamic and behavioral approaches.* New York: Plenum.

Wade, T. C., & Baker, T. B. (1977). Opinions and use of psychological tests: A survey of clinical psychologists. *American Psychologist, 32,* 874–882.

Washburn, S. L., & Moore, R. (1980). *Ape into human: A study of human evolution.* Boston: Little, Brown.

Watzlawick, P. (Ed.). (1984). *The invented reality: Contributions to constructivism.* New York: Norton.

Weimer, W. B. (1977). A conceptual framework for cognitive psychology: Motor theories of mind. In R. Shaw & J. Bransford (Eds.), *Perceiving, acting, and knowing.* Hillsdale, NJ: Erlbaum.

______. (1979). *Notes on the methodology of scientific research.* Hillsdale, NJ: Erlbaum.

______. (1982). Hayek's approach to the problems of complex phenomena: An introduction to the theoretical psychology of The Sensory Order. In W. B. Weimer & D. S. Palermo (Eds.), *Cognition and the symbolic processes* (Vol. 2). Hillsdale, NJ: Erlbaum.

______. (in press, a). *Rationalist constructivism, scientism, and the study of man and society.* Hillsdale, NJ: Erlbaum.

______. (in press, b). Spontaneously ordered complex phenomena and the unity of the moral sciences. In G. Radnitzky (Ed.), *Unity of the sciences.* New York: Paragon House.

Werner, H. (1948). *The comparative psychology of mental development.* New York: Science Editions.

Wiggins, J. S. (1981). Clinical and statistical prediction: Where are we and where do we go from here? *Clinical Psychology Review, 1,* 3–18.

Wiggins, J. S., & Hoffman, P. J. (1968). Three models of clinical judgment. *Journal of Abnormal Psychology, 73,* 70–77.

Wilson, P. J. (1980). *Man: The promising primate: New Haven:* Yale University Press.

Wundt, W. (1912). *An introduction to psychology.* New York: Macmillan.

Zeleny, M. (Ed.). (1980). *Autopoiesis, dissipative structures, and spontaneous social orders.* Washington, DC: American Association for the Advancement of Science.

9 | Reinterpreting the Transference

Jerome L. Singer

ONE of the great discoveries to emerge from Sigmund Freud's development of psychoanalysis was the transference phenomenon. The intense passions that surfaced in the daily encounters of the patients with their relatively "neutral" and businesslike analysts, Breuer and Freud (and which so embarrassed the senior in the practice that he withdrew from such work), gradually led Freud to the realization that their method was exposing a profound, basic characteristic of human mental life. Under the special circumstances of the quasi-hypnotic trappings of analysis (Wolstein, 1954) and the requirement for complete exposure of thoughts and recovery of childhood incidents, patients' long-standing childhood wishes, fantasies, and expectations not only surfaced in consciousness but became attached ("transferred") to the analyst. Eventually Freud saw in the "transference neurosis" the reenactment within the ongoing psychotherapeutic relationship of a persistent and self-defeating childhood conflict, an opportunity for the analyst to intervene directly in the patient's neurotic structure and to reshape the personality through insight and "working through" of this *in vivo* primal conflict (Chrzanowski, 1979; Fenichel, 1938; Gill, 1982; Sandler, Dare, & Holder, 1973; Schafer, 1977,1983). The analysis of transference became the touchstone of the specific "curative" effect of classical or neo-Freudian psychoanalysis.

Some of the material in this chapter appeared in an article in *Psychoanalytic Psychology*, 1985, *2*(3), 189–219.

Of special importance was Freud's observation that transference is not a phenomenon unique to the psychoanalytic situation. Rather, he came to see it as a general pattern of behavior so that many of the complexities of human relationships reflect the long-standing wishes and conflicts that each of us brings to new adult interactions with spouses, co-workers or authorities (Freud 1912/1958, 1925/1959, 1937/1959). Increasingly psychoanalysts, particularly the neo-Freudians, proposed that a major task of psychotherapy was identifying and helping patients to work through the maze of transferences with key figures in their lives outside of therapy (Bird, 1972; Chrzanowski, 1979; Schimek, 1983).

In this chapter I will examine some of the psychoanalytic "lore" about the transference phenomenon and relate this clinical material to important new developments in personality and social psychology. I propose that, on the one hand, our general grasp of the nature of interpersonal cognitions, emotions and interrelationships can be deepened by recognizing how pervasive are the transferences or "hidden agendas" that color all sorts of human interactions. On the other hand, our effectiveness as clinicians in all approaches can be strengthened by fusing the notions drawn from the traditional psychoanalytic literature with the new concepts and empirical data available from psychologists who deal with social cognition. In this chapter, I will demonstrate the importance of this fusion by discussing the psychoanalytic concept of the transference in the terms of investigators of social information processing.

A Personal Note: Transference and Modern Psychology

My continuing clinical work and active research on the psychology of imagination over about 35 years has confirmed again and again for me the importance of the "hidden agendas" we all bring to each new social situation. What has been less clear, however, is whether (a) a transference neurosis inevitably develops in therapy, (b) whether transference interpretation is crucial to producing change in patients and (c) whether transferential issues specific to the therapist are as pervasive in therapy or clinical work as some analysts such as Gill (1982) have proposed. My own experiences have made it clear that what often really matters to patients are their distorted expectations or interpretations of the "real people" in their daily lives (or their memories of family figures), and one can often help them to identify these distortions and to try new ways of perceiving and relating to others with only occasional identification of transferences in the analytic hour. Recently an unpublished paper by Murray Stern drawing on his own 30 years of experience as an analyst called attention to a similar recognition. He not only describes the faulty or hasty overemphasis on transference that often prevails in our work but examines the possibility that, for many patients, a good "therapeutic alliance" is there from the start of treatment. Such clients view analysts as trained professionals who are supposed to try to help them untangle their interpersonal difficulties by skillfully identifying their long-standing distortions; only occasionally do they spend much time thinking about therapists or even trying to appease, placate, or malign them.

The more I reflected on my work, reviewed the literature in psychoanalysis, and considered the research developments in cognitive, social, and personality psychology, the more I felt that it would be necessary to reexamine the tenets of psychoanalysis within the context of modern social science. A critical construct such as the transference phenomenon must be interpretable to some degree within the framework of a burgeoning experimental literature on how people process information, how they encode material for storage in some form of a memory system, and how they retrieve such memories, as well as on the role of social or physical context and of emotional arousal in memory retrieval, the role of expectation in construing the physical and social environment, the nature of the stream of consciousness, etc. Social psychologists, for example, after several decades of devising ingenious experimental methods for demonstrating social behaviors such as conformity, aggression, obedience, and attitudinal shift, have moved increasingly to a recognition that how people construe a social situation may be more predictive of their subsequent behavior than the "objective" characteristics of the setting. The emergent area of social cognition, replete with careful research and definitions, seems very close indeed to many of the issues posed initially by psychoanalysts in identifying transference phenomena, which are, after all, idiosyncratic interpretations of an interpersonal situation drawing on one's limited range of actual experience or on private fantasies derived from childhood. (See appendix for a tabular representation of relevant terminology, general and operational definitions, and specific bibliography, as well as the earlier chapter by Turk, Salovey, & Prentice.)

I then proceeded to a review of the recent psychoanalytic literature to determine if I could find a "handle" for developing an integration. And here, I must say, I confronted a distressing dilemma. The relevant literature consists essentially of a series of assertions and pronouncements. Each paper begins with its obligatory citation of one of Freud's writings, usually the case of Dora (Freud, 1905/1953), in which the concept of transference was first fully limned. Again and again the authors of these papers seek to tease out new meanings from such articles or to demonstrate the prescience of the old master, even as they propose subtle changes in application of the concept of transference. And yet, except for the historical interest in the origins of psychoanalytic thought, why waste more time in formulating a theory of transference on what we must recognize today was a botched case in which Freud unwittingly may have lent himself to a cynical manipulation of Dora by her father (Lewis, 1981)? Modern psychoanalysts continue to try to demonstrate by citation that their conceptions remain essentially continuous with the presumed views of the Viennese master.

More serious, however, than our collusion in a system of obeisance to an illusory father figure is the lack of solid evidence provided in recent writings to support the many assertions about the nature of the transference. One reads the "deepest" and often most scholarly of writers in this area such as Kohut (1984) or Gill (1982) and finds only scraps of clinical examples, a scattering of vignettes that at first seem to support the author's point but on closer scrutiny allow for many other interpretations or simply a Scottish verdict of "not proven." Each article is convincing in turn, but throughout the dozens of papers my assistant and I reviewed, I kept hearing an inner voice echoing the recent popular hamburger commercial, "Where's the data?"

A Cognitive–Affective Perspective

Since the 1960s we have witnessed a major paradigm shift in the way psychologists and many other behavioral scientists interpret human and other animal behavior. The emphasis on energy and hydraulic systems, on innate drives pressing for discharge, on all human beliefs and actions as reflections in symbolic form of recurring, peremptory, appetitive, aggressive, or erotic biologic impulses (Rapaport, 1960) has begun to disappear from psychoanalysis as well as from the psychological learning theories that prevailed from the 1930s through the 1950s. Important research evidence ranging from the findings of central-brain rewarding and punishing systems closely linked to emotion, the indications that drives like hunger, thirst, or sex are far more complex than had been realized and that they must be amplified by some emotional reaction to be motivating (Tomkins, 1962, 1963), the data from sensory deprivation and laboratory studies of night dreaming all point to a much more complex view of human behavior than psychologists held previously. The human being is increasingly regarded as an information-seeking, information-processing organism whose joys, sorrows, fears, rages, or excitements are closely tied to the novelty, variety, and complexity of the data presented from an external physical and social environment, from an environment of private thoughts or wishes generated from long-term memory, and from less easily decipherable signals emitted by the working machinery of the body.

The important developments in experimental cognitive psychology have made clear that we do not respond all at once to environmental stimuli but process new information in a temporal sequence, measurable in milliseconds to be sure, but characterized by complex yet definable steps. These include anticipation and expectancy, attention, search strategies, development in short-term memory of some kind of icon or echo (depending on whether material is visual or aural), matching of the material against some previous template of relevant memories before "assigning it" via an imagery or semantic encoding system (or a combination of both) to long-term memory for "permanent storage." I want to call attention to three particular features of information processing that highlight the link between basic cognition and the phenomenon of transference:

Expectancy

Anticipatory or expectancy processes are intrinsic to the way we deal with the information in our environment. That is, we draw on previously stored, more-or-less organized information in deciding what attracts us, where to look, how to explore a new situation, what to reverberate of that information in the shift from short- to long-term memory, and in what forms to encode the information for later retrieval. The extent and complexity of our previous knowledge, its accessibility at the moment, and our personal style of processing (e.g., emphasizing the most recent match versus a more extended search process [Broadbent, 1958]), all lead to differences in what we notice, retain, and eventually in how we reshape our organized bodies of beliefs and knowledge, which we call schemas.

Emotions and Incongruities

Our emotional system is closely linked to our cognitive system, so that it is almost impossible to identify situations in which information processing does not evoke the experience of an affect or of a valuing response (Neville, 1981; Rychlak, 1981; Singer, 1974; Tomkins, 1962,1963; Zajonc, 1980). Differential-emotions theory has developed and has been at least partially supported by research, in the work of Ekman and Friesen (1975), Izard (1977), Plutchik (1962), Schwartz, Weinberger, and Singer (1981), and Tomkins (1962,1963). Emotions are identified as limited cross-culturally to about six basic affects in humans. These are measurable along three dimensions: 1) self-reports; 2) facial expression; and 3) psychophysiological correlates in facial myography, cardiovascular patterning, and brain hemispheric excitation variations. The affects include *excitement–interest* and *joy* as positive emotions that, when invoked, are inherently rewarding. *Fear–terror, distress–sadness, anger,* and *shame–guilt–humiliation* are the negative affects that are inherently punishing experiences. As Tomkins (1962, 1963) has suggested, we are motivated not by biological drives but by the four possibilities of emotion: we seek to maximize experiences that we have found to generate positive emotions and to avoid or limit experiences that have aroused negative emotions. We also need to express emotions as fully as possible yet learn to control such expression. The specific tie of emotions to information processing has been hypothesized to relate to the suddenness with which we must process new information, e.g., a startle response, or to the novelty and complexity of the information, e.g., the demands made on established schemata for matching the new with the stored material; the elaborate associative networks aroused by new material; and the persistence over time of unresolved novel material that cannot readily be assimilated into previous schemata (Singer, 1974; Tomkins, 1962, 1963).

Emotions are differentially aroused by the rate, novelty, and complexity of information we process and by our preparation in anticipatory or easily available schemata for assimilating this information. If this is the case, one can begin to see how all of behavior involves some process of expectancy and a pattern of emotional reactivity as our anticipations are confirmed (joy), only partially confirmed (arousal of interest/curiosity), or grossly unconfirmed (arousal of fear, then anger or sadness). From this vantage point, transference phenomena seem less mysterious, indeed, but rather an inherent feature of the human search for organization and integration of novelty and ambiguity. Put another way, the incongruity between our wishes and expectations and the information provided in a specific situation is the key to emotional arousal (Mandler, 1984). If our expectations are fully confirmed, we experience relief, joy, or (in situations of minimal novelty) we simply are unaware of emotion—what Abelson (1983) has called "cold cognition" situations. If the situation is one of moderate incongruity, we feel the positive affect of interest and are motivated to move forward and to explore. If the situation is of gross incongruity, we are surprised or afraid, and if such incongruity persists, we become angry or distressed. Humor involves a period of moderate incongruity followed by a resolution that matches our previous expectations of a "punch line" or "explanation," and we respond with the emotion of joy or the smiling response. The emotions evoked in the transference, as we shall see, hinge on the range and extent of expectations for different situations that are already a part of the patient's repertory.

Ongoing Thought and the Stream of Consciousness

A third feature of the cognitive sequence that merits special attention is the fact that human experience involves processing information from at least two other sources of stimulation besides the physical or social environment. These sources are the continuous activity of our stream of thought and memory system and the concurrent activity of the body, which sends us often incomprehensible signals. In a sense we are in a perpetual state of choosing the stimulus source to which we wish to assign priority—the external physical or social milieu, our own private interior monologue and flow of images and anticipations, or the temperature shifts, momentary aches and pains, muscle strains, stomach gurglings, that are part of our body's working machinery (Singer, 1975a,b). Probably, as Rapaport (1960) put it in the psychoanalytic terminology of the '40s and '50s, "there is a permanent gradient of attention cathexis to the external environment" (p. 96). That is, normal adaptation and safety requires us to assign our highest priority of attention to the physical setting lest we bump into objects, be hit by automobiles, or offend those talking to us in a social situation by inattention. Yet the human condition puts us almost simultaneously in a situation of not only constantly playing and replaying mentally the new information from outside but also noticing thoughts in the form of interior commentary or visual or verbal images that bear no obvious resemblance to the external setting. Experimental studies show that as the novelty or complexity of an external setting is reduced, people begin to respond more and more to centrally generated imagery or to become more aware of wishes, fantasies, memories, etc. (Singer, 1974, 1984). Studies both of waking and sleep mentation carried on in laboratories suggest that a special characteristic of reverie or of the content and pattern of stage 1-rapid eye movement sleep (REM) dream reports reflects a reduced awareness of one's physical surroundings and a heightened sequence of associations to material from long-term memory. Indeed there is little evidence that the night dreams we recall are any different (except that we believe in their reality as they occur) from the kind of thought that characterizes normal waking reverie under relaxed conditions (Antrobus, Reinsel, & Wollman, 1987).

Although Freud clearly recognized the advantages of trying to capture ongoing thought through the use of free association under reduced stimulus novelty (e.g., patient on couch, looking at ceiling, therapist out of sight, etc.), it can be argued that he shifted too much from his earlier emphasis on imagery towards verbal associations and lost some of the potential effectiveness for evoking vivid memories, fantasies, and arousing emotions quickly (Reyher, 1978; Singer, 1974). Indeed Spence's astute analysis of Freud's personal dream interpretations and the more general method he advocated suggests the inherent dilemma for psychoanalysis when verbal summaries are accepted for the complex and rich visual or auditory imagery of dreams or memories (Spence, 1983).

The main point I wish to stress in relation to the waking thought stream is that, to the extent that we can capture it by experimental procedures (Klinger, 1978; Singer, 1975b, 1984), it is mainly characterized by a continuous pattern of *alogical* thought, internally associated *respondent* processes (Klinger, 1978) that involve imagery sequences, remembered conversations, potential future encounters or conversations. Continuing thought also includes *operant* processes that are self-monitored and have a specific, time-limited goal. Operant thoughts are more like what we specifically communicate to others in speech or in writing or when pursuing a defined problem in arithmetic or in repairing an appliance. Our ongoing respondent thought resembles Freud's primary-process thinking; however, it is not only drive-determined but much broader, characterized by replaying and reshaping memories, by awareness of a range of unfinished business or unfulfilled intentions, humorous or sardonic commentary on current situations, playful explorations of a range of futures (Pope & Singer, 1978a,b).

For some individuals awareness of this respondent aspect of their private reality is painful, and they seek to escape from conscious processing by a flight into processing external information or public reality. Such individuals have been characterized as defensive repressors, short-samplers, or simply extroverts (Singer, 1984). They may often be ill-prepared through anticipatory schemas to confront novel situations or they may react with terror or distress when, under conditions of reduced external stimulation, they become aware of their own images or memories. Individual differences in awareness, control and enjoyment of one's private thought stream, may account for the degree to which some patients may enter easily into an analytic mode or may be aware of thoughts about the therapist while others may be startled and frightened when images recur vividly in the redundant external informational setting of an analyst's office, linking the analyst to figures from one's past.

If we take cognizance of the nature of the stream of thought we must also consider that memories are constantly being rehearsed and, very likely, reshaped. The organized beliefs we have about ourselves or about others, our self-schemas and prototypes, are also being continuously modified as we match new inputs to earlier memories. It may well be, therefore, that the search for early critical memories that one seeks to elicit through transference may be, at least for some people, an exercise in futility, as Spence's distinction between historical truth and narrative truth suggests (Spence, 1983). On the other hand, for extroverts or hysterics, who have tried to avoid conscious awareness and control of ongoing thought, early memories may have remained encapsulated, not easily retrieved. Their recurrence in the contexts of childhood scenes created by the special properties of the psychoanalytic setting and process, may be vivid, powerful and lend increased credence to the narrative constructions that form the textual basis of psychoanalysis (Spence, 1983).

Knowledge Structures: Schemas and Scripts About Self and Others

Although the concept of schemas or schemata, as organizational structures that encapsulate knowledge about self or the world is traceable in psychology to the concepts of Piaget, Lewin, Tolman, Kelly ("personal constructs"), and, of course, reflect as well the psychoanalytic notions of unconscious fantasy, object representations (Blatt & Wild, 1976), and transference, it is only during less than the last decade that systematic efforts at operationalizing and experimenting with such notions have proliferated (Hollon & Kriss, 1984; Turk & Speers, 1983). Schemas may serve to filter the complex new information our senses confront, but they are also continuously strengthened when similar information is processes ("Dogs bark when someone is at the door") or when one reflects on new, slightly divergent information ("Why isn't Fido barking when the bell rings? Is he sick?").

Self-schemas as operationalized and investigated systematically by Markus (1977), Bandura (1977) and, in work with depressed patients, by Beck, Shaw, Rush, and Emery (1979) represent a special case of beliefs about one's self. Beliefs about other people, fuzzy set "prototypes," such as "a typical businessman" or "the usual politician," have also been identified and studied (Cantor & Mischel, 1979). The term "scripts," originally proposed by Tomkins (1962, 1963) has been developed by researchers in artificial intelligence in a specialized way to define organized belief systems about action sequences in the "real world," sequences that unroll relatively automatically like well-programmed series (Schank & Abelson, 1977). Indeed, a model for a similar schema in dealing with the imaging process was developed by Minsky (1975).

The recent theorizing of Tomkins has proposed that scripts about self or about especially important interpersonal interactions have been organized out of often fairly specific childhood "scenes" that were associated with either strong positive or negative emotions (Tomkins, 1979). The work of Carlson (1981) and L. and R. Carlson (1984) exemplifies the way in which positive or negative affective "scenes" and scripts are differentially influential in current behavior and in the interpretation of new information. The semantic and practical relationship of schemas, scripts, and prototypes to the transference phenomena identified in psychoanalytic sessions deserves much more extensive attention. It is increasingly clear that the long-standing dilemma of social psychology, "Why don't attitudes predict behavior?", has been resolved when careful measurement of schemas about self and about others are considered separately and combined to predict overt actions (Kreitler & Kreitler, 1976, 1982).

This very brief review of a major area of development in the lively field of social cognition is designed to suggest that if we wish to understand hidden agendas we will, first of all, have to seek them in the relatively automatic unrolling of scripts, the filtering processes of schemas, or in the inherent rules for evaluating information and making judgments described as *availability, representativeness,* and *anchoring with adjustment* heuristics by Tversky and Kahneman (1974). Yet so far such patterns of relatively automatic sequences have been explored chiefly in the framework of assigning individuals rather specific tasks to accomplish or problems to solve.

The thrust of my earlier presentation leads me to propose that schemas, scripts, or prototypes are not static, if moderately well-organized, structures. They are constantly subject to reexamination and reshaping during waking conscious thought or even in the course of rumination about night dreams, especially if one approaches such a process, as a psychotherapy patient might, with a particular schema for interpretation.

If we are ultimately to understand the workings of "the unconscious," we will have to "unpackage" the various individual schemas, prototypes, scripts, "core organizing principles" (Meichenbaum & Gilmore, 1984) or behavior heuristics through some types of systematic questioning or through various forms of thought sampling that can permit us to observe how they are used in ordinary daily life. Of course psychoanalysis has been engaged in such a task but, I suggest in an often unwitting and diffuse fashion. More recently, cognitive–behavior therapists have begun addressing this task quite directly in treatment (Meichenbaum & Gilmore, 1984; Singer, 1984). Luborsky's (1977) demonstration of reasonably reliable methods for identifying "core conflictual themes" (surely close relatives of schemas and scripts) within psychoanalytic sessions could also be applied to more extensive samples of nontherapeutic ongoing thought sequences in daily life or in laboratory settings as well as to samples of patients' communication in various forms of psychotherapy.

In view of the great importance assigned to beliefs about self both by psychoanalysts oriented towards object relations theory and cognitive researchers, special attention should be paid to how such schemata become organized through ongoing interior monologues. Tomkins's notion of positively or negatively laden nuclear scripts (Tomkins, 1979), which usually involve the self, implies differential filtering processes for new information in relation to expectancies based on such scripts, e.g., *hypersensitivity* to possible analogies in new settings for negative nuclear scripts, efforts to "reshape" new information to *enhance* its similarity to positive nuclear scenes.

Can we identify such processes through extended samples of thought or self-monitoring procedures? Certainly no one would seriously claim nor could they prove that the "objects" of psychoanalytic object relations are permanently crystallized in the original pregenital schemas. Very likely they emerge again and again into conscious ruminations, tested and elaborated in mental rehearsals or reminiscences, and also "acted out" in transferential encounters in daily life as well as in analysis (Singer, 1985). Indeed as we shall consider in the next section, they may also be replayed and reshaped further in what we remember of our sleep mentation. An individual stylistic variable worth exploring may be that "repressors" may have developed long-standing strategies to avoid extended attention to ongoing thought and thus may have differentiated and reshaped earlier schemas, prototypes, and scripts less than other individuals. The result: when such material emerges into consciousness it may indeed (a) surprise them more or seem alien and peremptory and (b) remain more global, child-like, and rigid in structure. Recent as yet unpublished work by Bowen suggests that such undifferentiated patterns may also be evident in their cardiovascular response to emotional arousal.

One of the most intriguing recent studies in the emerging field of life-span explorations of personality has been the work by Helson, Mitchell, and Moane (1984) on the "social clock." This term suggests both a social group's agreement about when certain events ought to occur in one's life (e.g., marriage before age 30) and one's own more personal set of goals (or "script") for achieving such states as intimacy, childbearing, career success or financial security. In this sense, the "social clock" can be thought of as an example of a knowledge or schema about the sequence events in one's life. In a 20-year follow-up of female college graduates, it was possible to identify those women adhering to a traditional feminine social clock, those willing to postpone but not give up such expectations of marriage and childrearing, and those women who early eschewed such a script or who, by age 28, had chosen career lines that conformed in the 1960s to a masculine social clock. The data point up the long-term predictive effect of scales on the California Personality Inventory and of personal social clocks in suggesting the patterns of adherence to these early scripts over the years and also the reactions of the women who, despite adherence, experienced divorce or other disruption of these scripts.

Reexamining the Transference

The Transference Neurosis

The concept of a transference neurosis, the gradual reevocation in the analytic situation of a skeletonized and identifiable basic neurotic structure that can then be examined and that becomes the foundation for cure, is an elegant conception, indeed. As presented by Fenichel (1938–39) for example, one can see how this view provides a rationale for avoiding the simplicity of a catharsis theory of therapeutic intervention in favor of a careful "surgical" model. But what evidence is there beyond wishful thinking for the regularity of occurrence or specific therapeutic value of the phenomenon? We can all attest to specific instances of transference behaviors, as Schimek (1983) has noted, but how often can we demonstrate a full-blown transference neurosis? There are only, as yet, a few reasonably careful research studies of the transference phenomenon in the framework of psychoanalytic therapy, all involving relatively short-term treatment (Luborsky et al., in press; Malan, 1980; Marziali, 1984). These studies identify clear instances of transference interpretations or of core familial conflicts that include similar reactions to the therapist but they provide no information supportive of the concept of transference neurosis. The fine study by Luborsky, Mellon, van Ranenswanny, Childress, Levine, Alexander, Cohen, Hole, and Ming (in press) has tracked a series of Freud's assertions about transference (e.g., its generalizability, relation to childhood schemas, etc.) through objective analyses of therapy protocols. It supports the evidence for a general transference phenomenon, but it does not address the special properties of transference neurosis and the specific hypothesized link of "cure" to transference neurosis analysis.

Indeed the relatively good results demonstrated in the Marziali (1984) and Luborsky et al. (in press) studies where transference interpretations are characteristic of better outcomes also indicate that the transference comments are most effective when they point to transference links to other important people in the patients' lives. For example, Marziali (1984) found that the highest and most consistent positive outcomes (based on outside judges' ratings of the patient's status on variables of *friendship, intimacy, assertiveness, capacity to use support,* and *self-esteem*) emerged when there was a higher frequency of interpretations specifically linking the patient's attitudes toward therapist-parent-sibling-and significant others together. These data point up what Schafer (1977) or Spence (1983) would call a mutually convincing narrative but say little about the emergence of a transference neurosis. Suggestive findings in a study of long-term treatment reported by Blatt (1984) indicate that for "anaclitic" patients who come to treatment with profound concerns about the disruptions of their interpersonal relationships (Blatt, 1984), the therapeutic relationship, as manifested in warmth, empathy, and provision of an alternative quasi-parental model may be critical for change in early therapy. For "introjective" patients (e.g., obsessives), interpretations seem associated with signs of change. The specific approach to transference may, therefore, involve differential responses for personality types rather than only the "transference interpretation" so often cited in the literature.

My own hypothesis, which could be tested from careful analyses of recorded psychoanalytic protocols following the methods pioneered by Luborsky, Malan, Marziali, Dahl, and Gill, among others, is that a full-blown transference neurosis, e.g., a pattern of recurrent, extreme dependency or, in the classic form, of erotic attachment, is a consequence of the specific stance of the therapist. As Gill (1982) and Stolorow and Lachman (1984) have carefully argued, the so-called neutral observer stance is already conveying some message to the patient. Indeed, even the Rorschach inkblots are not equally ambiguous; some of them evoke more animal responses, some more specific human forms than others. The extensive social psychological data provide ample evidence that the therapist's appearance, speech pattern, and personal expectancies (even if exploitative countertransference responses of "authority," "seductiveness," or "chicken-soup motherliness" are restrained) lead to special attitudes within the dyad. It might be argued that insistence on early childhood memories (or simply greater interest shown in them by the analyst) and the use of the couch (a posture that for adults revives an early childhood context of the bedtime ritual for where else, except in hospitals, do adults lie down while others sit up nearby?) all establish a script that fosters regression and that may, for some clients, play into such desperate dependency needs that a transference neurosis is created.

But is the transference neurosis and its analysis necessary for effective therapy? That question remains unanswered from the current state of our knowledge. My own guess is that, as the success of shorter psychodynamic and cognitive therapies has demonstrated in the recent evaluation literature, a more direct inquiry about nuclear scenes, nuclear scripts, schemata, or personal constructs can avoid the emergence of a full-blown transference neurosis and yet allow for effective use of transference material as an interpretative resource. The silence of the so-called neutral analyst can be taken quite differently by different patients. The important study of psychodynamic and behavior therapies by Sloane, Staples, Cristol, Yorkston, and Whipple (1975) found that patients actually rated behavior therapists as more empathic than psychodynamic therapists. I suspect this reflected the patients' experience that the curious, inquiry-oriented behavior therapist "cared more," while the neutral analysts often seemed remote and detached. A recent review of studies on the therapeutic relationship in behavior therapies points up the fact that therapists who are demanding, explicit, challenging but *also* warm, understanding and respectful have a better chance of good results using behavioral methods (Sweet, 1984).

Generality of the Transference Phenomenon

In this section I will address the issue of whether the traditional concept of transference can be interpreted and clarified using the language and experimental data of social cognition researchers. The main thrust of the cognitive perspective in experimental, personality, and social psychology supports Freud's general view of transference as a basic characteristic of the human condition. We are information-seeking and information-processing at all times, anticipating each new situation through the use of sets of schemas, prototypes, nuclear scripts or scenes, and inherent thought mechanisms (what Meichenbaum and Gilmore, 1984, termed *core organizing principles* and Kahneman and Tversky, 1982, *heuristics*). This paradigm shift, as Erdelyi (1985) has shown, reflecting a move from a "rat" model to a "computer" model, makes it possible to incorporate many of Freud's clinical insights about people's self-defeating and defensive thoughts or behaviors and seeming unawareness of their own intentions or purposes into a more precisely definable, testable format.

Our continuing search for meaning, for some explanations of our thoughts or behavior or the behavior of others—"man the scientist" in Kelly's (1955) phrase; the mode of continuing *cognitive orientation*—in the more recent theory and empirical work of Kreitler and Kreitler (1976, 1982) is expressed through an ongoing stream of consciousness. We play out and replay new information or stored memories in waking thought and in dreams; we try out possibilities for the future constantly, some of these close to immediate intentions or "current concerns" (Klinger, 1977, 1978), some reflecting a mixture of long-standing, unfulfilled intentions of the type psychoanalysts have emphasized, some of the possible scenarios representing an inherent human curiosity and exploratory trend (Singer, 1974, 1984). In the course of such activity we must, if the situation demands it, produce a specific overt act, a verbal or behavioral response that reflects only a very limited segment of our complex processing. Often such overt responses reflect the most overlearned, most thoroughly rehearsed schemas or scripts in our repertory and these seem, therefore, to have an automatic, "mindless" (Langer, 1978) quality that *appears* to reflect unconscious processes. As Erdelyi's

(1985) extensive research has shown even seemingly repressed or forgotten material emerges once one is given more time for reflection, for increased reliance on imagery processes as a method of retrieval rather than relying on rapid verbal responses.

Transference as identified in psychoanalysis originally can now be viewed as a phenomenon characteristic of all human encounters. We all bring our hidden agendas to each daily interaction, but sometimes the latent set of plans are hidden even from the subject as well as the others in a social situation, not so much buried in an unconscious geographical region but simply not immediately functional or at the center of conscious attention. Viewed from this vantage point, as Stolorow and Lachman (1984) have noted in a very stimulating analysis, the key role of *distortion* as an indicator of transference must be reexamined. It is inevitable that our efforts to give meaning and organization to social situations will look "erroneous" or distorted from the other's vantage point. Rather than focus on the patient's "mistake" ought we not, instead, to accept the fantasy as an inherent reality of the human condition, the search for organization and meaning, and try to help the patient identify those situations or circumstances where such a particular fantasy may be more or less adaptive?

Indeed Stolorow and Lachman (1984) urge upon the analyst a stance of the curious investigator sharing this role with the patient rather than as the subtle, somewhat authoritarian critic, a posture that so often seems to emerge when one points in interpretation to "transference distortions" as "regressions" or replays of childhood fantasies. Indeed they imply a resolution that seemed to have evaded Freud in his somewhat anguished last great paper on "Interminable Transferences" (Freud 1937/1959). Eliminating all transference is not only a futile effort for analysis, it is counterproductive. As Stolorow and Lachman write:

> When transference is viewed as an expression of a universal human organizing tendency, analysis aims . . . rather for the acceptance and integration of the transference experience into the fabric of the patient's analytically expanded psychological organization. (p. 25)

Even so-called "infantile" fantasies can be accepted as perhaps outmoded but, in some ways, creative efforts of a child that persist in memory and that can be used playfully in fantasy or even as a basis for a somewhat detached, humorous view of oneself.

As Schimek (1983) has also suggested, one major outcome of a valuable psychoanalytic experience is the awareness of the multiple meanings and multiple perspectives we all bring to situations. I would carry this further and propose that effective psychotherapy is a remarkable educational experience, sensitizing individuals to cognitive processes of expectancy, attention, causal attribution, and the search for meaning, which not only they but their friends and intimates bring to situations. Such broadened awareness of the possible meaningfulness or uses of one's dreams and imagery (Singer, 1974) as well as one's actions *transfers* the excitement *we* feel as psychoanalysts to our patients. We trust they will not become caricature analysts boring people at cocktail parties but rather that they will become inherently excited by their recognition of the rich possibilities for thought and interaction that are features of our human capacities. From an emotional standpoint, they will become curious and capable of surprise by recognizing multiple possibilities rather than startled, embarrassed, or terrorized by peremptory ideation or automatized impulsive actions. Where fear, shame, and anger were, there should excitement and curiosity be!

The Form and Content of Transference Interpretations

Gill (1982) has devoted considerable attention to the problem of what must be the focus of transference interpretation, but, as I suggested, he can adduce no evidence to support his decision to emphasize the more Sullivanian "here and now" interpretations. What research evidence we do have from studies by Malan (1980), Marziali (1984), and Luborsky (1984) does not support the position of the Kleinians about the key role of extreme pre-Oedipal interpretations. Most of the scoring examples for identifying core conflicts and transferences provided in the research protocols, if they involve early childhood memories, rarely go back before the family romance or Oedipal period and some involve sibling or juvenile period peer relationships, a confirmation of Lesser's (1981) and Sullivan's (1953) proposals that these sibling or peer influences on transference have been underemphasized. Admittedly these data are all from limited numbers of cases, some from short-term or early phases of psychodynamic therapy. But, it seems to me, the burden of proof for demonstrating that truly "mutative" or personality-change-producing nature of transference interpretations must involve links between the patient's attitude to the therapist and pre-Oedipal experience lies with those analysts following Strachey who have made such assertions. If psychoanalysis is to remain a form of treatment that falls within the scope of modern behavioral and biological science then it must move beyond acceptance of the assertions of authorities, as Spence (1983) and Edelson (1984) have argued.

I should like to propose several ways that transference interpretations may produce change. I believe these are testable from therapy protocols or at least supportable through current or potential future personality and social psychology research. The first step is a clear and convincing demonstration of some of the patient's core conflicts or nuclear scripts, scenes, or core personal constructs. Suppose a Ms. Dorianne O., in an imaginary encounter with a modern cigar-smoking Sigmund Freud, eventually managed to complain that his puffing away was a hazard to her health. Can she be helped to recognize that her hesitation and blocking prior to her forceful assertion of a legitimate request that Freud stop smoking may represent a long-standing pattern of fear of authorities? A gentle encouragement of her to take note of some extreme language she used to make her request may point to a continuing nuclear script that links inhibition of self-assertion with authority to a build-up of anger and then, in other less protected situations, an overresponse that may have self-defeating consequences. Other instances, similar transference reactions to teachers, bosses, parents of friends or lovers, can be gradually identified or even obtained by encouraging a series of partially directed images. In this way the inherent curiosity, the human need to give organization and meaning to seemingly random events, can be recruited as a basic feature of a therapeutic alliance and as a gradually developed *new* skill for understanding social interactions and one's own thought processes.

As I have already suggested, the strong emotion evoked in the transference response may be of great motivational value for enhancing the spirit of inquiry and the therapeutic alliance. I see no good evidence that emotions themselves are stored (Isaacs, 1984) or that strong emotional expression has an inherently curative effect. Rather it provides a further clue to the patient that the issue (in our example, the inhibition with authority) is a very important one and worth further pursuit. One also learns that, having expressed strong emotions, nothing drastic has occurred (a form of behavior technique of implosion or flooding) and one now gains a greater sense of control. Further instances of potential transference reaction need not be avoided out of fear but pursued actively with the emotion of interest-excitement that Tomkins has proposed is evoked by moderately novel or complex new information (Singer, 1974; Tomkins, 1962).

The continuing exploration of transference examples (whether with significant others in one's current life or in the "here and now" with the therapist) may also lead to a systematic desensitization of the intensity of response to the nuclear script. Tomkins's theory has shown that repetition where analogies to a basic script are formed from only "partial" fits with new situations can enhance and magnify the power of the script. But once the script has been identified and key nuclear scenes played and replayed with the therapist, the well-established therapeutic effect of emotional desensitization may follow. And since *in vivo* desensitization, that direct experience of the distressing situation, has been consistently found to be somewhat more effective than imagery or symbolic desensitization (Bandura, 1969), a series of direct responses to the therapist that mirror recurrent conflicts can gradually lead to a reduced intensity of emotion, especially where such emotional responsiveness is counterproductive or self-defeating. Such a procedure has, indeed, been recently proposed in a psychoanalytic paper by Silverman (1984).

Another special feature of transference occurrences in therapy has been signalled by Kohut (1984) as an opportunity for the therapist to demonstrate not only the recurrent conflict but to behave in such a way as to provide for the patient an alternative form of self-object or internalized representation that can be a recurrent feature of the patient's later thought. Occasionally this may mean breaking the old rule of abstinence or nongratification of long-standing neurotic needs. Such instances are necessary if one recognizes the genuine and long-standing failure of some patients to experience kindly or benevolent figures as part of their upbringing. More typically what may be necessary is that the rigid internalized personifications or prototypes of authorities that the individual may be carrying on continuous interior dialogues with (see James Joyce or Saul Bellow for good literary examples of this pattern) need to be recognized as outmoded. New "imaginary friends" can be developed, more in keeping with the broader society and adult life situation in which the patient currently participates.

Extremely suggestive data by Geller, Cooley, and Hartley (1981) on the memories and images of professionals who have undergone psychoanalysis indicate that those who reported less satisfactory outcomes were also characterized by images of their analysts as extremely positive or quite negative figures. Those whose results were more satisfactory preserved an ongoing image of the analyst as a therapeutic ally involved in continuous inquiry. In this sense, one might guess that a new Kohutian self-object has developed, a recurring fantasy companion who performs no magic but spurs one on to examining and reexamining the multiplicities of one's own and others' schemas and expectations before drawing hasty inferences or acting only on impulse. Such internalized new patterns of thought need not lead to obsessional rumination. As any practiced skill they may soon run themselves off smoothly and often with only minimal conscious awareness but produce a richer, more empathic human response. I believe that Geller's work points to a very useful further direction for studying how systematic transference interpretations may gradually be internalized so that, as analyses go on, we see, more and more, the patient carrying on the work of inquiry that is part of a natural therapeutic relationship. The message of the transference in psychoanalysis is that if we do our work well we will not stay in our clients' memories as saints, or parents, or magicians. Indeed, they may not think very much about us at all. But, if we succeed, we *will* live on in their thoughts as they confront the ever new complexities of their daily lives with a spirit of curiosity, excitement, and a sense of inquiry. We will be there as ghostly reminiscences in the clients' streams of consciousness, echoing the patient voices of their therapists as they encourage a further look at the multilayered nature of human experience.

Although I have devoted much of this chapter to detailing the importance and utility of the concept of transference, it should also be clear that this construct can be understood within the modern framework offered by researchers of social cognition. Moreover, this discussion should serve as an example of how classic psychoanalytic concepts—that previously have not lent themselves to empirical investigation—might now be more precisely defined and, hence, more systematically studied.

Acknowledgments

Support for research by the John D. and Catherine T. MacArthur Foundation is gratefully acknowledged.

The assistance of Annette Telgarsky for critical reading and for collaboration on preparation of the appendix to this book is gratefully acknowledged. Useful suggestions about the manuscript have come from Lisa Gornick, Silvan Tomkins, Jefferson Singer, Peter Salovey, Paul Crits-Cristoph, Lester Luborsky, and Mardi Horowitz.

References

Abelson, R. (1983). Whatever became of consistency theory? *Personality and Social Psychology Bulletin, 9,* 37–54.

Antrobus, J. S., Reinsel, R., & Wollman, M. (1987). Dreaming: Cortical activation and perceptual thresholds. In S. Ellman & J. S. Antrobus (Eds.), *The mind in sleep* (2nd ed.). Hillsdale, NJ: Erlbaum.

Bandura, A. (1969). *Principles of behavior modification.* New York: Holt, Rinehart & Winston.

———. (1977). Self-efficacy: Toward a unified theory of behavioral change. *Psychological Review, 84,* 191–215.

———. (1978). The self-system in reciprocal determinism. *American Psychologist, 33,* 344–358.

———. (1982). Self-efficacy mechanism in human agency. *American Psychologist, 37,* 122–147.

Bargh, J. A., & Pietromonaco, P. (1982). Automatic information processing and social perception. The influence of trait information presented outside of conscious awareness on impression formation. *Journal of Personality and Social Psychology, 43,* 437–439.

Bartlett, F. C. (1932). *Remembering: A study in experimental and social psychology.* New York: Cambridge University Press.

Beck, A. T., Rush, A. J., Shaw, B. F., & Emery, G. (1979). *The cognitive therapy of depression.* New York: Guilford Press.

Bird, B. (1972). Notes on transference: Universal phenomenon and hardest part of analysis. *Journal of the American Psychoanalytic Association, 20,* 267–301.

Blatt, S. J. (1984). *Object-relations theory and the therapeutic process: The study of change in the intensive treatment of seriously-disturbed young adults.* Presented at the annual meeting of the American Psychological Association, Toronto.

Blatt, S. J., & Wild, C. M. (1976). *Schizophrenia: A developmental analysis.* New York: Academic Press.

Cantor, N., & Mischel, W. (1979). Prototypes in person perception. In L. Berkowitz (Ed.), *Advances in experimental social psychology* (Vol. 12). New York: Academic Press.

Cantor, N., Mischel, W., & Schwartz, J. (1982). A prototype analysis of psychological situations. *Cognitive Psychology, 14,* 45–77.

Carlson, L., & Carlson, R. (1984). Affect and psychological magnification: Derivations from Tomkins' script theory. *Journal of Personality and Social Psychology, 52,* 36–45.

Carlson, R. (1981). Studies in script theory: I. Adult analogs of a childhood nuclear scene. *Journal of Personality and Social Psychology, 40,* 501–510.

Chrzanowski, G. (1979). The transference–countertransference transaction. *Contemporary Psychoanalysis, 15,* 458–471.

Edelson, M. (1984). *Hypothesis and evidence in psychoanalysis.* Chicago: University of Chicago Press.

Ekman, P., & Friesen, W. V. (1975). *Unmasking the face.* Englewood Cliffs, NJ: Prentice-Hall.

Erdelyi, M. (1985). *Psychoanalysis: Freud's cognitive psychology.* San Francisco: Freeman.

Fenichel, O. (1938–9). *Problems of psychoanalytic technique.* Albany: Psychoanalytic Quarterly Inc.

Freud, S. (1962). The psychotherapy of hysteria. *Standard Edition, 2:* London: Hogarth. (Originally published, 1895.)

______. (1962). *The interpretation of dreams. Standard Edition, 5.* London: Hogarth. (Originally published, 1900.)

______. (1953). Fragment of an analysis of a case of hysteria. *Standard Edition, 7:* 7–122. London: Hogarth. (Originally published, 1905.)

______. (1958). The dynamics of transference. *Standard Edition, 12:* 99–108. London: Hogarth. (Originally published, 1912.)

______. (1959). An autobiographical study. *Standard Edition, 20:* 7–74. London: Hogarth. (Originally published, 1925.)

______. (1959). Analysis terminable and interminable. *Standard Edition, 23:* 216–253. London: Hogarth. (Originally published, 1937.)

______. (1953). An outline of psycho-analysis. *Standard Edition, 23:* 144–207. London: Hogarth. (Originally published, 1940.)

Geller, J. D., Cooley, R. S., & Hartley, D. (1981). Images of the psychotherapist: A theoretical and methodological perspective. *Imagination, Cognition and Personality, 1,* 123–146.

Gill, M. (1982). Analysis of transference: I. Theory and technique. *Psychological Issues, 53,* 1–17.

Gill, M., & Hoffman, I. Z. (1982). A method for studying resisted aspects of the patient's experience in psychoanalysis and psychotherapy. *Journal of the American Psychoanalytic Association, 30,* 137–167.

Helson, R., Mitchell, V., & Moane, G. (1984). Personality and patterns of adherence and nonadherence to the social clock. *Journal of Personality and Social Psychology, 46* 1079–1096.

Hollon, S. D., & Kriss, M. (1984). Cognitive factors in clinical research and practice. *Clinical Psychology Review, 4,* 35–76.

Horowitz, M. (1978). *Image formation and cognition* (2nd ed.). New York: Appleton-Century-Crofts.

Isaacs, R. (1984). Feeling bad and feeling badly. *Psychoanalytic Psychology, 1,* 43–60.

Izard, C. E. (1977). *Human emotions.* New York: Plenum.

Kahneman, D., & Tversky, A. (1973). On the psychology of prediction. *Psychological Review, 80,* 237–251.

———. (1982). Intuitive prediction: Biases and corrective procedures. In D. Kahneman, P. Slovic, & A. Tversky (Eds.), *Judgment under uncertainty: Heuristics and biases.* New York: Cambridge University Press.

Kelly, G. A. (1955). *A theory of personality: The psychology of personal constructs.* New York: Norton.

Klinger, E. (1977). *Meaning and void: Inner experience and incentives in people's lives.* Minneapolis: University of Minnesota Press.

———. (1978). Modes of conscious flow. In K. S. Pope & J. L. Singer (Eds.), *The stream of consciousness.* New York: Plenum.

Kohut, H. (1984). *How does psychoanalysis cure?* Chicago: University of Chicago Press.

Kreitler, H., & Kreitler, S. (1976). *Cognitive orientation and behavior.* New York: Springer.

———. (1982). The theory of cognitive orientation: Widening the scope of behavior prediction. In B. Maher (Ed.), *Experimental personality research.* New York: Springer.

Langer, E. (1978). Rethinking the role of thought in social interaction. In J. Harvey, W. Ickes, & R. Kidd (Eds.), *New directions in attribution research* (Vol. 2). Hillsdale, NJ: Erlbaum.

Lesser, I. (1981). A review of the alexithymia concept. *Psychosomatic Medicine, 43,* 531–543.

Lewis, H. (1981). *Freud and modern psychology.* New York: Plenum.

Luborsky, L. (1977). Measuring a pervasive psychic structure in psychotherapy: The core conflictual relationship theme. In N. Freedman & S. Grand (Eds.), *Communicative structures and psychic structures.* New York: Plenum.

———. (1984). *Principles of psychoanalytic psychotherapy: A manual for supportive-expressive treatment.* New York: Basic Books.

Luborsky, L., Mellon, J., van Ravenswany, P., Childress, A. R., Levine, F. J., Alexander, K., Cohen, K. D., Hole, A. V., & Ming, S. (in press). A verification of Freud's grandest clinical hypothesis: The transference. *Clinical Psychology Review.*

Malan, D. H. (1980). *Toward the validation of dynamic psychotherapy.* New York: Plenum.

Mandler, G. (1984). *Mind and body: Psychology of emotion and stress.* New York: Norton.

Markus, H. (1977). Self-schemata and processing information about the self. *Journal of Personality and Social Psychology, 35,* 63–78.

______. (1983). Self-knowledge: An expanded view. *Journal of Personality, 51,* 543–565.

Marziali, E. A. (1984). Prediction of outcome of brief psychotherapy from therapist interpretive interventions. *Archives of General Psychiatry, 41,* 301–304.

McCoy, M. M. (1981). Positive and negative emotion: A personal construct theory interpretation. In H. Bonarius, R. Holland, & S. Rosenberg (Eds.), *Personal construct psychology.* New York: St. Martin's Press.

McGuire, W. J. (1973). The yin and yang of progress in social psychology: Seven Koans. *Journal of Personality and Social Psychology, 26,* 446–456.

Meichenbaum, D., & Gilmore, J. B. (1984). The nature of unconscious processes: A cognitive–behavioral perspective. In K. Bowers & D. Meichenbaum (Eds.), *The unconscious reconsidered.* New York: Wiley.

Minsky, M. (1975). A framework for representing knowledge. In P. H. Winston (Ed.), *The psychology of computer vision.* New York: McGraw-Hill.

Neisser, U. (1976). *Cognition and reality.* San Francisco: Freeman.

Neville, R. C. (1981). *Reconstructions of thinking.* Albany: State University of New York Press.

Piaget, J. (1951). *Play, dreams and imitation in childhood.* (C. Gattegno & F. M. Hodgson, Trans.). New York: Norton.

Plutchik, R. (1962). *The emotions: Facts, theories and a new model.* New York: Random House.

Pope, K. S., & Singer, J. L. (1978a). (Eds.), *The stream of consciousness.* New York: Plenum.

______. (1978b). Determinants of the stream of consciousness. In J. Davidson & R. Davidson (Eds.), *Human consciousness and its transformations.* New York: Plenum.

Posner, M. (1981). Cognition and personality. In N. Cantor & J. F. Kihlstrom (Eds.), *Personality, cognition and social interaction.* Hillsdale, NJ: Erlbaum.

Rapaport, D. (1960). *The structure of psychoanalytic theory: A systematizing attempt.* New York: International Universities Press.

Reyher, J. (1978). Emergent uncovering psychotherapy: The use of imagoic and linguistic vehicles in objectifying psychodynamic processes. In J. L. Singer & K. S. Pope (Eds.), *The power of human imagination.* New York: Plenum.

Roseman, I. J. (1982). *Cognitive determinants of emotions.* Unpublished doctoral dissertation, Yale University.

Rychlak, J. (1981). Logical learning theory: Propositions, corollaries, and research evidence. *Journal of Personality and Social Psychology, 40,* 731–749.

Salso, R. (1979). *Cognitive psychology.* New York: Harcourt Brace Jovanovich.

Sandler, J., Dare, C., & Holder, A. (1973). *The patient and the analyst: The basis of the psychoanalytic process.* New York: International Universities Press.

Schafer, R. (1977). The interpretation of transference and the conditions for loving. *Journal of the American Psychoanalytic Association, 25,* 471–490.

______. (1983). *The analytic attitude.* New York: Basic Books.

Schank, R. C., & Abelson, R. P. (1977). *Scripts, plans, goals, and understanding.* Hillsdale, NJ: Erlbaum.

Schimek, J. G. (1983). The construction of the transference: The relativity of the "here and now" and the "there and then." *Psychoanalysis and Contemporary Thought, 6,* 435–456.

Schwartz, G., Weinberger, D., & Singer, J. A. (1981). Cardiovascular differentiation of happiness, sadness, anger and fear following imagery and exercise. *Psychosomatic Medicine, 43,* 343–364.

Shevrin, H. (1984). *Unconscious conflict: A convergent psychodynamic and electrophysiological approach.* Paper presented at conference sponsored by MacArthur Foundation on emotional and cognitive factors in unconscious processes. Palo Alto, CA.

Silverman, L. H. (1984). Beyond insight: An additional necessary step in redressing intrapsychic conflict. *Psychoanalytic Psychology, 1,* 215–234.

Singer, J. L. (1974). *Imagery and daydreaming: Methods in psychotherapy and behavioral motivation.* New York: Academic Press.

———. (1975a). *The inner world of daydreaming.* New York: Harper & Row.

———. (1975b). Navigating the stream of consciousness: Research in daydreaming and related inner experience. *American Psychologist, 30,* 727–738.

———. (1984). The private personality. *Personality and Social Psychology Bulletin, 10,* 7–30.

———. (1985). Transference and the human condition: A cognitive-affective perspective. *Psychoanalytic Psychology, 2,* 189–219.

Sloane, R. B., Staples, F. R., Cristol, A. H., Yorkston, N. J., & Whipple, K. (1975). *Psychotherapy versus behaviour therapy.* Cambridge, MA: Harvard University Press.

Spence, D. (1983). *Narrative truth and historical truth.* New York: Basic Books.

Stolorow, R. D., & Lachman, F. M. (1984). Transference: The future of an illusion. *Annual of Psychoanalysis, 12,* 28–49.

Strachey, J. (1934). The nature of the therapeutic action of psycho-analysis. *International Journal of Psychoanalysis, 15,* 128–129.

Sullivan, H. S. (1947). *Conceptions of modern psychiatry.* Washington, DC: William Alanson White Foundation.

———. (1953). *The interpersonal theory of psychiatry.* New York: Norton.

Sweet, A. A. (1984). The therapeutic relationship in behavior therapy. *Clinical Psychology Review, 4,* 253–272.

Tomkins, S. S. (1962). *Affect, imagery, consciousness* (Vol. 1). New York: Springer.

———. (1963). *Affect, imagery, and consciousness* (Vol. 2). New York; Springer.

———. (1979). Script theory: Differential magnification of affects. In H. E. Howe, Jr. & R. A. Dienstbier (Eds.), *Nebraska Symposium on Motivation, 1978,* (Vol. 26). Lincoln: University of Nebraska Press.

Tulving, E. (1983). *Elements of episodic memory.* Oxford, England: Oxford University Press.

Turk, D. C., & Speers, M. A. (1983). Cognitive schemata and cognitive processes in cognitive-behavioral interventions: Going beyond the information given. In P. C. Kendall (Ed.), *Advances in cognitive-behavioral research and therapy* (Vol. 2). New York: Academic Press.

Tversky, A., & Kahneman, D. (1974). Judgment under uncertainty: Heuristics and biases. *Science, 185,* 1124–1131.

Wolstein, B. (1954). *Transference: Its meaning and function in psychoanalytic therapy.* New York: Grune & Stratton.

Zajonc, R. B. (1980). Feeling and thinking: Preferences need no inferences. *American Psychologist, 35,* 151–175.

Zajonc, R. B., & Markus, H. (1984). Affect and cognition: The hard interface. In C. E. Izard, J. Kagan, & R. B. Zajonc (Eds.), *Emotions, cognition and behavior.* New York: Cambridge University Press.

PART IV

Overcoming Limitations in Clinical Information Processing

10 Identifying and Reducing Causal Reasoning Biases in Clinical Practice

Lynn H. Arnoult
Craig A. Anderson

THINKING about causes is a fundamental part of clinical practice. Both causes of clients' problems and therapeutic interventions (i.e., potential causes of desired change) must be considered. Why is Mr. Jones having anxiety attacks? And what experiences are most likely to alleviate his problem? In answering such questions clinicians make use of available evidence and previously acquired general knowledge to understand the causes of behavior. Unfortunately, there is much room for bias to enter into the deliberations, and obviously, the negative consequences of biased causal judgments could be serious. Of course, clinicians are aware of the possibility of bias in clinical judgment. Trainees are reminded to be objective and to look at an issue from more than one perspective. Yet recent research provides evidence that biased thinking is prevalent among both novices and experienced practitioners (Cantor, Smith, French, & Mezzich, 1980; Chapman & Chapman, 1967, 1969; Horowitz, Post, French, Wallis, & Siegelman, 1981; Temerlin, 1968).

Although we recognize that it is not possible to totally avoid bias, we believe that a reduction of biased thinking is possible. In this chapter we offer two approaches to reducing biases in thinking about causes: (a) increased awareness of potential sources of bias, and (b) activities designed to promote more normative causal inference. We will begin by reviewing research on sources of bias that might be present whenever causal judgments are made. Then we will consider sources of bias specific to clinical practice. We can mention only a few of the innumerable potentials for bias in clinical judgments. Our purpose is to increase awareness, and we suggest that readers draw from their personal experiences to add to our list as they go along.

Next, we will suggest some bias-reducing activities. The general directives customarily given trainees to be objective and to avoid bias may be ineffective because they are *too* general. That is, the practitioner may be unable to relate such general directives to specific instances on the job. With this in mind, we will suggest a number of specific training procedures and exercises designed to help clinicians (and student clinicians) develop bias-reducing thinking habits that will remain operative in day-to-day practice. Again, we can mention only a few of many possible strategies, and we encourage readers to invent others.

Sources of Bias in Causal Reasoning

Among the major potential sources of bias in causal reasoning are the decision maker's causal beliefs, the structural features of situations, and the information available about the people involved in those situations. These factors affect the decision maker's expectations, which in turn guide the selection of a cause to explain a given outcome. In the following sections we will consider a number of these factors, beginning with causal beliefs.

Causal Beliefs

Causal beliefs take many forms. They range from specific beliefs about why a particular event occurred (e.g., attributions), through fairly broad conceptions about how two or more variables are related (e.g., social theories), to general beliefs about the meaning of life (e.g., philosophical or religious beliefs). Our causal beliefs influence a wide variety of thoughts, feelings, and behaviors. They influence motivation, emotional reactions, performance, assessments of new information, and judgments about future performance, as discussed earlier in this volume by Snyder and Thomsen.

Lord, Ross, and Lepper (1979) demonstrated that people who hold different social theories may evaluate new data relevant to those theories in a biased fashion. Subjects who initially held different beliefs about the efficacy of capital punishment laws as deterrents to murder evaluated two purportedly authentic studies on this issue. Studies that supported subjects' views were evaluated as methodologically superior to those that contradicted them. Furthermore, having seen a mixed set of studies (one supporting and one contradicting their initial views), the subjects did not moderate their initially extreme views; instead, they became even more convinced that their initial causal beliefs were correct.

In the attribution domain, researchers have found that prior beliefs about the abilities of a target person (self or other) influence attributions made for success and failure at tasks related to those abilities. For example, Feather and Simon (1971a,b) showed that people tend to attribute expected outcomes to the target, and unexpected outcomes to factors external to the target. So if Jane is believed to be a competent and responsible worker, then loss of her job (an unexpected outcome) is more likely to be attributed to economic recession than to inadequate job performance. (Other theoretical bases for these ideas are described earlier in this volume by Jordan, Harvey, and Weary.)

Although there are many studies showing effects of causal beliefs on interpretation of new information, such effects are not found universally. Anderson and Sechler (1986) manipulated subjects' causal beliefs about the relation between a personality trait and subsequent behavior (a social theory). Subjects later were given new information about the trait–behavior relation and were asked to evaluate this new information. There was no biasing effect of prior causal belief. Subsequent research in a similar paradigm also has failed to yield a biased evaluation effect (Anderson & Kellam, in preparation).

Thus, prior causal beliefs sometimes do and sometimes do not lead to biased evaluation of new information. But the conditions that give rise to the effect are not yet clear. Anderson and Sechler (1986) speculated that biased evaluation may occur primarily when the causal belief is strongly held, is ego involving, is extreme, is connected to other cognitive systems, or when a justifiable rationale for selectively valuing and devaluing new information is available. Despite the lack of evidence about which of these variables is (are) important in producing the effect, clinical judgments are at risk because several of these factors could be present.

Social theories and attributions also have been shown to influence judgments about future performances. In the Anderson and Sechler work, subjects also made judgments about future outcomes in situations related to the social theories manipulated earlier in the experiments. In domains as varied as child abuse, delay of gratification, and job performance of firefighters, manipulated causal beliefs affected judgments.

Similarly, attributions for prior outcomes affect future success expectancies. For instance, people led to attribute initial failure at an interpersonal persuasion task to lack of effort or to use of an ineffective strategy are more optimistic about their future performances than those led to attribute initial failure to lack of ability or to interfering personality traits (e.g., Anderson, 1983a; Anderson & Jennings, 1980; Anderson, Jennings, & Arnoult, 1987). Similar effects occur with attributions and expectations about others. (See Weiner, 1985, for a review and theoretical integration.)

The links between causal beliefs and motivation, performance, and emotion are also well established. In the Anderson (1983a) study cited above, people who were led to attribute initial task failures to effort or strategy problems persisted longer at the task and eventually obtained higher success rates than those in the ability/trait attribution conditions. Weiner, Russell, and Lerman (1979) showed that many emotions are linked to specific attributions and to attribution-outcome combinations. For instance, an achievement failure attributed to others' interference produces anger, a failure attributed to one's own lack of ability produces feelings of incompetence, and a success attributed to ability produces pride (see also Weiner, 1982). Indeed, developmental research reveals that even young children understand many of the relations between attributions and emotional reactions in others, and that they will modify their reported attributions to produce the desired emotions in others (Weiner & Handel, 1985).

Given the importance of causal beliefs, it would be helpful to know more about how those beliefs are derived and how errors might occur. These questions have been the subject of extensive research, a review of which is beyond the scope of this chapter. Interested readers may want to refer to classic works by Heider (1958), Jones and Davis (1965), Kelley (1967), and Weiner (1974). For a sampling of more recent work see Harvey, Ickes, and Kidd (1976, 1978, 1981) and Nisbett and Ross (1980, especially chap. 6). One principle of interest to the present discussion is that people tend to infer causal relations between events that occur together. For example, if John is nervous when he goes to the doctor, it might be inferred that going to the doctor makes John nervous. Although this type of reasoning is often useful, it can lead to inference errors. Correlations do not always represent causal relations, and even when they do, the direction of causality may be unclear. For instance, John may go to the doctor *because* he is nervous.

Causal Structure of Situations

Recent research has yielded further insights into factors that affect the selection of causes. It has been shown, for example, that the selection of a cause for a particular outcome can be affected by certain structural features of the situation in which the outcome occurred.

The notion of causal structure of situations actually derives from a larger two-stage model of attributions (Anderson, 1983b, 1985; Anderson & Slusher, 1986). The first stage is an information-gathering one. The features of the situation (including the type of situation, the outcome, and the goals of the attributor) are matched to available guiding knowledge structures. The one that best matches is selected and used to guide further information search. For example, it will suggest what kinds of information are needed to arrive at a sufficient explanation. In a sense, the guiding knowledge recruits other knowledge from the past (e.g., other knowledge structures about the attributional target) and from the present situation. It also suggests the most likely causes or causal candidates for the situation and the information needed to test these candidates. In the second stage, the attributor uses the recruited information to test the most likely causal candidates, one at a time. The search is best characterized as a truncated search (Shaklee & Fischhoff, 1982). That is, as soon as a sufficiently reasonable fit between a causal candidate and the recruited information is found, the search is abandoned and an attribution is made. Thus, the most salient causal candidates (those thought of first) have the best chance of being selected even if they do not provide the best fit to the information. If the first candidate does not fit well, then the second is considered. This continues until a candidate fits, or until all candidates have been tested. At that point, the attributor will either abandon the search, or will attempt to use a different guiding knowledge structure with a different set of causal candidates and different sets of relevant information.

The idea of causal structure of situations is that different causes are listed as causal candidates for different types of situations. Indeed, one way of changing which guiding knowledge structure is selected at the outset is to make a particular type of cause salient. This essentially primes those knowledge structures that contain that cause. It is through this process that seemingly innocuous attribution manipulations, such as having a confederate mention a particular type of cause prior to any task engagement, have robust effects on success expectancies, motivation, performance strategy, and performance quality (Anderson, 1983a; Anderson Jennings, 1980, Anderson, Jennings, & Arnoult, 1987; Jennings, 1980; Kiesler, Nisbett, & Zanna, 1969).

This model applies to self-attributions, other attributions, and to more general explanation processes (cf. Kruglanski, 1980). The major difference between self and other attributions, from this perspective, is the kinds of information (in knowledge structures) available for use. Actors typically have a much greater store of target-relevant information than do observers (see Jones & Nisbett, 1972; Monson & Snyder, 1977). When this is the case, we expect final attributions (result of the second stage) to be more closely related to causal structure for observers than for actors. This is because observers have relatively little information to contradict the causal candidates suggested by the causal structure of the situation, whereas actors have relatively more information to force attributions away from the causal structure candidates. This predicted difference between actor and observer attributions has been obtained by Anderson (1985). (See also chapter by Jordan, Harvey, and Weary, this volume, for more information on actor–observer differences in attribution.)

Argument Availability

Because of the potential for error in the formulation of causal beliefs, our ability to determine the validity of our beliefs is of great importance. Unfortunately, there is evidence that people do not always use effective criteria in evaluating their beliefs. Sometimes, for example, they rely too heavily on judgmental heuristics such as the availability of arguments, the ease or readiness with which arguments for or against a particular belief come to mind.

A long series of studies of social theories has supported the idea that argument availability (or accessibility) often is used to judge the validity of social theories. More specifically, we seem to use the availability of supporting causal arguments relative to the availability of causal arguments for alternative social theories in judging theory validity (Anderson, 1982, 1983d; Anderson, Lepper, & Ross, 1980). For instance, whether we think the best placement policy (in general) for abused children is to remove them from their abusing parents permanently or to reintegrate them depends upon whether we have created causal theories in favor of removal or in favor of reintegration (Anderson & Sechler, 1986). The most direct support for the argument availability hypothesis comes from Anderson, New, and Speer (1985). In that study, subjects were led to believe, via two case histories, that either a positive or a negative relation exists between a person's risk preference (as measured by a paper and pencil test) and his or her subsequent performance as a firefighter. This procedure leads most subjects to create causal social theories linking risk preference and firefighting ability (Anderson, 1983d). Later, the subjects were informed that the initial case histories were totally fictitious. Subjects' personal beliefs about the true relation between the two variables were then assessed. Finally, subjects were asked to write out causal arguments in favor of each of the two competing social theories (positive and negative). Within-cell correlations and covariance analyses revealed that subjects' personal beliefs were significantly correlated with the availability of competing causal arguments. Those who could create more arguments in favor of the positive theory than the negative theory tended to believe the positive theory was correct, and made social judgments in line with that belief (and vice versa).

So we see that decision makers may overestimate the validity of particular causal beliefs due, in part, to their inability to generate arguments opposing those beliefs. But what if they encountered opposing arguments without having to generate them? What if they were presented with strong evidence that their causal beliefs were unfounded? Then could we expect a revision of the beliefs? Unfortunately, the answer is "not always," as other research on belief perseverance has shown.

Belief Perseverance

Perseverance of beliefs in this domain usually means the *unwarranted* persistence of beliefs in the face of empirical or logical challenges. The phenomenon was first popularized by Ross, Lepper, and Hubbard (1975), who showed that both self- and social impressions can persist to a normatively unwarranted extent. In particular, they showed that beliefs about one's own or others' social perceptiveness can survive even the total discrediting of the evidential base that gave rise to those beliefs. Subsequent research demonstrated this effect in the domain of social theories, beliefs about how variables in the social environment are related to each other (Anderson et al., 1980). The processes underlying the perseverance effect have been the target of much investigation. Perhaps the most consistent finding is that some type of explanation process underlies the effect. The results for self-beliefs have been somewhat equivocal, perhaps because people may develop quite different explanations for outcomes when they are actors rather than observers. The different explanations may, in turn, have quite different implications for subsequent judgments.

The results of studies on social theories have been more consistent. For instance, the type of data that induces the initial theory influences the amount of perseverance. Concrete data (as in case histories) induce more causal processing than do abstract data (as in statistical summaries). A consequence of this is that concrete data lead to stronger perseverance biases than do abstract data, even when the abstract data are logically superior (Anderson, 1983d). This phenomenon supports the notion that the availability of causal explanations or arguments is a primary determinant of social theories.

Other support comes from work that showed the effect of forcing people to consider alternative explanations or arguments or to take an opposing perspective. Several lines of work have shown that such "counterexplanations" reduce (and sometimes eliminate) the bias (Anderson, 1982; Anderson & Sechler, 1986; Koriat, Lichtenstein, & Fischhoff, 1980; Lord, Lepper, & Preston, 1984; Slovic & Fischhoff, 1977). Anderson (1982) showed that this type of procedure works both when introduced before the initial data are encountered (an inoculation procedure) and after the data have been examined and explained (a counterexplanation procedure). The strength of this debiasing procedure did not differ as a function of timing (before or after data examination), but the way it worked did differ with timing. The inoculation procedure led subjects to be more cautious in interpreting the subsequent data, whereas the counterexplanation procedure had its entire effect after the data had been examined and interpreted.

The research on the effects of counterexplanations is reminiscent of earlier work concerned with the effects of counterattitudinal role playing on attitude change. Sometimes, role playing led to attitude change, but not always (see Elms, 1967; McGuire, 1966, for reviews). Several different counterattitudinal role-playing paradigms were used. For example, in one paradigm subjects enacted emotional scenes that contradicted their attitudes, as in playing the role of a smoker who discovers that he or she has cancer (Janis & Mann, 1965). The paradigm most relevant to our current discussion involves writing counterattitudinal essays. Several findings from this research tradition parallel the explanation/counterexplanation work quite closely.

The main findings of interest were that: (a) When people expect to defend their own opinion, they tend to accept supporting arguments as valid and reject opposing arguments as invalid, but do not show this evaluation bias when they expect to defend the opposing opinion (Greenwald, 1969); (b) People assigned to improvise arguments in favor of one or the other side of an issue (e.g., the desirability of generalized vs. specialized undergraduate education) change their opinions in the direction of assignment. They also remember personally improvised arguments better than experimenter-presented arguments (Greenwald & Albert, 1968); and (c) Counterattitudinal essay writing does not produce attitude change when people are provided an opportunity to consider and reject the counterattitudinal arguments prior to being assigned to defend that position, but the attitude change effect does occur when the assignment to defend the position occurs before the opportunity to consider and reject arguments (Greenwald, 1970).

The counterattitudinal studies did not look at the specific nature of the arguments being considered or improvised. Specifically, they did not address the notion that *causal* explanations seem to be particularly important. That is, people seem to be particularly concerned about understanding causal relations (Heider, 1958). And we might speculate that counterattitudinal arguments that are causal in nature are likely to have stronger effects on subsequent attitudes than are other kinds of counterattitudinal arguments. It is also important to note that in Greenwald's work the opinions were very similar to social theories, whereas in others' work (e.g., Janis & Mann, 1965) the opinions were less theory-like.

Imagination

Some of the early work on emotional counterattitudinal role playing (e.g., Janis & Mann, 1965) suggested that imagined visual scenes may be causal in nature and may have strong effects on expectations and behavior.

More recent work has explicitly tested the effects of imagining scenes on expectations and behavior.

Self-judgments and social judgments concerning the likelihood of a person engaging in certain behaviors are based to a great extent on how easy it is to imagine the person doing the behaviors. There is a visual quality to many such judgments, as reflected in everyday language. Consider statements such as "I can't imagine myself doing (x)," or "I see myself doing (y) five years from now," or "It is difficult to visualize her doing (z) on her own."

Recent research suggests that imagining behavioral scenarios (i.e., multiple scene scripts) is used to make several kinds of probability judgments, including self-expectations (Anderson, 1983c; Anderson & Godfrey, in press; Gregory, Cialdini, & Carpenter, 1982; Sherman & Anderson, in press) and social expectations (Anderson & Godfrey, in press). In addition, imagining single scenes affects likelihood judgments about the self and others (Carroll, 1978; Sherman, Cialdini, Schwartzman, & Reynolds, 1985) and stereotype-based frequency estimates (Slusher & Anderson, 1987).

The determining factor seems to be the ease of imagining behaviors. To the extent that a particular behavioral scenario is easy to imagine, one judges the likelihood of the main characters in the scenario actually performing the behaviors to be relatively high. Thus, by inducing people to create such scenarios, thereby making them cognitively available, one can change likelihood estimates (expectations) about the main character, whether oneself or another (Anderson, 1983c; Anderson & Godfrey, in press). Similarly, because people imagine stereotype-congruent scenes when complete information is lacking and then confuse imagined features with presented ones, people's expectations and judgments about others tend to be biased in favor of the relevant stereotypes (Slusher & Anderson, 1987).

In summary, we have seen that causal beliefs (both verbal and imagined) can be important determinants of expectations, judgments, and behaviors. Of particular interest to the present discussion is the influence of causal beliefs on the handling of information, including the inference of cause–effect relations. Unfortunately, causal beliefs are not always valid, and effective validity criteria are not always applied. Further, there is a tendency to persist in erroneous beliefs despite contrary evidence, though recent research has given us some ideas about how to counteract this tendency. Because causal beliefs influence the selection of specific causes to explain specific outcomes, invalid beliefs can introduce bias into the selection process. So far we have discussed possible sources of bias in causal reasoning that might occur regardless of the context in which the causal judgments are made. We turn now to sources of bias specific to clinical practice.

Sources of Bias Specific to Clinical Practice

Just as causal beliefs can introduce bias into causal reasoning, so too can certain elements of clinical practice contribute to error. The therapy setting itself, client characteristics, and other therapists are among the variables that can bias thinking. Generally, such factors affect the derivation of causes, just as causal beliefs do, through their influence on expectations. In the following sections we will examine some of these factors. Again, our purpose is to raise awareness of the potential for bias. We hope that readers will go beyond the instances given here to search out other sources of bias, paying particular attention to idiosyncratic aspects of their own practice environments.

The Therapy Setting. Many features of the therapy setting can influence thinking about the likely causes of client problems or about the possible causes of desired changes. For example, if a client reports repeated failures at work and difficulty getting along with co-workers, then lack of motivation is one possible cause. But this potential cause may be more salient to inner-city practitioners than to others working in suburban settings, simply because of the setting. Of course, it may be that lack of motivation really *is* more common among the clients seen at some inner-city facilities, but thinking is biased if this cause is accepted too readily at the expense of overlooking other possible causes. Another problem is that the kinds of services most frequently provided in a given setting may become the most salient forms of treatment, possibly leading the therapist to define the client's treatment needs in terms of those services while overlooking less salient treatment alternatives (cf. Kadushin, 1969).

Client Characteristics and Unrepresentative Client Behaviors. Expectations about clients are affected by demographic variables (age, sex, race, ethnicity, marital status, education, occupation, and general socioeconomic status), the client's apparent desire for treatment (e.g., is treatment voluntary?), and his or her physical appearance (health, dress, and grooming). All of these factors can activate stereotypes and bias the therapist toward typical cause–effect relations. The causes that immediately come to mind when a 45-year-old man, happily married for 20 years, reports loss of interest in his marriage are likely to be quite different from those first thought of when a recently married 20-year-old reports the same problem. Similarly, available information from the client's past, such as recordings about client characteristics and previous diagnoses, if any, can lead the therapist too quickly to the conclusion that the current problems are repetitions of previous ones.

On the other hand, one striking but unrepresentative instance of behavior, directly observed, may bias thinking against information from the past. The observed instance may not be typical of the client's behavior. But being more concrete and vivid, it is more likely to make a strong impression and to be remembered easily than is more abstract information, such as that found in case records. Several studies of memory provide evidence that concrete information is more likely to be remembered than is abstract information (e.g., D'Agostino, O'Neill, & Paivio, 1977; Richardson, 1974). Further, social psychologists have demonstrated that concrete information has more impact on decisions than does abstract information (Borgida & Nisbett, 1977). Also, Anderson (1983d) found more perseverance of beliefs when they were based on concrete rather than abstract data. So one observation of a woman dramatically escalating conflict can overshadow more pallid recordings about repeated conflict avoidance, and a need for conflict may be judged a likely cause of her inability to keep friends. In all of these cases, bias arises from the practitioner's overdependence on generally useful guidelines. Certainly direct observations of current behavior are important. The problem stems from overweighting these observations despite less salient but, perhaps equally valid, data. Maybe the woman's major problems actually are more closely related to low self-esteem, which usually leads her to avoid conflict in an effort to retain her friends.

Therapy Modalities, Therapy Specializations, and Other Therapists. Therapy modalities (e.g., behavioral, humanistic, analytic) represent different theoretical approaches to understanding behavior and effecting behavior change. And theoretical approaches to behavior are, in large part, statements of cause–effect relations. There is danger, therefore, that causal explanations consistent with the therapist's own orientation will be so readily accepted that other possibilities are given insufficient consideration.

Closely related to biases arising from therapy modalities are those arising from therapy specializations. If one has acquired a reputation for successfully treating communication problems, then a client's communication style may receive an unfair share of one's attention.

Instructors, supervisors, colleagues, even famous therapists can contribute to bias in much the same way as therapy modalities and therapy specializations can, by providing strong statements about cause–effect relations. Practitioners may think back to something a respected teacher used to say, perhaps overestimating the relevance of the teacher's words to the judgment at hand.

The Clinician's Personal Experiences. Therapists are not immune to subjectivity. Biases originating within the therapist may be among the most difficult to recognize. One potential source of such biases is the therapist's personal psychological experiences. If the clinician once suffered from fear of rejection or has experienced anxiety over career decisions, then the causes of the clinician's own problem are likely to come to mind when clients with the same problem are encountered. Similarly, therapists can be biased by their experiences with former clients. Certain former clients and the causes of their problems may be especially memorable. If, for example, a former client's problem was constant teasing of others, and the teasing turned out to be an expression of hostility, then hostility may be immediately suspected when a new client teases constantly. The new client's lack of skill in expressing affection appropriately (another possible cause of the teasing) may be neglected.

To summarize, potential sources of bias specific to clinical practice include the therapy setting, client characteristics, striking but unrepresentative client behaviors, theoretical orientations, treatment specializations, other therapists, and the practitioner's personal experiences. These factors can cause biased causal reasoning chiefly through their effects on the therapist's expectations. If such errors were easily corrected by exposure to specific case data, then we would have somewhat less reason for concern. However, a large body of work from a variety of areas of psychology demonstrates that such expectation-based errors are extremely difficult to correct. New information may be sought and interpreted through expectation-confirmation processes (e.g., Lord et al., 1979; Snyder & Swann, 1978). Or the initial guess may get fixed and other information totally ignored (e.g., Anderson, 1983c; Shaklee & Fischhoff, 1982). Finally, there are numerous personal, situational, and social forces at work that tend to make initial expectations rigid. For instance, internal consistency pressures as well as social pressures to maintain group solidarity can interfere with rational inference change processes (e.g., Festinger, 1957; Janis, 1972).

Thus, the presence of these various sources of bias raises concern about the probability of error in judging the causes of behavior problems and finding the most likely route to adaptive behavior change. Practitioners should be alert to biasing influences in their own milieus and within themselves. Although awareness is a useful first step in reducing bias, much more can be done. In the remainder of this chapter we suggest a number of activities aimed at the development of bias-reducing thinking habits.

Bias-Reducing Procedures and Exercises

An effective general strategy for reducing bias in causal inference is to hypothesize more than one cause–effect relation. That is, for any given outcome consider as many possible causes as can be generated. Chamberlin (1897) first suggested the formulation of multiple working hypotheses as a means of avoiding bias in scientific inquiry, and scientists in fields as diverse as physics and psychology still value this method. As mentioned above, it has been proposed that in everyday causal inference people do, in fact, generate several causal candidates and then try to select the one that provides the best explanation for the outcome in question (Anderson, 1983b; Kruglanski, 1980). However, there is evidence that people tend to seize upon the first cause that provides a reasonable (though not necessarily the best) explanation and fail to complete a thorough search for alternatives (Shaklee & Fischhoff, 1982). The activities we will suggest for reducing bias in causal reasoning are designed to encourage the routine generation of alternative causes and the careful evaluation of alternatives. We will present our suggestions in the order that they might be used in making causal inferences.

Gathering Information

Generating as many causes as possible requires gathering as much information as possible. Reviewing case records, if any, and interviewing clients are the first steps. Further information might be gained by examining clients' functioning in all of their roles and in various settings. For example, if a man is having difficulty concentrating at work because he believes that his co-workers are plotting to destroy his career, then it would be useful to know if he has any similar suspicions about family members, friends, neighbors, and so on. Are there times at work when he is not bothered by such ideas? If so, what is distinctive about those times? How is he functioning in other roles, as a father, for example, or as a son? What information might be gained from the people in his various environments? It may be possible to interview some of these people or to observe the client in various settings.

Another approach to gathering information is to make separate assessments of the different aspects of the client's psychological functioning. Lazarus (1976), for example, suggests assessments of behavior, affect, sensation, imagery, cognition, interpersonal relations, and need for medication, as a means of both specifying problems and determining appropriate treatments.

In addition to these methods, we suggest that clinicians make a list of questions to ask themselves about each case. For instance, "What information is missing, and how might it be relevant?" or, "Have I given enough consideration to possible environmental constraints on the client's behavior?" Research has shown that attributing too much responsibility to the actor in a situation while discounting external factors is a common error. (See, for example, discussion of the "fundamental attribution error" in Nisbett & Ross, 1980; Ross & Anderson, 1982.) The list of questions should be reviewed and expanded periodically throughout the course of treatment. Such lists also could be reviewed in supervisory sessions or group training sessions.

After every effort has been made to collect as much relevant information as possible, there remains the problem of keeping that information available to the therapist as treatment proceeds. Because information can be forgotten, or remembered inaccurately, clinicians should not be dependent on their own memories. More efficient means of keeping data available are needed (cf. Arkes, 1981). Therapists should work on designing recording instruments that are systematic and not too time consuming. As an example, a chart could be made of the client's behaviors, listing specific statements and actions, with a column for recording the frequency of the behaviors on different occasions. More behaviors could be added as needed. Therapists should pay attention to occasions when the behaviors do not occur as well as occasions when they do. They also might share their recording methods with colleagues, who could try using them for their own cases. Then the advantages and the disadvantages of the various methods could be reviewed by all, and the best features of each method might be incorporated into some new recording instruments. Procedures such as these should help put practitioners in a better position to handle the next step in clinical causal inference: determining the causes of clients' problems and the most promising causes of change.

Determining Causal Relations

Recall that the general strategies underlying our suggestions are the generation of alternative causes for a given outcome (behavior problem or behavior change) and the effective evaluation of alternatives. In the following sections we will describe a number of activities designed to develop clinicians' abilities to generate and evaluate alternatives.

Multiple Judges. One way to generate alternative causes is to use multiple judges. That is, provide a group of clinicians with the available information from one case, and have each of them independently generate as many causes as possible for particular outcomes. Then participants could share the causes they have generated. If students are included in the group, the more experienced practitioners could be the last to share their ideas, as it is likely that they could generate some causes that students had not. The emphasis in this exercise would be not on thinking of *good* causes, but rather on generating as many *reasonable* causes as possible. Causes would first be shared without any explanation of how they had come to mind. After all participants had stated their causes, each could describe as far as possible how the causes were generated. Repeated use of this activity should help clinicians develop a more exploratory approach to considering available information.

Empathy. Another means of generating multiple causes is to apply one of the basic clinical tools, empathy. Looking at case data from another's point of view could lead the clinician to think of causes that would otherwise be overlooked. An obvious alternative perspective to try is that of the client. What would the client say about the cause(s) of the behavior problems? What does the client think might create the desired behavior changes? Assuming the client's perspective also could provide a challenge to the therapist's tentative causal theories. For example, if the therapist thinks the client's poor performance is due to lack of motivation, then taking the client's point of view could help make the therapist aware of what the client has tried to do about the problem and of how much effort the client has applied. After this exercise, the therapist might decide that the motivation factor is not as important as it had seemed to be. On the other hand, the exercise might provide support for the motivation–performance hypothesis. Other perspectives that clinicians might assume include those of the client's family members, friends, and co-workers; the clinician's various instructors, supervisors, and colleagues; and other therapists whose theoretical orientations differ from the clinician's own.

Recall that imagining behavioral scenarios can affect one's expectations, which may in turn affect one's causal explanations. Imagining scenarios related to the client's problems from different perspectives could give further insights into the etiology and possible resolution of the problems.

Role Playing. Assuming another person's perspective can be made a more vivid experience by actually acting out the role of the other person. Some clinicians have used role playing to help clients gain new perspectives. For instance, married couples in conflict might enact each other's role to improve their understanding of the other's point of view. Also, clients sometimes are able to change their behaviors, thinking, and affective reactions by acting out unfamiliar behaviors, as is done, for example, in assertiveness training. Similarly, role playing might help clinicians break away from their habitual approaches to causal judgments. As an example, pretending to be a therapist whose theoretical orientation is different from one's own could direct attention to information that might be neglected when reviewing evidence from one's own perspective. Attending to such information could, in turn, lead to the generation of alternative causal hypotheses that might otherwise have been overlooked.

Another way to use role playing would be to have a group of clinicians who know each other well generate alternative causes, with each participant approaching the problem as he or she thinks one of the others might. This would be followed by comments from other group members. This exercise could give clinicians insight into biases that they share with others in the group as well as their own idiosyncratic biases.

Videotapes. There are a number of ways to use videotapes of client interviews or of clients interacting with each other to reduce biases in causal reasoning. One simple method is for therapists to view a videotape and then simply reproduce (preferably in writing) as much information as they can recall. Then the film would be viewed again, and comparisons made between actual and recalled information. This could alert therapists to any inaccuracies in memory that might have resulted from biased perception or interpretation of data, the evidence on which any future causal inferences would be made. Recall could follow immediately after the first viewing, or after a delay (perhaps one week), or both. Generally, memory inaccuracies due to biases can be expected to increase over time.

Another way to use videotapes to improve causal reasoning is to have several therapists view the same tape, independently generate causes, and then share their conclusions. Alternatively, therapists could watch one film repeatedly, assuming a different perspective each time and generating causes from each perspective. Again, possible perspectives include those of other therapists, the client's family members, and so on.

Statistics. Courses in statistics are a routine part of the clinician's training. However, statistics often are viewed exclusively as research tools, and the potential for applying statistical logic to clinical judgments may be unrecognized. In causal inference problems the application of knowledge about concepts such as probability (e.g., consideration of base rates), correlation, and regression can help the clinician with the appropriate sampling and weighting of evidence and can prevent several kinds of errors in identifying causal factors. Use of base-rate information, for instance, can reveal how likely an outcome is (was) to occur regardless of the presence or absence of a particular hypothesized cause. An understanding of correlation can prevent the common error of inferring a causal relation when only covariance exists. And knowledge of regression can aid in evaluating the relevance of extreme behaviors and correctly identifying the causes of both extreme and more typical behaviors. A common error is to attribute a change from an extreme to a more typical behavior to an event immediately preceding the change; in fact, such a change frequently is due to normal regression toward the mean and is totally unrelated to the intervening event. (See Kahneman &

Tversky, 1973, for a discussion of this and related issues.) Because clinicians may fail to recognize the relevance of statistical concepts to their work with clients, it would be helpful to incorporate examples from clinical practice into statistics courses, to have the students provide examples, and to incorporate statistical thinking into clinical practica. Besides improving clinical judgments (including causal judgments), this procedure could increase interest in studying statistics.

Rating Scales. One way that use of rating scales can reduce bias in causal reasoning is by helping clinicians to resist the tendency to stereotype clients and to infer cause–effect relations that fit such stereotypes. For example, if many of the therapist's clients are very similar in some way (e.g., ethnicity, socioeconomic status) or have similar psychological problems, there might be a tendency to overlook a particular client's distinguishing characteristics or behaviors. This tendency could be counteracted by rating the client for similarities to and differences from typical clients encountered. Rather than one global similarity rating, multiple ratings of specific traits and behaviors should be made. Use of this procedure lessens the chance of hypothesizing an erroneous, stereotype-based causal relation. The need for alternative causes becomes more apparent.

Rating scales also could be used to lessen the tendency to think in terms of dichotomies. People tend to ask whether a potential cause was present or absent, or whether a factor caused or didn't cause an outcome. Use of rating scales might reveal that a potential cause was present *to some degree,* or that a particular factor had *some* but not *total* influence on the outcome. Again, the need to generate alternatives may be more easily recognized.

Balance Sheets. A balance sheet offers a systematic way to evaluate evidence for and against a hypothesis about the cause of a psychological problem. A balance sheet might list each item of evidence (pro and con), accompanied by ratings of various kinds. Balance sheets could be constructed for each of several causal hypotheses, so that the relative merit of each alternative could be assessed. Therapists could invent several different formats for balance sheets, share their inventions with colleagues, and try formats designed by others. Similarly, balance sheets could be used to evaluate one or more choices for treatment (i.e., proposed causes of behavior change).

Graphics. Graphics of several kinds (e.g., flowcharts, organization charts) can be used to illustrate hypothesized causal relations and to generate alternatives. Clinicians should be innovative in drawing graphic illustrations, perhaps using symbols to represent various kinds of relations and writing or drawing in several colors. Use of graphics can help clarify the relevance or centrality of a proposed cause to the outcome in question, possibly forcing implicit assumptions to be made explicit. Graphic illustrations also can help identify items of evidence that do not fit easily into the picture. Studying items that don't seem to fit might provide valuable insights and suggest alternative causal scenarios.

Graphics can be used to clarify the direction of causality in relations. For example, one might ask if a particular symptom is an effect, a cause, or both. Illustrations could help to identify relations that are unidirectional, bidirectional, or cyclical. They can reveal mediating causes, spurious correlations, or multiple causes of an outcome. They also can help to distinguish among predisposing, precipitating, and maintaining causes. Like other methods discussed earlier, use of graphics can help the clinician evaluate proposed causes of both problems and desired changes.

Questions. In the section on information gathering we suggested that clinicians make a list of questions to ask themselves as a means of assessing the adequacy of their data collection efforts. We suggest also that a list of questions concerning the generation and evaluation of causes be prepared and periodically updated. The list might include questions similar to the following:

Have I examined the problem from several perspectives?
Have I given careful thought to the direction of causality?
Have I considered the possibility of regression effects?
Have I given equal attention to each alternative cause?

Such questions can be used by clinicians individually and reviewed in consultation with others. Questions that cannot be answered satisfactorily indicate a need for further efforts to generate alternative causes or for more thorough evaluation of proposed causes.

Written Explanations. Putting hypothesized causal explanations into writing is an excellent way to clarify thinking about causal relations. Written explanations might delineate causes, effects, directions of causality, and other interrelations. They also should include the rationale behind the proposed causal hypotheses. In writing the explanations, vague ideas may become sharper, and ideas that remain vague may be discarded. This procedure could help clinicians identify faulty assumptions, logical errors, and inconsistencies. It could reveal gaps, such as missing data or unaccounted-for effects. Also, putting proposed causal relations into writing could bring to mind new alternative causes. In the case of several competing hypothesized causes, written explanations could help the clinician assess the relative worth of each. A therapist's written explanations could be reviewed by colleagues, whose objectivity might enable them to recognize any flaws that the therapist has overlooked.

In the preceding sections we have presented several methods for generating and evaluating alternative causes. As far as possible, clinicians should suspend final judgments (i.e., selecting specific causes for specific outcomes) until they have applied the methods that they believe will be helpful. Eventually, though, a decision will be made about the cause(s) of a particular outcome. And when a judgment is made, that judgment should be evaluated. In the next section we offer some suggestions for the evaluation of causal judgments.

Evaluating Causal Judgments

Even carefully made causal judgments can be inaccurate, and therefore, they should be questioned. Working alone, therapists can apply the counterexplanation procedure described above. That is, if the therapist thinks that X causes Y, then he or she should try to explain (perhaps in writing) why X might not cause Y; why Z, A, B, or C might cause Y. In other words, therapists should argue with themselves, questioning their own reasoning. Readers familiar with Ellis's rational-emotive therapy will notice a similarity between this method and Ellis's method of teaching clients to dispute the rationality of their dysfunctional beliefs (e.g., Ellis, 1977). In group sessions, the therapist's colleagues could help by providing additional counterexplanations. Group members also could take turns playing devil's advocate, raising every possible objection to the therapist's judgment. Recall that people appear to judge the validity of their theories by the relative availability of arguments for and against the theories. Once clinicians have made causal judgments, they have arguments *for* their theories. Use of counterexplanations and devil's advocates can expose them to arguments *against* the theories.

In the event that causal theories are shown to be inaccurate, instructors and supervisors can help clinicians resist tendencies to cling to the discredited theories by reminding them of the perseverance phenomenon and how it operates. (Ross et al., 1975, found that awareness of the mechanisms of perseverance can reduce the effect.) And there is yet another way that instructors can help their students. Most experienced clinicians can recall cases in which their own causal judgments were proven wrong. That is, they thought they understood the cause(s) of a client's problem, only to be surprised by the surfacing of an unexpected causal factor. Supervisors and instructors can probably give vivid examples from their own experiences to illustrate the folly of overconfidence in one's own causal inferences.

If a causal judgment seems quite satisfactory to a therapist, and colleagues can find no serious objections, the therapist still should continue to test the judgment against new evidence as it becomes available. Care should be taken to avoid overemphasizing evidence that confirms the causal theory or discounting conflicting evidence. The methods discussed above can be used to avoid these errors—for example, adding new evidence to balance sheets, graphic illustrations, or written explanations; testing the judgment for consistency with each alternative causal hypothesis.

Even if a causal judgment is correct, continued reevaluation is necessary, as the cause of a behavior problem can change over time. For example, a problem could be precipitated by one cause and maintained by another; or the problem could be maintained first by one cause and then by another. The same is true of the causes of desired behavior change. That is, a treatment strategy that is effective at one stage of therapy may need to be replaced at a later stage. So ongoing evaluation of causal judgments is a habit that should be firmly established.

Summary and Concluding Comments

In this chapter we have offered suggestions for reducing biases in clinical causal judgments, suggestions particularly designed to help clinicians become more aware of potential sources of bias and to acquire bias-reducing thinking habits. We first discussed both general sources of bias in causal reasoning and sources of bias specific to clinical practice. Then we described several bias-reducing procedures and exercises applicable to the various stages of causal inference: gathering information, determining causal relations, and evaluating causal judgments. We suggest that clinicians go beyond the present discussion to look for other potential sources of bias and to invent additional bias-reducing techniques.

We realize that use of the methods we have suggested may seem a bit excessive. Can clinicians really be expected to devote so much time to every causal judgment? Considering the consequences of erroneous judgments, we believe they should. Causal inference errors can decrease the probability of discerning true causal relations and can lead to the expenditure of much time and effort on ineffective interventions. Ultimately, such errors can lower therapy success rates. We believe the solution is extensive practice with methods such as these, so that the principles underlying them become internalized and resistance to biases becomes habitual. With practice, less biased causal judgments can become increasingly cost-effective.

Unfortunately, the efficacy of our suggestions has not been empirically tested in clinical settings. However, the suggestions are consistent with research findings about bias in causal reasoning. Clearly, more communication between clinicians and researchers is needed. Research in clinical settings could enhance our understanding of causal reasoning problems and provide practitioners with improved methods for handling complex causal judgments.

References

Anderson, C. A. (1982). Inoculation and counterexplanation: Debiasing techniques in the perseverance of social theories. *Social Cognition, 1,* 126–139.

______. (1983a). Motivational and performance deficits in interpersonal settings: The effect of attributional style. *Journal of Personality and Social Psychology, 45,* 1136–1147.

______. (1983b). The causal structure of situations: The generation of plausible causal attributions as a function of type of event situation. *Journal of Experimental Social Psychology, 19,* 185–203.

______. (1983c). Imagination and expectation: The effect of imagining behavioral scripts on personal intentions. *Journal of Personality and Social Psychology, 45,* 293–305.

______. (1983d). Abstract and concrete data in the perseverance of social theories: When weak data lead to unshakeable beliefs. *Journal of Experimental Social Psychology, 19,* 93–108.

______. (1985). Actor and observer attributions for different types of situations: Causal structure effects, individual differences, and the dimensionality of causes. *Social Cognition, 3,* 323–340.

Anderson, C. A., & Godfrey, S. (in press). Thoughts about actions: The effects of specifity and availability of imagined behavioral scripts on expectations about oneself and others. *Social Cognition.*

Anderson, C. A., & Jennings, D. L. (1980). When experiences of failure promote expectations of success: The impact of attributing failure to ineffective strategies. *Journal of Personality, 48,* 393–407.

Anderson, C. A., Jennings, D. L., & Arnoult, L. H. (1987). *The validity and utility of the attributional style construct at a moderate level of specificity.* Unpublished manuscript.

Anderson, C. A., & Kellam, K. L. (Manuscript in preparation). *Hypothetical explanation of social theories and evaluation of new data.*

Anderson, C. A., Lepper, M. R., & Ross, L. (1980). The perseverance of social theories: The role of explanation in the persistence of discredited information. *Journal of Personality and Social Psychology, 39,* 1037–1049.

Anderson, C. A., New, B. L., & Speer, J. R. (1985). Argument availability as a mediator of social theory perseverance. *Social Cognition, 3,* 235–249.

Anderson, C. A., & Sechler, E. S. (1986). Effects of explanation and counterexplanation on the development and use of social theories. *Journal of Personality and Social Psychology, 50,* 24–34.

Anderson, C. A., & Slusher, M. P. (1986). Relocating motivational effects: A synthesis of cognitive and motivational effects on attributions for success and failure. *Social Cognition, 4,* 270–292.

Arkes, H. R. (1981). Impediments to accurate clinical judgment and possible ways to minimize their impact. *Journal of Consulting and Clinical Psychology, 49,* 323–330.

Borgida, E., & Nisbett, R. (1977). The differential impact of abstract vs. concrete information on decisions. *Journal of Applied Social Psychology, 7,* 258–271.

Cantor, N., Smith, E., French, R., & Mezzich, J. (1980). Psychiatric diagnosis as prototype categorization. *Journal of Abnormal Psychology, 80,* 181–193.

Carroll, J. G. (1978). The effect of imagining an event on expectations for the event: An interpretation in terms of the availability heuristic. *Journal of Experimental Social Psychology, 14,* 88–96.

Chamberlin, T. C. (1897). Studies for students. *Journal of Geology, 5,* 837–848.

Chapman, L. J., & Chapman, J. P. (1967). Genesis of popular but erroneous psychodiagnostic observations. *Journal of Abnormal Psychology, 72,* 193–204.

______. (1969). Illusory correlations as an obstacle to the use of valid psychodiagnostic signs. *Journal of Abnormal Psychology, 74,* 271–280.

D'Agostino, P. R., O'Neill, B. J., & Paivio, A. (1977). Memory for pictures and words as a function of level of processing: Depth or dual coding? *Memory & Cognition, 5,* 252–256.

Ellis, A. (1977). The basic clinical theory of rational-emotive therapy. In A. Ellis & R. Grieger (Eds.), *Handbook of rational-emotive therapy.* New York: Springer.

Elms, A. C. (1967). Role playing, incentive, and dissonance. *Psychological Bulletin, 68,* 132–148.

Feather, N. T., & Simon, J. G. (1971a). Attribution of responsibility and valence of outcome in relation to initial confidence and success and failure of self and others. *Journal of Personality and Social Psychology, 18,* 173–188.

______. (1971b). Causal attributions for success and failure in relation to expectations of success based upon selective or manipulative control. *Journal of Personality, 39,* 527–541.

Festinger, L. (1957). *A theory of cognitive dissonance.* Stanford, CA: Stanford University Press.

Greenwald, A. G. (1968). Cognitive learning, cognitive response to persuasion, and attitude change. In A. G. Greenwald, T. C. Brock, & T. M. Ostrom (Eds.), *Psychological foundations of attitudes.* New York: Academic Press.

______. (1969). The open-mindedness of the counterattitudinal role player. *Journal of Experimental Social Psychology, 5,* 375–388.

______. (1970). When does role playing produce attitude change? Toward an answer. *Journal of Personality and Social Psychology, 16,* 214–219.

Greenwald, A. G., & Albert, R. D. (1986). Acceptance and recall of improvised arguments. *Journal of Personality and Social Psychology, 8,* 31–34.

Greenwald, A. G., Pratkanis, A. R., Leippe, M. R., & Baumgardner, M. H. (1986). Under what conditions does theory obstruct research progress? *Psychological Review, 93,* 216–229.

Gregory, W. L., Cialdini, R. B., & Carpenter, K. M. (1982). Self-relevant scenarios as mediators of likelihood estimates and compliance: Does imagining make it so? *Journal of Personality and Social Psychology, 43,* 89–99.

Harvey, J. H., Ickes, W. J., & Kidd, R. F. (Eds.) (1976). *New directions in attribution research* (Vol. 1). Hillsdale, NJ: Erlbaum.

______. (Eds.). (1978). *New directions in attribution research* (Vol. 2). Hillsdale, NJ: Erlbaum.

______. (Eds.). (1981). *New directions in attribution research* (Vol. 3). Hillsdale, NJ: Erlbaum.

Heider, F. (1958). *The psychology of interpersonal relations.* New York: Wiley.

Horowitz, L. M., Post, D. L., French, R., Wallis, K. D., & Siegelman, E. Y. (1981). The prototype as a construct in abnormal psychology: 2. Clarifying disagreements in psychiatric judgments. *Journal of Abnormal Psychology, 90,* 575–585.

Janis, I. L. (1972). *Victims of groupthink.* Boston: Houghton Mifflin.

Janis, I. L., & Mann, L. (1965). Effectiveness of emotional role-playing in modifying smoking habits and attitudes. *Journal of Experimental Research in Personality, 1,* 84–90.

Jennings, D. L. (1980). Effects of attributing failure to ineffective strategies. *Dissertation Abstracts International, 408,* 5461B. (University Microfilms No. 80–11, 654)

Jones, E. E., & Davis, K. E. (1965). From acts to dispositions. In L. Berkowitz (Ed.), *Advances in experimental social psychology* (Vol. 2). New York: Academic Press.

Jones, E. E., & Nisbett, R. E. (1972). The actor and the observer: Divergent perceptions of the causes of behavior. In E. E. Jones, D. E. Kanouse, H. H. Kelley, R. E. Nisbett, S. Valins, & B. Weiner (Eds.), *Attribution: Perceiving the causes of behavior.* Morristown, NJ: General Learning Press.

Kadushin, C. (1969). *Why people go to psychiatrists.* New York: Atherton.

Kahneman, D., & Tversky, A. (1973). On the psychology of prediction. *Psychological Review, 80,* 237–251.

Kelley, H. H. (1967). Attribution theory in social psychology. In D. Levine (Ed.), *Nebraska Symposium on Motivation.* Lincoln: University of Nebraska Press.

Kiesler, C. A., Nisbett, R. E., & Zanna, M. P. (1969). On inferring one's beliefs from one's behavior. *Journal of Personality and Social Psychology, 11,* 321–327.

Koriat, A., Lichtenstein, S., & Fischhoff, B. (1980). Reasons for confidence. *Journal of Experimental Psychology: Human Learning and Memory, 6,* 107–118.

Kruglanski, A. W. (1980). Lay epistemo-logic—process and contents: Another look at attribution theory. *Psychological Review, 87,* 70–87.

Lazarus, A. A. (1976). Multimodal behavior therapy: Treating the BASIC ID. In A. A. Lazarus (Ed.), *Multimodal behavior therapy.* New York: Springer.

Lord, C. G., Lepper, M. R., & Preston, E. (1984). Considering the opposite: A corrective strategy for social judgment. *Journal of Personality and Social Psychology, 47,* 1231–1243.

Lord, C., Ross, L., & Lepper, M. R. (1979). Biased assimilation and attitude polarization: The effects of prior theories on subsequently considered evidence. *Journal of Personality and Social Psychology, 37,* 2098–2109.

McGuire, W. J. (1968). The nature of attitudes and attitude change. In G. Lindzey & E. Aronson (Eds.), *The handbook of social psychology* (Vol. 3). Reading, MA: Addison-Wesley.

Monson, T. C., & Snyder, M. (1977). Actors, observers, and the attribution process: Toward a reconceptualization. *Journal of Experimental Social Psychology, 13,* 89–111.

Nisbett, R., & Ross, L. (1980). *Human inference: Strategies and shortcomings of social judgment.* Englewood Cliffs, NJ: Prentice-Hall.

Richardson, J. T. E. (1974). Imagery and free recall. *Journal of Verbal Learning and Verbal Behavior, 13,* 709–713.

Ross, L., & Anderson, C. A. (1982). Shortcomings in the attribution process: On the origins and maintenance of erroneous social assessments. In D. Kahneman, P. Slovic, & A. Tversky (Eds.), *Judgment under uncertainty: Heuristics and biases.* New York: Cambridge University Press.

Ross, L., Lepper, M. R., & Hubbard, M. (1975). Perseverance in self perception and social perception: Biased attributional processes in the debriefing paradigm. *Journal of Personality and Social Psychology, 32,* 880–892.

Shaklee, H., & Fischhoff, B. (1982). Strategies of information search in causal analysis. *Memory and Cognition, 10,* 520–530.

Sherman, R. T., & Anderson, C. A. (in press). Decreasing premature termination from psychotherapy. *Journal of Social and Clinical Psychology.*

Sherman, S. J., Cialdini, R. B., Schwartzman, D. F., & Reynolds, K. (1985). Imagining can heighten or lower the perceived likelihood of contracting a disease: The mediating effect of ease of imagery. *Personality and Social Psychology Bulletin, 11,* 118–127.

Snyder, M., & Swann, W. B. (1978). Behavioral confirmation in social interaction: From social perception to social reality. *Journal of Experimental Social Psychology, 14,* 148–162.

Slovic, P., & Fischhoff, B. (1977). On the psychology of experimental surprises. *Journal of Experimental Psychology: Human Perception and Performance, 3,* 544–551.

Slusher, M. P., & Anderson, C. A. (1987). When reality monitoring fails: The role of imagination in stereotype maintenance. *Journal of Personality and Social Psychology, 52,* 653–662.

Temerlin, M. K. (1968). Suggestion effects in psychiatric diagnosis. *Journal of Nervous and Mental Disease, 147,* 349–353.

Weiner, B. (1974). *Achievement motivation and attribution theory.* Morristown, NJ: General Learning Press.

———. (1982). The emotional consequences of causal attributions. In M. S. Clark & S. T. Fiske (Eds.), *Affect and cognition: The 17th Annual Carnegie Symposium on Cognition.* Hillsdale, NJ: Erlbaum.

———. (1985). An attributional theory of achievement motivation and emotion. *Psychological Review, 92,* 548–573.

Weiner, B., & Handel, S. (1985). Anticipated emotional consequences of causal communications and reported communication strategy. *Developmental Psychology, 21,* 102–107.

Weiner, B., Russell, D., & Lerman, D. (1979). The cognition–emotion process in achievement-related contexts. *Journal of Personality and Social Psychology, 37,* 1211–1220.

11 Judgment, Inference, and Reasoning in Clinical Perspective

Robert R. Holt

HERE I am, a judgmentalist called to sit in judgment and to be judged, a student of evaluation asked to evaluate the work of other such students and in turn to be evaluated by book reviewers and readers. Nothing could be more appropriate, from the standpoint I have been urging for some years: Judgment is an inevitable as well as desirable and necessary, albeit humanly frail, process, hence one that should be studied and improved, not merely condemned for its errors.

Happily, as the research assiduously collated here testifies, a good many psychologists and others have indeed been busily at work studying judgment and related processes, many of them inspired by the emerging framework of information processing. The contributors to this volume have collected a great body of research and have supplied many hypotheses about ways the phenomena studied may apply to cognitive processes of the diagnostician and therapist. I previously knew little or nothing about a lot of this work, and suspect that practicing clinicians may be similarly enlightened. The present book offers an opportunity to see what has been learned from a perspective undreamed of half a century ago, when the controversy over clinical and statistical prediction started up. When this controversy came to its first great culmination, the index of Meehl's (1954) masterly review contained no entries for *information processing, cognitive science, heuristics,* not even for *computers*!

The result of this attention given to the process of judgment has been good. With this book, the topic of clinical and statistical prediction moves to a new level of sophistication and, I believe, more productive discussion. For the first few decades after the primary works (Allport, 1942; Horst et al., 1941; Meehl, 1954), the literature was dominated by a series of relatively sterile demonstrations—mostly demonstrations that clinicians without special training in the difficult and specialized task of predicting behavior (or future judgments about people) don't do a very good job and that increasingly sophisticated, mechanical-statistical, predictive systems were being designed.

Much of the early polemical writing stated or implied that human clinical judgment was a messy anachronism shortly to be displaced by neat formulas. Oddly enough, though, despite the dominance of this school of thought in many universities and other training centers, and despite the growing availability of microcomputers capable of ingenious and complex computational feats with large data bases, the mechanists' dream has not come true. Recent generations of clinical psychologists have a trained iconoclastic attitude that many an old-timer would call anticlinical, yet they have found themselves using clinical judgment constantly in most aspects of their work because there simply are no formulas in existence.

Happily, this book largely takes for granted that clinical psychology is and remains a judgmental realm. Subjective cognitive operations, whether called *attribution, thinking, information processing, inference,* or *clinical judgment,* occupy a great part of the practicing psychologist's time—as well as that of most physicians, including but by no means limited to psychiatrists—and that of many other human service professionals. We have long known how difficult it is to do this kind of cognitive work well; now, thanks to a variety of scattered lines of research that have been helpfully surveyed and summarized here, we are beginning to see, in some concrete detail, what kinds of pitfalls await the unwary. An increase in wariness stimulated by books like this one may help the next generation of clinicians to function more effectively. If so, that should ultimately redound to the decrease of human suffering and the promotion of health and happiness.

It won't do so automatically, however. As usual, diagnosis is easier than treatment. Here I must point out an irony that should have a sobering effect upon all of us. The authors have illustrated or demonstrated for us, in the very act of reflecting about the cognitive errors against which they warn, many of these same defects in judgment and reasoning. There could hardly be a more convincing demonstration that learning about a phenomenon does not suffice to protect against it in ourselves. Yet one of the big lessons of recent advances in cognitive science is that we must apply problem-solving strategies to ourselves: we must decenter, or learn to get out of strange loops by going to a meta-level (Hofstadter, 1979). I shall begin, therefore, by reviewing some of the main themes of the book, attempting to apply these strategies to the very chapters that deal with these issues.

Some Cognitive Errors Exemplified

Expectancy Effects and the Need for Cost/Benefit Analysis

In the initial overview chapter, the third paragraph warns that

> Many judgments are made before the clinician and client have met for the first time. A clinician's initial encounter with a client is influenced by his or her preconceptions and prior expectations. For example, one of the most basic expectations of clinicians is that they will observe pathology. This expectancy may reduce judgmental accuracy, or at least introduce systematic biases in the direction of overestimating pathology.

The same point applies to the initial contact of reader and author. Here, in the paragraph preceding the one I have quoted, the reader has been led to expect to observe error in clinical judgment, the functional equivalent of pathology, by the mention of *pitfalls, human biases,* and *cognitive limitations* with no counterbalancing reference to any of the desirable or beneficial aspects of human judgment. This paragraph also makes one question the expectations with which the contributors were chosen and the literature reviewed, a process that perhaps introduced systematic biases in the direction of overestimating the *pathology* of clinical judgment.

You may well ask what harm there is in that. Is there no place for a book that raises alarms and points to dangers? Must every critique be compulsively balanced by praise? Certainly not, but balance is not always compulsive; it can and should be judicious. And it does not seem too much to hope for judiciousness in a book on human judgment.

The implicit objective of the present book is to affect the practice of the mental health disciplines, thus, ultimately, to bring about social change. In the realm of public policy, no acceptable substitute has yet been found for a complete cost/benefit analysis of any proposed change, one that balances the good and the bad of what exists against the likely good *and* bad of what is proposed. The usual political approach to policy change relies instead upon rhetoric: it stresses what is bad about current practices and highlights the benefits promised by the proposed change. Rhetoric works, hence it continues to surround us; but as scientists, we should beware of slipping into it when our intent is to inform, not to win arguments.

At this point, I notice that I am presenting primarily the drawbacks of rhetoric, myself making a case by rhetorical devices. Let me take note of the fact that, like the authors of other chapters in this book, I am an advocate as well as a scientist. Rhetoric not only is the natural language of advocacy but also was the predecessor of the scientific method as an attempt at disciplined thought and the pursuit of truth. Yet an enlightened advocate does not want to win by whatever means work, without regard to the side effects. (There you have a small exercise in self-observation and the attempt to take one's own advice, incidentally demonstrating that it is possible to do so even if difficult to sustain.)

Perhaps I can make my point about cost/benefit analysis clearer by reference to a specific instance, the "pseudopatient" study by Rosenhan (1973), which was cited favorably by Turk, Salovey, and Prentice (Chapter 1 of this volume). That exercise demonstrated the reliance of everyday working clinicians on shortcuts, heuristics, and other assimilative methods of coping with heavy work loads. In such a state of affairs, it is easy to show that diagnostic errors can be and undoubtedly are made. Whenever a person relies on a base rate, or on the continuation of a strong correlation between a sign and a clinical syndrome, you have a setup for anyone who wants to fool the practitioner by deliberately breaking the expected links through the use of manufactured data. A sane person *can* present himself to a state hospital complaining of auditory hallucinations, and be admitted as schizophrenic; does it follow that any specifiable proportion of patients on our psychotic wards must be sane? Not at all. What is worse, however, is that those who staged this charade seem to have given no thought to the social costs of the implicit alternative: an intake/diagnostic/discharge procedure proof against such ecologically implausible errors as someone's trying to bluff her way into being committed and then demanding to be released. Granted, diagnosticians can develop slovenly habits of working; is that any great discovery? Did the investigators weigh the benefits of holding inadequate personnel up to public scorn against the harm done, for example, by decreasing public trust and faith in the professionals to whom people must entrust their psychopathologically suffering relatives?

The position of conservatives has always been, "Go slow on criticizing what exists; it must be there for a good reason. Your newfangled schemes will probably do more harm than good." Anything but a political conservative myself, I don't wish to be misunderstood as advocating a similar foot-dragging approach in the present scientific and professional area. Where there are known errors in contemporary policy or practice and no obvious pitfalls in a promising alternative, my prejudice is always to experiment rather than stand pat. We must strive to take our prejudices, however, and to restrain rash enthusiasm by prudent methods of taking into account the full spectrum of risks and benefits in both the old and the new.

Carried to its logical optimum, a risk (or cost)/benefit analysis becomes a decision analysis, well explained and illustrated by Elstein in his altogether exemplary chapter: "Decision analysis can help. . . by requiring decision-makers to be explicit about perceived benefits and risks of all options and by offering a technique for combining competing risks and benefits."

Therefore, when someone points out a flaw in a prevailing method of clinical procedure, one of the first questions to ask is: How *serious* is the danger? It pains me to report that, with the notable exception of Elstein, few of this book's contributors seem to have asked that question, in their zeal to discover more possible sources of error. Consider, for example, the chapter our editors themselves have contributed, on the effects of mood on the memory and judgment of clinicians. They have assembled a number of interesting experimental demonstrations that "clinicians *may* [emphasis added] be more likely to recall and therefore inquire about issues consistent with their current moods." That is not obvious and is surely worth knowing—*if and only if* the effect can be demonstrated to be clinically significant. Yet I searched the chapter in vain for any indication of effect size. If a phenomenon can be shown, under laboratory conditions, to be statistically reliable, then admittedly it could be true in the consulting room and might have unwanted effects. Even so, one could form a slightly better idea about how seriously to take the danger if some idea had been conveyed of the proportion of subjects in any given study who showed the effect, especially the number for whom it was large enough to support a plausible extrapolation to clinical practice.

Heuristics and Biases

The editors begin their chapter on the effects of affects (Chap. 6) with a concrete though hypothetical example about a clinician whose moods are said to have marked and clinically significant influences on his diagnostic and therapeutic activity. Their declared intent is merely to illustrate how various experimentally demonstrated effects *might* operate in the working situation. Yet, they present a worst-case scenario as if it were the norm; and the work of Tversky and Kahneman (1974) on the availability heuristic teaches us the danger of such a device. By making the possibility of undemonstrated extrapolations concrete and visualizable, one biases the reader's subjective estimation of the probability of such effects.

Another frequently encountered heuristic, with obvious dangers of introducing bias, is the seeking of order through the procrustean means of imposed dichotomies. In his philosophical chapter, Mahoney often makes use of it. Take his initial contrast of "traditional" realism and rationalism: the attempt to fit the great variety of ontologies into a dichotomy "may be oversimplifying the matter," he admits; but the damage to clear conceptualization is more serious than that. Many a reader may get the impression that a sophisticated modern realism could not exist or would have the same difficulties as the kind Mahoney calls *traditional.* The constructivist approach that he favors is far from the only available alternative to his dichotomy. Again, though realists and rationalists are initially presented as antithetical, in Mahoney's Table 1 we find them combined, now pitted against "developmentalists" in another dichotomy.

Cognitive Effects of Philosophical Commitments

I applaud the inclusion of a philosophical chapter, as for some time I have believed that the underlying source of disagreement in the clinical–statistical controversy is not in the facts but in the assumptions held by irreconcilable antagonists (Holt, 1970, 1978a,b). Those who have read my own brief attempt to elucidate the metaphysical issues (Holt, 1986) will recognize that I see them quite differently from Mahoney. There is of course no point in arguing about one's axioms; they are matters of volitional decision, made at a level unaffected by disputation.

In my preferred terminology, Mahoney's position is a form of contextualism, which is an advance over the simpler views he opposes and a more adequate metaphysical base for psychology than idealism or mechanism. Nevertheless, it has the disadvantage of being committed to relativism and having difficulty in accounting for the enduring structure of reality—problems not shared by systems philosophy (see below).

Overgeneralization and the Problem of Sampling

In a content area long dominated by the dogma of immaculate perception, it was theoretically important to demonstrate (as Salovey and Turk do in Chap. 6) that moods can have measurable effects on cognitive processes once thought to be autonomous and impervious. That is what is accomplished by a statistically significant result obtained under carefully controlled conditions. In the real world of the clinic, however, the same phenomenon may be negligible.

Arnoult and Anderson begin their chapter by a statement that "recent research provides evidence that biased thinking is prevalent among both novices and experienced practitioners," citing seven references. Are these references to studies that systematically assessed the thinking of random, representative samples of the population of (presumably, contemporary American) neophyte and experienced practitioners of clinical profession(s)? No, the referenced researchers all used as their subjects available samples of clinical psychologists and psychiatrists, drawn by methods that do not allow rational extension to practitioners at large. The evidence generated, therefore, does not support the conclusion that "biased thinking is *prevalent* among practitioners" (emphasis added).

Likewise, the research on the so-called illusory correlation demonstrates only the fact that clinicians tend to use projective test data in "theory-driven" ways, not that they thereby commit errors, since the validity of their theories has rarely if ever been satisfactorily tested. Jorden, Harvey, and Weary (Chap. 5) also cite the Rosenthal effect as if it were regularly true that experimenters find what they expect and as if there had not been a great many unsuccessful attempts to replicate Rosenthal's original findings.

Chicken Little was not hallucinating; something did fall from the sky onto her head. Her error was to generalize imprudently. The story is memorable partly because the generalization was so ridiculous and her followers so credulous; but then, barnyard animals are not trained in the scientific method. Turk and Salovey's authors do not generalize so grandiosely, and probably no more incautiously than their peers; moreover, I have no doubt that their education in the scientific method was as good as they could get. Some years ago (Holt, 1973), I noted how widespread is this anomaly: excellent, well-trained researchers who perform elegant experiments often seem to lose much of their scientific caution in generalizing their findings—in the Discussion section. The most plausible hypothesis I have been able to come up with is that their scientific training took them only to the end of Results and quit there, as if the whole job had been done by teaching how to ward off threats to internal validity without concern for external validity. We have to begin teaching our students the basic rules of drawing implications from scientific findings! Not an easy task, since there was not much methodological literature about it before the publication of Cook and Campbell (1979; see also Holt, 1978a). I should like to add that, in this book, a notable exception to the tendency to overgeneralize is Elstein, whose chapter contains a valuable section on the validity of research findings from the point of view of generalizability or external validity.

An error related to overgeneralizing is accepting purported evidence uncritically. In this book, as in so many others, one finds extensive *cita-*

tions of research, but very little critical consideration of the varying probative utility of the evidence provided. I have read only a small proportion of the hundreds of papers and books cited, but even that small sample includes several investigations I consider seriously flawed. It is hard to resist the interpretation that when a finding fits one's preconceptions or one's need of the moment, critical judgment tends to be set aside.

Such was the conclusion of Mahoney's (1977) study of journal referees, whose methodological objections seemed predictable largely by the degree to which papers' findings agreed with their own predilections. All of us (I wildly generalize), regardless of our level of experience and training, are vulnerable to wishful thinking. We accept purported demonstrations of what we already believe much too uncritically and generalize it much too incautiously. I am grateful to Snyder and Thomsen for informing me, in a generally excellent chapter, about Mahoney's study, and hope that every reader of this book will carry away its lesson in the need for self-discipline.

Attributional Biases

Jordan, Harvey, and Weary's chapter is a useful compilation of suggestive findings from the vast literature of attribution research, a good set of hypotheses many of which are plausible, but may be limited by not being backed up by relevant data. These authors also attribute clinicians' great tendency to explain behavior intrapsychically (or, as they put it, in *trait* terms) to biases growing out of the actor–observer difference. Note that in doing so, they themselves exemplify the tendency to account for behavior by attributing it to a characteristic of the actor rather than looking for situational causes.

Perhaps the current emphasis on situational determination of behavior, a valuable supplement if not carried to extremes (as by Mischel, 1968), will help clinicians realize that any attempt to predict behavior from no matter how intensive and accurate a study of the individual must be inherently limited by the lack of information about critical determinants of behavior in the larger systems of which this person is a part. (That is my restatement of Einhorn's point that clinicians typically err in trying to predict too much instead of accepting the error obviously entailed by a simple formula which seems to pay attention to too little.)

It is worth noting, however, that mental illness may be virtually defined as behavior that is (or seems) unresponsive or not appropriately responsive to the person's environment and the occasions of everyday life. Much more than its normal counterpart, abnormal behavior is *trait behavior*, determined by intrapersonal factors. Professionals who devote their careers to studying the mentally disturbed can be expected to lose sight of the great dependence of normal behavior on its setting and context, unless—like behavior therapists—they have been extensively trained to believe in the control of behavior by "stimuli."

Overall Comments

Our volume, in using as its data base the predominantly experimental literature of the past 15 years, incurs that literature's remarkable lack of historical and cross-cultural perspective and its corresponding lack of attention to effects of emotion and motivation on thought or information processing (Sorrentino & Higgins, 1986). When I edited a book on *Emotions and Thought* a couple of decades ago (Holt, 1968), a rich body of experimental and clinical-observational data was available, presenting many striking effects of motivation, emotions, and defenses on such processes as perception, inference, and judgment, effects about which the present book is silent. That whole area is represented here only by one chapter on effects of experimentally evoked moods on judgments and inferences. One would hardly guess that clinicians as well as patients are vulnerable to the tendencies to maximize what is pleasing and self-confirmatory and to minimize whatever threatens important values.

Another important stream of work which I miss here explores the inexhaustible variety of individual differences in information processing, the area that my late colleague George Klein (1970) called *cognitive style.* Inspired by Rapaport's teaching about diagnostic testing, much of our research agenda during two fruitful decades at the Research Center for Mental Health was devoted to elucidating how people differ in their ways of inputting information and processing it to form percepts, memories, judgments, attributions, inferences, and so forth. Klein and colleagues (see, for example, Gardner, Holzman, Klein, Linton, & Spence, 1959) found not only a great range on either side of population mean tendencies, but many reliable techniques of predicting a person's inclination (for example) to level out differences in an informational domain or to sharpen distinctions among differences (Holzman, 1954), to conceptualize in broad or in narrow categories (Gardner, 1953), to narrow awareness and keep experiences discrete or allow them to interpenetrate (Schlesinger, 1954), and other cognitive control principles.

Let me remind you also of the work of Witkin and his collaborators (1954, 1962) on what they originally called *field-dependence,* later *psychological differentiation.* There even exists some literature on the implications of cognitive styles for diagnostic and prognostic judgments (e.g., Austrian, 1976/1977; Cooper, 1967; Winkler, 1981/1982; Wolitzky, 1973).

These beginnings could be greatly extended if the people who are working actively on inferential and judgmental processes would take them into account. I believe that this neglected body of literature has a great deal to offer theoretically also. Social and cognitive psychology tends to share with experimental mainstream psychology too great a preoccupation with the general case, a tendency that perhaps originated in a desire to discover general laws of nature.

It is striking how much evidence is cited in several of the chapters indicating the widespread belief that one can test hypotheses by the logically flawed means of seeking confirmation, when the only sure way of gaining knowledge is to disconfirm prior conjectures (Popper, 1962). To be sure, there is a joker in Popper's deck, the little word *sure.* He writes as if knowledge consists only of universally valid propositions, whereas the very nature of the human sciences requires that they deal in probabilistic, not absolute, truths. Everyone ought to know that there are exceptions to virtually any generalization in psychology, and that the best we can hope for is statistical, not nomological laws; yet I constantly encounter colleagues whose methodological position implies the search for hard, universally valid laws. In this book, the authors frequently write as if the conclusions of the studies they cite *are* universally applicable. To take an example almost at random, "A great deal of evidence indicates that therapists exhibit a general tendency to form initial impressions of clients *very* quickly" (Snyder & Thomsen, p. 131). *All* therapists? *Any* clients? The authors would probably hasten to deny that they intended such sweeping statements, and might even say that the qualification of their statement is obvious though implicit. I simply wish to state my conviction that it should be more explicit.

Thus, it would have been helpful if more of the chapters had contained warnings that such phenomena as *behavioral confirmation* (the tendency of patients to behave in ways that confirm therapists' expectations) are by no means universal and that the discovery of such trends is merely the beginning of knowledge. The fact that they apply only to a majority of the instances studied poses a challenge: Can we find ways of distinguishing the positive from the negative cases, either in some attributes of the persons involved, in some aspect of situation, or in properties of their interactions? Snyder and Thomsen do report some research of this kind, but more is urgently called for if the challenging hints and hypotheses with which this book is rife are to become clinically useful.

For a good many years, we have known better than to make the naive assumption that the central tendency of a small group of available experimental subjects represents anything like a law of human nature, even a statistical one. People can, in a truly astonishing variety of ways, organize their worlds, solve problems, come to conclusions, and so forth, and we are only beginning to get an idea of the subtle and profound cognitive differences across the world's contemporary cultures (not to mention those of bygone eras).

Consider the controversy over Whorf's (1950) celebrated thesis, that language has a far-reaching determinative influence on thought (see Kluckholn, 1954). Human beings speak a huge number of tongues that linguists have grouped into several quite unrelated families. These languages categorize experience along such different dimensions that it is often impossible to find word-to-word equivalences (or translations) across languages from mutually alien cultures. Nevertheless, undoubtedly some psychological laws are applicable to all cultures. Only a beginning has been made toward mapping them, but meanwhile it behooves us not to ignore the little that is known about the other (non–United States) 95 percent of humankind!

As we develop more knowledge about the errors to which human judgment is prone, it helps us to understand the difference between natural and artificial intelligence (AI). That is a necessary bit of knowledge, because though the latter is free of certain biases and vulnerabilities, it is markedly lacking in common sense and other, as yet vaguely defined, attributes that constitute good clinical judgment. Even so, expert systems offer an immediately useful adjunct to the clinician, and should be *cautiously* encouraged. They should be kept off the unrestricted general market, at least for a while: We need more intensive study and discussion of the ethical problems they raise, and we need to learn how to train clinicians to use these systems effectively and wisely, not just lean on them.

One distinct possibility is that artificial intelligence differs from natural, human intelligence—especially that form we call *judgment*—in lacking affect. Such basic judgments as "this place is safe," "this person can be trusted," or "this thing seems good to eat" are all evaluations based on emotional responses, with obvious implications for survival and hence for natural selection. None of them can be programmed in such a fashion as: "If cues a, b, . . . x are present, approach, lift corners of mouth, and emit words 'like wow, fantastic!' " It would not be difficult to program a robot to simulate phony, merely enacted affect (ironically, an otherwise purely human or at least simian response), but it would add nothing to the purely cognitive part of the algorithm, its beginning. When Freud (1900/1953, chap. 7) noted that affect cannot be eliminated from effective, adaptive thought, only restricted to a minimal signaling function, he implicitly recognized that there is a simple but profound biological wisdom in our emotional reactions, which give color and depth to Yes! and No! Without them, we all too easily find ourselves in the obsessive's dilemma, counting items on lists of pluses and minuses, beset with doubts about whether their weights have been properly calculated and unable to make simple decisions. Such homely basic elements are major constituents of common sense, that elusive, intuitive possession of humble, limited human beings that supercomputers wholly lack. This affective component of judgment is the experiential repository of countless ancestral generations, stretching back to our prehuman mammalian forebears, their evolutionary legacy to our ability to survive in an ever-changing, unpredictable world.

Yet (as noted above) I found this book disappointing in its all-too-meager treatment of the many ways in which emotions can disrupt and dislocate thought. We say of the impetuous lover, the manic over-enthusiast, the panicky seller, or the enraged recipient of an insult, "They lost their heads," recognizing that intense affect usually overwhelms normal judgment and precipitates decisions that can be disastrous. Experimental research about such phenomena has not been done, because it is not ethically feasible to arouse such passions in the laboratory. Yet it is important to consider them anyway, as not only matters of general knowledge but the most important instances of a phenomenon under scientific scrutiny, even though they have not been replicated under conventionally controlled conditions.

Notice the paradox: The very way in which human judgment excels AI is also its greatest vulnerability. There is an important lesson here, and it can be summed up in a caution: *For every type of error found, consider the possibility that it results from a human capacity with important adaptive advantages.* If that were not the case, any consistent tendency to cognitive error would probably be eliminated through natural selection. The tragic flaw in human nature, but also its glory, is that we are *not* machines, not even computers of extraordinary complexity, but organisms. Without our capacity to be crazy we would not be creative; without susceptibility to despair we could not know ecstasy. Perhaps some of the very ways in which our rationality is normally bounded make genius possible.

All of which is not to suggest that the appropriate response for a psychologist is a reverent helplessness. I have little patience with those who feel that wisdom, for instance, is such a precious gift that it must remain unexamined. To suggest that there may be severe limits on what can be learned about human inference and judgment by attempts to program them on computers only means that we must redouble the ingenuity with which we study them in other ways. We will do well not to limit ourselves to the laboratory, but to make judicious use of clinical and naturalistic observation as well and to draw selectively on the wealth of suggestive ideas contributed by philosophers, literary critics, and other humanistic scholars, for hypotheses to be tested as rigorously as possible. Disciplined thought, which is not the exclusive domain of scientists, has a similar structure and uses similar means regardless of the thinker's academic department (Holt, 1961).

Here is another example of the paradox: In an average expectable environment of clinical practice, it probably *is* adaptive to process data in an assimilative way, and in a busy practice with case-finding (or sampling) methods that do not change much, it probably does not lead to many serious errors. I found Snyder and Thomsen's discussion of this point convincing—no doubt in part because I already believed it. Yet such procedures can and at times do get us into trouble, which makes a case for backing up diagnostic clinicians by expert systems or some other such nonjudgmental or at least automated device. I am less convinced that clinicians need to make radical changes in their ways—not until we have a lot more evidence that what *could* be true *is* true and that alternative methods do not have other, unsuspected, and possibly even more deleterious consequences. For it is a great and by now avoidable mistake to assume that if an existing method has flaws that can be obviated by an alternative, the latter is automatically to be preferred. It should be common knowledge by now and part of the assumptive base of all professionals in human service and public policy that, as R. K. Merton (1936/1976) long ago observed, all purposive social acts are likely to have unanticipated consequences, often as deleterious as the evils they were designed to correct. (For example, the Aswan dam was built to increase the supply of water for irrigation, but brought about a proliferation of snails and a consequent scourge of bilharziasis.)

That in turn follows from the systems point of view: human behavior takes place in complex social systems and is a function of system effects that are difficult even to notice, much less to predict. A contrary (and by now dangerously) anachronistic viewpoint of nineteenth-century mechanism shows up in the seemingly innocent substitution of the term *stimulus* for *information.* If the orientation is indeed to be that of information processing, it should be clear that a bit/byte of information is not defined in the same way as a stimulus even though it may initiate or alter a sequence of behaviors. By the same token, an information-processing network cannot process *stimuli.* They are indeed inappropriate leftovers, linguistic clues to the writer's previous incarnation as a stimulus–response behaviorist. It takes more than the mastery of a new vocabulary and set of formulas to enter the new information age. Ultimately, in my opinion, it requires a study and embrace of the systems point of view (see, for example, Laszlo, 1972).

Implications for Training Clinicians

We must not forget that any book devoted to criticism of prevailing clinical processes and practices inevitably finds itself in the realm of public policy. This book is being written at a time when the American system of caring for the ill is in profound crisis. It is growing crushingly expensive and cumbersome while providing grossly inequitable levels of care for the rich and the poor and for the metropolitan and the less urban parts of our population. It would take a bold person indeed to predict the shape of education for the clinical professions in the next few decades; clearly, a great deal will depend on our society's general level of commitment to social justice as against continuing to smooth the way for those who already have wealth and power. Should primary emphasis be put on training adequate *numbers* of physicians and psychotherapists to cope with the expectable problems of physical and mental health in our entire population, or on improving the *quality* of the professionals we turn out? My value system urges me to choose the former alternative, though my professional work has been aimed primarily at the latter. In any event, I want to call attention to this previously unmentioned social and political context looming behind and clearly relevant to the issues addressed here.

In the main chapter of this book that deals with implications for training, the first strategy Arnoult and Anderson suggest for reducing bias in causal inference is to "consider as many possible causes as can be generated." Although they cite no data, these authors assure us that this is "an effective general strategy." Of course, this procedure "requires gathering as much information as possible." The advice is, I fear, impractical for clinical trainees in a real-life setting, with a limited amount of time for each case. I doubt its effectiveness, along with that of these authors' suggestions to make many lists and charts, supplemented by group brainstorming, in an attempt to know everything that might be true and to forget nothing. Further, such perfectionism is likely to be countermanded by simple economic reality.

An underlying assumption seems to be that the most important ingredients of effective psychotherapy are cognitive and informational. If the spontaneity and human warmth of the therapeutic atmosphere must be sacrificed, the authors seem to say, so be it; accuracy is all-important. I suspect, on the contrary, that a confident but flexible therapist who dares to make mistakes and correct them via feedback from the client may do more good than a supercautious, self-doubting one who never makes an erroneous interpretation and never bases a treatment plan on a mistaken hypothesis. Nowhere here is there any indication of an awareness of what Glover (1931) called "the therapeutic effect of inexact interpretations" or even the commonsense idea that therapists should model realistic and reasonable behavior, not a compulsive pursuit of being right. Until we know just how much harm is done to psychotherapy by erroneous causal judgments and cognitive errors generally, and know that it exceeds the harm done by attempts to extrapolate from scientific research procedures to therapy, we should go very slowly in advocating any widespread use of the suggestions so earnestly laid out here.

One of the hidden dangers of emphasizing the weaknesses of clinical judgment so unrelentingly is that it probably makes it harder for our students to gain and retain respect for what's good about judgment. That is especially a problem for the trainee, who has to learn to sharpen and deepen intuition, to develop observational skills, and to act decisively yet judiciously, blending caring and ethical concern with hardheaded calculation. If future clinical psychologists, diagnosticians, and therapists of all kinds are going to have to have expertise in statistics and computers added to what they already need, that is a threat to our ability to produce good practitioners in large enough numbers.

Much as I admire Elstein's chapter, I do not wholly agree with its implications for clinical training. In the past, the problem may have been overvaluation of clinical judgment and intuition; today, I see a good deal of evidence that they are being undervalued. Indeed, part of my past criticism of the literature on clinical and statistical prediction was that the framing of the issues as a contest, forcing a dichotomous choice, tended to undermine respect for judgmental processes to a dangerous extent. It is so hard for people, even distinguished psychologists, who have been raised in our culture of violence and competition, to avoid structuring complex issues as fights! Be that as it may, all too many psychologists who hold major policy-making roles in universities seem convinced that any attempt to encourage the development of good clinical judgment is antiscientific, a failure to know or appreciate the results of research.

Actually, of course, no one of us is in a good position to make recommendations about how to make constructive changes in the ways we educate clinical psychologists, psychiatric social workers, and psychiatrists. Education is like psychotherapy in being an extraordinarily complex system of efforts to change behavior or affect growth. Both are arts, attempts to apply poorly developed sciences, by people who mostly learn their trade by practicing it. Having begun my career by several years spent studying the selection and training of psychiatrists, for a long time I was astonished by my academic colleagues from experimental psychology. They looked down on us "applied" folks as reprehensibly neglecting what we knew about the scientific method in our attempts to help people, yet when it came to their own practice of teaching—also an attempt to change behavior—they were equally indifferent to the lack of hard evidence that methods they passionately defended had any value. Before long, I learned to be tolerant and to realize that with all the best intentions it is still extraordinarily difficult to get good data on teaching methods, almost as hard as doing decent research on psychotherapy.

I still think it is worthwhile to encourage younger generations of educators to study evaluation research and try to apply it to their own work. A great deal has been learned in recent years about this kind of research (see, for example, Guttentag & Struening, 1975; Struening & Guttentag, 1975), and there is even a healthy trend among some funding agencies to require that part of the money granted for efforts at social change be spent on systematic attempts to evaluate them. So, let's have lots of experimentation on new ways to help clinicians learn to make inferences and judgments about the people they are trying to help; but we surely know by now that that unsystematic and uncontrolled efforts merely to learn from experience work no better in education and training than they do in diagnosis and prognosis.

Acknowledgment

Preparation of this chapter was supported by a U.S. Public Health Service Research Career Award (No. 5-K06-MH-12455) from the National Institute of Mental Health.

References

Allport, G. W. (1942). *The use of personal documents in psychological science.* New York: Social Science Research Council Bulletin, No. 49.

Austrian, R. (1977). Differential adaptation of field independent and field dependent subjects to therapy-analogue situations varying in degree of structure (Doctoral dissertation, New York University, 1976). *Dissertation Abstracts International, 38,* 885B.

Cook, T. D. & Campbell, D. T. (1979). *Quasi-experimentation: Design and analysis issues for field settings.* Boston: Houghton Mifflin.

Cooper, L. W. (1967). The relationship of empathy to aspects of cognitive control. *Dissertation Abstracts, 27,* 4549B-4550B. (University Microfilms No. 67-7003)

Freud, S. (1953). The interpretation of dreams. In J. Strachey (Ed. and Trans.), *The standard edition of the complete psychological works of Sigmund Freud* (Vols. 4 & 5). London: Hogarth Press. (Original work published 1900)

Gardner, R., Holzman, P. S., Linton, H., & Spence, D. P. (1959). Cognitive control: A study of individual consistencies in cognitive behavior. *Psychological Issues, 1*(4, Monograph No. 4).

Gardner, R. W. (1953). Cognitive styles in categorizing behavior. *Journal of Personality, 22,* 214–233.

Glover, E. (1931). The therapeutic effect of inexact interpretation: A contribution to the theory of suggestion. *International Journal of Psycho-Analysis, 12,* 397–411.

Guttentag, M. & Struening, E. L. (1975). *Handbook of evaluation research* (Vol. 2). Beverly Hills, CA: Sage.

Hofstadter, D. R. (1979). *Gödel, Escher, Bach: An eternal golden braid.* New York: Basic Books.

Holt, R. R. (1961). Clinical judgment as a disciplined inquiry. *Journal of Nervous and Mental Disease, 133,* 369–382. Also in Bobbs-Merrill Reprint Series in the Social Sciences, P-480, 1966. Reprinted in Holt (1978a).

———(Ed.) (1968). Motives and thought: Psychoanalytic essays in honor of David Rapaport. *Psychological Issues, 5*(2-3, Monograph No. 18/19).

———. (1970). Yet another look at clinical and statistical prediction; or, is clinical psychology worthwhile? *American Psychologist, 25,* 337–349. Reprinted in Holt (1978a).

———. (1973). *Methods of research in clinical psychology.* Morristown, NJ: General Learning Press. Reprinted in Holt (1978a).

———. (1978a). *Methods in clinical psychology, Vol. 2. Prediction and research.* New York: Plenum.

———. (1978b). A historical survey of the clinical-statistical prediction controversy. In Holt (1978a).

———. (1986). Clinical and statistical prediction: A retrospective and would-be integrative perspective. *Journal of Personality Assessment, 50,* 376–386.

Holzman, P. S. (1954). The relation of assimilation tendencies in visual, auditory, and kinesthetic time-error to cognitive attitudes of leveling and sharpening. *Journal of Personality, 22,* 375–394.

Horst, P. et al. (1941). *The prediction of personal adjustment.* New York: Social Science Research Council Bulletin, No. 48.

Klein, G. S. (1970). *Perception, motives, and personality.* New York: Knopf.

Kluckholn, C. (1954). Culture and behavior. In G. Lindzey (Ed.), *Handbook of social psychology, Vol. 2. Special fields and applications.* Reading, MA: Addison-Wesley.

Laszlo, E. (1972). *The systems view of the world.* New York: Braziller.

Mahoney, M. J. (1977). Publication prejudices: An experimental study of confirmatory bias in the peer review system. *Cognitive Therapy and Research, 1,* 161–175.

Meehl, P. E. (1954). *Clinical vs. statistical prediction.* Minneapolis: University of Minnesota Press.

———. (1978). Theoretical risks and tabular asterisks: Sir Karl, Sir Ronald, and the slow progress of soft psychology. *Journal of Clinical and Consulting Psychology, 46,* 806–834.

Merton, R. K. (1976). The unanticipated consequences of social action. In R. K. Merton, *Sociological ambivalence and other essays.* New York: Free Press. (Originally published 1936).

Mischel, W. (1968). *Personality and assessment.* New York: Wiley.

Popper, K. R. (1962). *Conjectures and refutations: The growth of scientific knowledge.* New York: Basic Books.

Rosenhan, D. L. (1973). On being sane in insane places. *Science, 171,* 250–258.

Schlesinger, H. J. (1954). Cognitive attitudes in relation to susceptibility to interference. *Journal of Personality, 22,* 354–374.

Sorrentino, R. M. & Higgins, E. T. (1986). Motivation and cognition: Warming up to synergism. In R. M. Sorrentino & E. T. Higgins (Eds.), *Handbook of motivation and cognition: Foundations of social behavior.* New York: Guilford.

Struening, E. L. & Guttentag, M. (1975). *Handbook of evaluation research* (Vol. 1). Beverly Hills, CA: Sage.

Tversky, A. & Kahneman, D. (1974). Judgment under uncertainty: Heuristics and biases. *Science, 185,* 1124–1131.

Whorf, B. L. (1950). An American Indian model of the universe. *International Journal of American Linguistics, 16,* 67–72.

Winkler, M. M. (1982). *Field dependence: The effect on clinicians' impressions of videotaped patient analogs.* Unpublished doctoral dissertation, New York University.

Witkin, H. A., Dyak, R. B., Faterson, H. F., Goodenough, D. R., & Karp, S. A. (1962). *Psychological differentiation: Studies of development.* New York: Wiley.

Witkin, H. A., Lewis, H. B., Hertzman, M., Machover, K., Meissner, P. B., & Wapner, S. (1954). *Personality through perception: An experimental and clinical study.* New York: Harper & Row.

Wolitzky, D. L. (1973). Cognitive controls and person perception. *Perceptual and Motor Skills, 36,* 619–623.

Afterword: Research and Clinical Practice

Dennis C. Turk
Peter Salovey

As we indicated in our preface, the primary aim of this volume was to bring together investigators from diverse areas whose research and theoretical conceptualizations are applicable to the practice of clinical psychology, especially the two central activities of clinical practice, diagnosis and psychotherapy. From our perspective as educators of clinical psychology graduate students, the tremendous amount of research on judgment and decision making in the areas of medicine, law, business, risk management, prediction of climatic trends, international relations, political science, and public policy is rarely considered. This research devotes a great deal of attention to the difficulties encountered in making decisions under conditions of extreme uncertainty. Investigators from these diverse areas all acknowledge the problems in decision making for all individuals regardless of training or discipline, and seek strategies to improve the quality of the decision-making process. As we stated earlier:

> It is our contention that, as Meehl (1954) noted: "... psychologists should be sophisticated about errors of observing, recording, retaining, and recalling to which the human brain is subject. We, of all people, ought to be highly *suspicious of ourselves*. We have no right to assume that entering the clinic has resulted in some miraculous mutation and made us singularly free from ordinary errors." [pp. 27–28, emphasis added]

It behooves us to be aware of the general principles of decision making that are currently being examined and to apply them to our own work. Ignorance may be bliss for the clinician, but what about the client?

Our charge to the contributors to this volume was to discuss their specific areas of research (e.g., social cognition, person perception, and decision making) and to extrapolate from these general areas themes that might be relevant to clinicians. Our hope was that these chapters would generate discussion among clinical scientists, practitioners, and students of the implications of these themes for their activities. Moreover, we hoped that the issues raised would provide an impetus to clinical research and that the applicability of such efforts would be directly examined and, where relevant, integrated into the training of new clinicians. We asked Robert Holt to comment critically on the material presented, from his unique vantage point. According to Holt's commentary, we obviously achieved our primary aim: his comments clearly led us to believe that we have created a provocative volume indeed.

The following dilemma is always inherent in bringing together laboratory research from diverse domains and attempting to extrapolate to the day-to-day activities of clinical practice: Will pointing out the potential biases in clinical judgment lead to reduction in support of clinical practice? If the contributors to this volume had generalized from the research presented to question the efficacy of psychotherapy, then, in fact, we would be quite concerned. Rather than focusing on treatment outcome, however, the chapters raise questions about potential difficulties that might influence the psychotherapeutic process. If laboratory research can be generalized at all to the consulting room, then attending to common problems discovered through such research might improve treatment and lead to greater support for various clinical activities. This "if" is a major concern: psychotherapists often wonder whether the results of laboratory-based studies really do generalize to direct clinic service. The goal of the chapters was to draw on diverse literature and methodologies and to suggest *potential* clinical applications. We do not suggest that the results of laboratory research on judgment and decision making are "facts" that should be accepted wholesale by clinical practitioners. The actual impact of the findings on clinical practice needs to be demonstrated, since most research in this area was not conducted in clinical settings. Clinical practitioners may choose to conduct the relevant research, and the beauty of specifying the results is that they are subject to refutation. The alternative is to argue from anecdote. The burden of proof would seem to be on clinicians to demonstrate that they are different regarding judgment and decision making from physicians, lawyers, political scientists, public policy makers, weather forecasters, as well as all human beings.

What are the merits of sensitizing clinicians to the issues raised in this volume? Is the cure suggested worse than the disease? Some of the strategies offered as having potential utility for "debiasing" clinicians might be easily challenged as impractical because time is so limited in clinical practice. But what is the alternative—continuing to muddle through despite potentially useful alternatives that may improve judgment? Are *all* the suggestions time-consuming? We worry about complacency and what we might characterize as "know-nothingism": If we don't attend to a problem then it cannot harm us. Clinicians often suggest that in practice it may be appropriate to rely on intuition and judgment because, as Holt states, "it probably does not lead to many serious errors." That may be true, but how do we know that serious errors do not occur? If we were considering whether or not to have bypass surgery, given the seriousness of the consequences we would be likely to invest the time needed to make the most informed and best decision possible. Is psychiatric diagnosis or psychotherapy so much less worthy of considerate care than hiring a cardiovascular surgeon?

Will identification of the potential sources of bias undermine clinical psychology students and make it harder for them to retain respect for what is good about judgment and clinical work in general? We submit that making students aware of the problems that they (as well as all humans) face in the domain of judgment and inference should sensitize them to the issues. Perhaps forewarned will be forearmed (Turk & Salovey, 1986). We believe that knowledge should be enlightening, not stultifying; open for discussion, challenge, and refutation. We want our students to read the results section of journal articles, not just the discussion (in fact, we want them to read and reflect on the issues raised here, even if they *are* uncomfortable and disagree with the conclusions). Our intention in this volume was to contribute to the falsification of the notion that decision research is irrelevant for clinical practice. Thus, contributors presented data to challenge claims that clinicians have made regarding their unique abilities in this domain. Although we can be accused of creating the expectancy that clinical decision makers are fallible, we are willing to accept this burden if the results lead to dialogue and research rather than neglect, benign or otherwise. This is what science is about: moving from the nonempirical polemic and the unfalsifiable anecdote to the specification of hypotheses that are testable and capable of being disconfirmed. How else can one pursue truth?

The laboratory research and speculations are presented here with the desire to foster further research to determine if the results are clinically relevant. If such possibilities are never raised, then clinical relevance can never be confirmed or refuted. Many of the contributors to this volume have generalized from the results of laboratory studies to the clinic. Although caution is appropriate, we must not disregard the *potential* utility of the research and findings. It is true that one must generalize *appropriately* from any research, laboratory as well as clinical. But disregarding a body of research because you do not like its conclusions is hardly a practice that we would endorse. The research cited and conclusions drawn can and should be challenged; but to be criticized, they must first be read and pondered. We hope that this volume will inspire a lively and much needed debate among clinicians as well as clinical researchers.

References

Meehl, P. E. (1954). *Clinical vs. statistical prediction.* Minneapolis, MN: University of Minnesota Press.

Turk, D. C. & Salovey, P. (1986). Clinical information processing: Bias inoculation. In R. E. Ingram (Ed.), *Information processing approaches to clinical psychology*. Orlando, FL: Academic Press.

Appendix

Jerome L. Singer
Annette D. Telgarsky

THE following table represents a rough chronological grouping of the various forms of schemas, or schemata, and related constructs about self and others that can be identified in the research literature of psychology and psychoanalysis. Note that in addition to definitions we have included brief examples of the kinds of evidence adduced by the proponents of these terms in support of their positions. It is important to keep in mind from a psychoanalytic standpoint that these groupings reflect basically unconscious processes, i.e., people don't consciously think, "My personal construct of fathers is. . . " Presumably the various schemas, scripts, prototypes, or the organizing principles of thought operate in an almost instantaneous fashion. We would argue that much of the "work" by which these schemas are formed does take place in the conscious ruminations that characterize the stream of thought, the mental play of daydreams, the reshaping of memories, etc. But the special property of these constructs is that, however formed, they become relatively "automatic" and, hence, efficient information-organizing structures. It is in this fashion that the transference phenomena that emerge in psychoanalysis must presumably be constructed.

Reference	*Terms*	*Definition*	*Evidence*
Cantor & Mischel, 1977	"prototypes" (person perception)	A prototype is a natural classification schema for grouping people that is based on personality attributes inferred from everyday behavior and social interaction. This network of traits and behavior patterns characteristic of a particular "type" of person (e.g., an "extrovert") are "conceptual prototypes, analogous to visual-pattern prototypes or scripts for everyday episodes" (p. 38).	The authors cite relevant theoretical and experimental literature related to the concept of the prototype: "The unifying and often biasing influence of conceptual prototypes has been discussed and studied in the context of free-recall paradigms that make use of well-learned or naturalistic material (e.g., Bartlett, 1932; Bransford & Johnson, 1972; Minsky, 1975; Schank & Abelson, 1977)" (p. 39). The authors report the results of a study utilizing a recognition memory paradigm which support the "hypothesized operation of personality traits as conceptual prototypes" (p. 38).
Cantor & Mischel, 1979	"prototypes" "fuzzy sets"	The definition is the same as above; however, the authors also discuss "fuzzy sets" (i.e., this concept recognizes that category decisions are probabilistic and that there is a continuum of category membership).	The authors cite numerous experimental studies in both cognitive psychology and social cognition. They report the results of a study in which undergraduates were asked to generate lists of features common to exemplars of a variety of different personality categories and were able to do so quite readily.
Cantor, 1981	"prototypes" (person perception and	The author discusses "personality" as being at "the dynamic interface be-	Cantor cites numerous experimental studies in both cognitive psychology

	perception of social situations)	tween . . . self-inferences and cognitive generalizations and the contextual structure of situations" (p. 41).	and social cognition. The author provides a theoretical analysis of a vignette involving riding on the New York City subways in terms of the interaction between "prior expectations and current perceptions."
Kelly, 1955	"personal constructs"	"Man looks at his world through transparent patterns or templates which he creates and then attempts to fit over the realities of which the world is composed. The fit is not always very good. Yet without such patterns the world appears to be such an undifferentiated homogeneity that man is unable to make any sense out of it" (pp. 8–9). *Personal constructs* are the name given to these "patterns that are tried on for size" (p. 9). "In general man seeks to improve his constructs by increasing his repertory, by altering them to provide better fits, and by subsuming them with superordinate constructs or systems. In seeking improvement he is repeatedly halted by the damage to the system that apparently will result from the alteration of a subordinate construct. . . . It may take a major act of psychotherapy or experience to get him to adjust his construction system to the point where the new and more precise construct can be incorporated" (p. 9).	Kelly developed the Role Construct Personality Test (REP) to identify the important constructs an individual uses to construe significant individuals in his life. Much of the empirical literature dealing with Kelly's concept of "personal constructs" involves the REP. Epting (1981) cites numerous studies that have used various modifications of the REP to study different clinical populations including schizophrenic patients, obsessive compulsive patients, alcoholic patients, depressed patients, and psychopathic patients. Epting (1981) also reviews studies that investigate psychotherapies derived from personal construct theory. These include fixed role therapy, personal construct group therapy, serial validation therapy, therapy for stuttering, and REP interaction technique (RIT), developed by Bonarius (1977).

(*continued*)

Reference	*Terms*	*Definition*	*Evidence*
Frank, 1974	"assumptive world"	A set of more or less implicit assumptions about oneself and the nature of the world in which one lives that are developed out of one's personal experiences. These "highly structured, complex, interacting set of values, expectations, and images of oneself and others, which guide and in turn are guided by a person's perceptions and behavior . . . are closely related to his emotional states and feelings of well being" (p. 27).	Frank bases the concept of the "assumptive world" on the writings of several theoreticians, including Kelly (1955), and on clinical examples. He cites Imboden (1957) when he describes how "the assumptive world starts as soon as the infant enters into transactions with his environment" (p. 31).
Piaget, 1951	"affective schemas"	"All those with whom the child lives give rise to a kind of 'affective schema,' a summary or blending of the various feelings aroused by them, and it is these schemas which determine the main secondary symbols, as they often determine later on certain attractions or antipathies for which it is difficult to find an explanation except in unconscious assimilation with earlier modes of behavior." (p. 176).	Piaget bases the concept of affective schemas on developmental studies and observations of children.
Tomkins, 1979	"scenes" "scripts" "nuclear scenes" "nuclear scripts"	A "scene" is the basic unit of analysis in Tomkins's theory. It is an organized whole that includes persons, place, time, action, and feelings. "Scripts" deal with "the individual's rules for predicting, interpreting, re-	Script theory builds on Tomkins's earlier theoretical and empirical work on affect and cognition (Tomkins, 1962, 1963, 1979) and on research in developmental psychology. Clinical illustrations of nuclear scenes

		sponding to, and controlling a magnified set of scenes" (p. 217). Scripts involve the connection of one affect-laden scene with another affect-laden scene. "Through memory, thought, and imagination, scenes experienced before can be coassembled with scenes presently experienced, together with scenes which are anticipated in the future" (p. 217). "Nuclear scripts" involve construing present situations in terms of their similarity to affect-laden childhood "nuclear scenes." Positive scenes are characteristically magnified by the production of "variants," the detection of differences around a stable core. Negative affect scenes are usually magnified by the formation of "analogs," the detection of similarities in different experiences. Analogs involve a vigilant stance in which new situations are scanned for old dangers. Thus, individuals can be "victimized" by their own "high-powered ability to synthesize ever-new repetitions of the same scene" without knowing that they are doing so (p. 231).	and nuclear scripts are provided in the article. Research by Carlson (1981) and by L. Carlson and R. Carlson (1984) lends support to Tomkins's script theory by demonstrating the way in which positive and negative affective scenes and scripts are differentially influential in the interpretation of new information.
Markus, 1977	"self-schemata"	"Self-schemata" are "cognitive generalizations about the self, derived from past experience, that organize and	The concept is related theoretically to literature on schemata (e.g., Bartlett, 1932; Kelly, 1955; Piaget, 1951);

(*continued*)

Reference	*Terms*	*Definition*	*Evidence*
		guide the processing of self-related information contained in the individual's social experience" (p. 64).	frames (Minsky,1975); and scripts (Schank & Abelson, 1977). A questionnaire study and an experimental study are reported in which individuals' self-schemata are compared to a number of specific empirical referents. The results indicate that "self-schemata facilitate the processing of information about the self (judgments and decisions about the self), contain easily retrievable behavioral evidence, provide a basis for the confident self-prediction of behavior on schema-related dimensions, and make individuals resistant to counterschematic information" (p. 63).
Markus & Smith, 1981	"self-schemata"	Same as above; however, the authors argue that self-schemata also "provide an anchor or frame of reference for judgments and evaluations of others" (p. 256).	The authors review several studies and report a recent study in which an assessment is made of individuals' self-schemata and then compared to the way in which they perceive others. These studies suggest that "individuals will differentially process information about others that is relevant to their own schematic domains" (p. 256).
Kuiper & Rogers, 1979	"self" as "prototype" or "schema"	The authors cite the the definition of self-schemata set forth by Markus (1977). The authors note that not	Current cognitive psychology and social cognition literature on biasing and facilitating effects of schemata

		only does "a person's organization, summation, and explanation of personal data" involve self-schemas, but that these schemas are thought to interact with incoming data and produce both facilitating and biasing effects in information processing (pp. 499–500).	are reviewed. The authors report studies in which self–other differences in processing personal information were investigated by having subjects make self-referent or other-referent ratings of personal adjectives. The results from five studies indicate that "unknown-other referent processing involves a relatively inefficient rehearsal or effort strategy, whereas self-referent processing involves the self as a highly organized and efficient schema" (p. 499).
Rogers, 1981	"self-schemata," or "self-as-prototype," described as a "hierarchical category structure"	Rogers states that "the elements of the prototype are self-descriptive terms such as traits, values, and possibly even memories of specific behaviors and events. These terms are ordered hierarchically, becoming more concrete, distinctive, specific, and less inclusive, with increasing depth into the hierarchy" (p. 196).	The author reviews several experimental studies which provide evidence for a "self-prototype." Modelled on cognitive psychology research on schemata, these studies show that "false alarm effects," the "prototype effect," and "enhanced memory for self-descriptive words" all occur. The occurrence of these effects is reported as evidence that "the self really is structured as a prototype" (p. 197). Rogers reviews two cognitive models for the self-referent process. These are Bower and Gilligan's (1979) use of Anderson and Bower's (1973) HAM model and an availability/computation model. Rogers develops a theoretical model that adds affect to the cognitive model for self-referent processing.

(*continued*)

Reference	*Terms*	*Definition*	*Evidence*
Bandura, 1978	"self-system"	Based on social learning theory, Bandura describes a "self-system" which refers to "cognitive structures that provide reference mechanisms and to a set of subfunctions for the perception, evaluation, and regulation of behavior" (p. 348). Thus the self-system is *not* a psychic agent that controls behavior. Rather, "behavior, internal personal factors, and environmental influences all operate as interlocking determinants of each other" (p. 346) in what Bandura has labeled the "process of reciprocal determinism."	Bandura bases the concept of the "self-system" on research based on social learning theory and on laboratory investigations of self-regulatory processes. Bandura argues that the concept of the self-system and its role in the process of reciprocal determinism can be applied to both intrapersonal development and interpersonal behavior. At the intrapersonal level, e.g., "people's conceptions influence what they perceive and do, and their conceptions are in turn altered by the effects of their actions and the observed consequences to others" (p. 356).
Cantor, Mischel, & Schwartz, 1982	"prototype" (applied to social situations)	"Knowledge about any given category is structured around, and represented in long-term memory as, a *prototype* which captures the meaning of the category. The prototype serves as a symbol and reference point for the category" (p. 46). The authors review three possible forms a prototype may take according to various studies of perception and categorization. The form the authors study is "an abstract set of features commonly associated with members of a category, with	The authors review cognitive psychology and social cognition research on the concept of the prototype. They report the results of three studies they conducted to study how the "naive perceiver construes, categorizes, and gives meaning to classes of social situations (e.g., parties, work, therapy sessions)" (p. 45). Free description, imagery reaction time, and structured rating paradigms were used to analyze structural, processing, and content properties of a sample of

		each feature assigned a weight according to degree of association with the category" (pp. 46–47).	everyday situation categories. The results of the studies indicated that people share relatively orderly and easily retrievable prototypes for the 36 situation categories studied. The situations were often characterized by typical person–action combinations expected in them. Naive perceivers appeared to share knowledge of most prototypic behaviors and general personality types associated with different classes of situations.
Hamilton, 1979	"stereotype"	"The term 'stereotype' is in essence a cognitive structural concept, referring to a set of expectations held by the perceiver regarding members of a social group" (p. 65). "A stereotype can also be thought of as a structural framework in terms of which information about another person is processed and hence has the properties of a schema" (p. 65).	Hamilton reviews recent literature on cognitive biases (experimental studies in cognitive and social psychology) and argues that "stereotypes, as cognitive schemas, can influence the encoding, interpretation, retention, and retrieval of subsequently obtained information about members of stereotyped groups, as well as the perceiver's causal attributions regarding the target person's behavior" (p. 80).
Nisbett & Ross, 1980	"personae"	"Personae" are "cognitive structures representing the personal characteristics and typical behaviors of particular 'stock characters.' Some personae are the unique products of one's own personal experience. . . . Others are shared within the culture or subculture" (p. 35). "The	The book reviews cognitive-psychology and social-cognition literature on knowledge structures and judgmental heuristics as well as the literature on normative principles in inferential tasks and "causes, consequences, and cures" of inferential errors. The concept of personae is based on

(*continued*)

Reference	*Terms*	*Definition*	*Evidence*
		persona constitutes a knowledge structure which, when evoked, influences social judgments and behaviors. Once the principal features or behaviors of a given individual suggest a particular persona, subsequent expectations of and responses to that individual are apt to be dictated in part by the characteristics of the persona" (p. 35).	research literature on knowledge structures and social cognition. The authors state that the term "personae," while essentially the same as "stereotype," is preferable because it lacks the pejorative implications of "stereotype." They note that "persona" is also similar to the concept of a "person-prototype," proposed and investigated by Cantor and Mischel (1977).
Tversky & Kahneman, 1974	"availability heuristic" "representativeness heuristic"	The "availability heuristic" is employed in situations "in which people assess the frequency of a class or the probability of an event by the ease with which instances or occurrences can be brought to mind" (p. 1127). Thus an individual may inaccurately assess the risk of heart attack among middle-aged people by recalling such occurrences among acquaintances. That is, based on an individual's past experiences, certain events are likely to be more salient and may serve as a source of cognitive bias. Using the "representativeness heuristic" can also lead individuals to make inaccurate judgments. Individuals tend to judge people or events by how representative of, or similar	The concepts are based on numerous experimental studies of decision making and situations in which individuals are required to draw inferences from limited information. The authors provide several examples of problems which the reader can try before reading the authors' analysis of biases in judgments that individuals might have with such problems.

		to, a particular stereotype they are. Important distinctions are often ignored. Thus every patient who hallucinates is not necessarily schizophrenic, yet because a patient reports hallucinations, one may think of the ways in which the patient is similar to rather than different from a schizophrenic.	
Abelson, 1981	"script"	A script is "a hypothetical cognitive structure that when activated organizes comprehension of event-based situations" (p. 715). It is one type of schema.	The script concept is based on empirical research in cognitive psychology, social cognition, and artificial intelligence. Numerous examples "suggesting the psychological reality of scripts" are provided in an earlier book by Schank and Abelson (1977). Abelson notes that scripts are close to what Tomkins (1979) calls "nuclear scenes." These are described by Abelson as "the repeated construction of present situations in terms of *preemptive metaphor,* that is, an inappropriate similarity to a kernel situation from the past" (p. 724).
Meichenbaum & Gilmore, 1984	"core organizing principles" ("cops")	"Cops" are theoretical superordinate cognitive structures that explain and predict present and future behavior. "Cops" represent a "tacit knowledge" that guides and influences thoughts, feeling, and behaviors. "Cops" often operate, and influence behavior, with-	The first half of the article reviews theoretical and experimental literature on cognitive structures and cognitive processes, including such processes as the "confirmation bias" (Snyder & Swann, 1976, 1978; Taylor & Crocker, 1981), which may contrib-

(*continued*)

Reference	*Terms*	*Definition*	*Evidence*
		out any conscious awareness of them by the individual. A clinical illustration of a "cop" is provided in the case of a client whose presenting problem of becoming overly upset at a variety of daily hassles developed from a preoccupation with a need for "justice" (idiosyncratically defined, beginning with childhood experiences of perceived injustices). Each new social interaction was evaluated by the client in terms of his peremptory ideas about equity and was exacerbated by his rigidity in not being open to disconfirmatory data and to other competing hypotheses.	ute to the perseveration of maladaptive schemas. The authors base the "cops" concept on an integration of the literature mentioned above as well as on clinical case material. In describing how "cops" function, the authors cite Wachtel (1982), who describes a similar process as "the cumulative skewing of experiences through the course of development. These experiences lead to patterns which, whatever their origins in the person's history, are maintained in the present by their present consequences" (p. 287). The authors also point out the similarity between "cops" and Tomkins's (1979) concept of a nuclear script.
Luborsky, 1977	"core conflictual relationship theme"	In looking at segments of cases of 20 different patients, it was discovered that certain "themes" appeared to be repeated across the patients' interpersonal relationships. While the specific theme varied among individuals, it seemed to be "similar across virtually all types of objects" (p. 384). These themes were labeled "core conflictual relationship themes."	The themes were identified by analyzing four 20-minute segments of transcribed therapy sessions of 20 different patients. The "core conflictual relationship theme" is compared to the "main transference theme" in discussion (p. 386) and also to Freud's (1912) concept of "recurrent conflictual patterns" and "repetition compulsion."
Blatt & Lerner, 1983	"object relations" "object representations"	"Object relations, through the processes of internalization, result in the formation of intrapsychic structures	This work draws upon object relations theory, ego psychology, and the cognitive developmental theories of

		(ego functions and cognitive structures such as object- and self-representations) that regulate and direct behavior" (p. 192). "The organization of concepts of self and other are psychological structures that are the consequence of the internalization of formative interpersonal interactions with significant figures. These concepts or representations of self and others in turn shape and direct subsequent interpersonal relationships" (p. 192). "Broadly defined, object representation refers to the conscious and unconscious mental schemas—including cognitive, affective, and experiential components—of objects encountered in reality" (pp. 194–195).	Piaget and Werner. The authors cite several studies "based on the principle that when a stimulus is consistently ambiguous, its image is shaped by the organizing characteristics of the individual's representational world" that have investigated the structure and content of early memories, manifest dreams, the human response on the Rorschach, and open-ended descriptions of significant figures (p. 195). The article describes the work of Mayman and his colleagues, who have focused on the thematic elements of object representations utilizing a variety of projective test procedures, and the work of Blatt and his colleagues, who have focused primarily on the structural dimensions of object representation utilizing projective test data as well as the manifest content of dreams and open-ended descriptions of significant figures.
Kohut, 1971	"self-representation" "selfobject"	The self-representation, described as "quite analogous to the representations of objects, is a content of the mental apparatus but is not one of its constituents, i.e., not one of the agencies of the mind" (p. xv). The "selfobject" is the representation of objects—images of others—"which are experienced as part of the self" (p. xiv).	Kohut cites the work of Freud, Hartmann, and numerous other psychoanalytic writers. Many clinical examples of the concepts are provided.

(*continued*)

Reference	*Terms*	*Definition*	*Evidence*
Bandura, 1977	"self-efficacy"	In his analysis of behavior change, Bandura hypothesizes that individuals must have both a positive sense of outcome expectations and self-efficacy to carry out a particular course of action. An outcome expectancy is a person's belief that a given behavior will produce certain outcomes. A self-efficacy expectation is the belief that one can successfully execute the behavior required to produce the outcome.	The concept is based on evidence derived from studies in social learning theory and studies on mediating cognitive processes in behavioral change. Bandura states that self-efficacy theory is "based on the principal assumption that psychological procedures, whatever their form, serve as a means of creating and strengthening expectations of personal efficacy" (p. 193).
Bandura, 1982	"self-efficacy"	The definition is the same as above; however, this article extends the concept of self-efficacy to include the effect of significant others' beliefs about an individual's self-efficacy on the individual and the concept of perceived "collective efficacy" and its role in social change. Bandura extends the definition of self-efficacy by stating that "self-percepts of efficacy influence thought patterns, actions, and emotional arousal. In causal tests the higher the level of induced self-efficacy, the higher the performance accomplishments and the lower the emotional arousal" (p. 122).	Several lines of experimental research that support the concept of self-efficacy are reviewed in detail. Studies are reviewed which indicate that "perceived self-efficacy helps to account for such diverse phenomena as changes in coping behavior produced by different modes of influence, level of physiological stress reactions, self-regulation of refractory behavior, resignation and despondency to failure experiences, self-debilitating effects of proxy control and illusory inefficaciousness, achievement strivings, growth of intrinsic interest, and career pursuits" (p. 122).

Review Articles

Reference	*Terms*	*Synopsis*
Goldfried & Robins, 1983	"self mastery" "self-efficacy" "schema" "self-schemata" "cognitive bias" "heuristics"	Reviews theoretical and experimental literature on concepts of self-mastery, self-efficacy, schema, and self-schemata. Emphasizes ways in which cognitive structures such as schemata can lead individuals to distort their environments and their interpersonal interactions. Also reviews literature on ways in which self-schemata can serve to make individuals resistant to counter-schematic information, often creating a "negative self-bias." Reviews literature on "negative self-schemata." Following a review of the concepts mentioned above, the authors then review the literature on ways to modify schemata, focusing especially on cognitive bias and the processing of therapeutic information. Specific therapeutic techniques are reviewed and clinical examples are provided, including transcriptions of illustrative segments of therapy sessions. Finally, the authors discuss the current status of research in this area as well as raising questions for future research.
Hollon & Kriss, 1984	"cognitive structures" "cognitive processes" "cognitive products" "schemata" "confirmatory bias" "self-fulfilling prophecy" "heuristics"	Reviews theory and research on basic cognitive and social cognitive processes and their relation to clinical theory, research, and practice, particularly theories of psychopathology, theories of therapeutic change, and theories of clinical inference. The role of knowledge structures (including schemata and related concepts), processing heuristics, biases, and cognitive products such as self-statements (Meichenbaum, 1977) and "automatic thoughts" (Beck, 1976) are explored with particular emphasis on their role in the clinical change process. Specific treatment components are discussed with regard to their different loci of action. The role of the clinician in the therapeutic process is discussed, especially the role of cognitive

(*continued*)

Reference	*Terms*	*Synopsis*
		bias in clinicians. Suggestions for refinements in clinical practice and research are offered.
Turk & Speers, 1983	"cognitive schemata" "cognitive processes" "attention" "confirmatory bias" "prototypes" "biases of clinicians" "self-schemata" "self-efficacy" "scripts"	Provides brief review of key cognitive concepts. Defines "cognitive schemata" as "the set of hypothetical constructs that include all the individual's knowledge at any given moment about himself or herself and his or her world" (p. 4). Reviews basic cognitive processes and cognitive biases. Briefly reviews the role of cognitive schemata and cognitive processes in maladaptive behavior of clients and clinicians. Briefly discusses the implications of cognitive schemata and cognitive processes in cognitive–behavioral interventions.
Turk & Salovey, 1985a	"cognitive structures" "cognitive processes" "schemata" "self-schemata" "person prototype"	The authors review theoretical and experimental literature on various cognitive structures and cognitive processes that are of clinical importance. They review Bartlett's (1932) and Taylor and Crocker's (1981) definition of schemata. They also review and discuss literature on self-schemata with particular empha-

	"self-efficacy" "selective attention" "confirmatory bias" "egocentric bias" "heuristics"	sis on aspects that are relevant to clinical work. Various problems that can occur in information processing related to cognitive structures of schemata and self-schemata are discussed. Biases and heuristics arising from schemata processing are described, including selective attention, schema-confirming biases, egocentric biases, availability and representativeness heuristics, and illusory correlation. Also described is the role of affect in cognitive processing and the importance of metacognitive strategies for generalization and maintenance of therapeutic change.
Turk & Salovey, 1985b	"schemata" "confirmatory bias" "prototype matching" "availability heuristic" "representativeness heuristic" "illusory correlation"	The authors review and discuss some of the cognitive processes involved in clinical decision making. Common shortcomings in human information processing that might affect the clinician are discussed. Potential problem areas include confirmatory bias and prototype matching, use of the availability and representativeness heuristics, and problems with illusory correlation. Ways in which clinicians can minimize the biasing effects of cognitive structures and resulting cognitive processes are suggested.

References for Appendix

Abelson, R. P. (1981). Psychological status of the script concept. *American Psychologist, 36,* 715–729.

Anderson, J. R., & Bower, G. H. (1973). *Human associative memory.* Washington, DC: Winston.

Bandura, A. (1977). Self-efficacy: Toward a unified theory of behavioral change. *Psychological Review, 84,* 191–215.

———. (1978). The self-system in reciprocal determinism. *American Psychologist, 33,* 344–358.

———. (1982). Self-efficacy mechanism in human agency. *American Psychologist, 37,* 122–147.

Bartlett, F. C. (1932). *Remembering: A study in experimental and social psychology.* London: Cambridge University Press.

Beck, A. T. (1976). *Cognitive therapy and the emotional disorders.* New York: International Universities Press.

Blatt, S. J., & Lerner, H. (1983). Investigations in the psychoanalytic theory of object relations and object representations. In J. Masling (Ed.), *Empirical studies of psychoanalytic theories.* New York: Analytic Press.

Bonarius, J. C. J. (1977). The interaction model of communication: Through experimental research towards existential relevance. In A. W. Landfield & J. K. Cole (Eds.), *1976 Nebraska Symposium on Motivation* (Vol. 24). Lincoln: University of Nebraska Press.

Bower, G. H., & Gilligan, S. G. (1979). Remembering information related to one's self. *Journal of Research in Personality, 13,* 420–432.

Bransford, J. D., & Johnson, M. K. (1972). Contextual prerequisites for understanding: Some investigations of comprehension and recall. *Journal of Verbal Learning and Verbal Behavior, 11,* 717–726.

Cantor, N. (1981). A cognitive-social approach to personality. In N. Cantor & J. K. Kihlstrom (Eds.), *Personality, cognition, and social interaction.* Hillsdale, NJ: Erlbaum.

Cantor, N., & Mischel, W. (1977). Traits as prototypes: Effects on recognition memory. *Journal of Personality and Social Psychology, 35,* 38–48.

———. (1979). Prototypes in person perception. In L. Berkowitz (Ed.), *Advances in experimental social psychology* (Vol. 12). New York: Academic Press.

Cantor, N., Mischel, W., & Schwartz, J. (1982). A prototype analysis of psychological situations. *Cognitive Psychology, 14,* 45–77.

Carlson, L., & Carlson, R. (1984). Affect and psychological magnification: Derivations from Tomkins' script theory. *Journal of Personality, 52,* 36–45.

Carlson, R. (1981). Studies in script theory: I. Adult analogs of a childhood nuclear scene. *Journal of Personality and Social Psychology, 40,* 501–510.

Epting, F. R. (1981). An appraisal of personal construct psychotherapy. In H. Bonarius, R. Holland, & S. Rosenberg (Eds.), *Personal construct psychology: Recent advances in theory and practice.* New York: St. Martin's Press.

Frank, J. (1974). *Persuasion and healing.* (2nd ed.). New York: Schocken.

Freud, S. (1912). The dynamics of transference. *Standard Edition, 12:* 99–108. London: Hogarth.

Goldfried, M. R., & Robins, C. (1983). Self-schema, cognitive bias, and the processing of therapeutic experiences. In P. C. Kendall (Ed.), *Advances in cognitive–behavioral research and therapy* (Vol. 2). New York: Academic Press.

Hamilton, D. L. (1979). A cognitive-attributional analysis of stereotyping. In L. Berkowitz (Ed.), *Advances in experimental social psychology* (Vol. 12). New York: Academic Press.

Hollon, S. D., & Kriss, M. (1984). Cognitive factors in clinical research and practice. *Clinical Psychology Review, 4,* 35–76.

Imboden, J. B. (1957). Brunswick's theory of perception: A note on its applicability to normal and neurotic personality functioning. *Archives of Neurology and Psychiatry, 77,* 187–192.

Kelly, G. A. (1955). *A theory of personality: The psychology of personal constructs.* New York: Norton.

Kohut, H. (1971). *The analysis of the self.* New York: International Universities Press.

Kuiper, N. A., & Rogers, T. B. (1979). Encoding of personal information: Self-other differences. *Journal of Personality and Social Psychology, 37,* 499–514.

Luborsky, L. (1977). Measuring a pervasive psychic structure in psychotherapy: The core conflictual relationship theme. In N. Freedman & S. Grand (Eds.), *Communicative structures and psychic structures.* New York: Plenum.

Markus, H. (1977). Self-schemata and processing information about the self. *Journal of Personality and Social Psychology, 35,* 63–78.

Markus, H., & Smith, J. (1981). The influence of self-schemata on the perception of others. In N. Cantor & J. F. Kihlstrom (Eds.), *Personality, cognition, and social interaction.* Hillsdale, NJ: Erlbaum.

Meichenbaum, D. H. (1977). *Cognitive behavior modification: An integrative approach.* New York: Plenum.

Meichenbaum, D., & Gilmore, J. B. (1984). The nature of unconscious processes: A cognitive–behavioral perspective. In K. S. Bowers & D. Meichenbaum (Eds.), *The unconscious reconsidered.* New York: Wiley.

Minsky, M. (1975). A framework for representing knowledge. In P. H. Winston (Ed.), *The psychology of computer vision.* New York: McGraw-Hill.

Nisbett, R. E., & Ross, L. (1980). *Human inference: Strategies and shortcomings of social judgment.* Englewood Cliffs, NJ: Prentice-Hall.

Piaget, J. (1951). *Play, dreams and imitation in childhood.* (C. Gattengno & F. M. Hodgson, Trans.). New York: Norton.

Rogers, T. B. (1981). A model of the self as an aspect of the human information processing system. In N. Cantor & J. F. Kihlstrom (Eds.), *Personality, cognition, and social interaction.* Hillsdale, NJ: Erlbaum.

Schank, R. C., & Abelson, R. P. (1977). *Scripts, plans, goals, and understanding.* Hillsdale, NJ: Erlbaum.

Snyder, M., & Swann, W. (1976). When action reflects attitude: The politics of impression management. *Journal of Personality and Social Psychology, 34,* 1034–1042.

______. (1978). Hypothesis testing processes in social interaction. *Journal of Personality and Social Psychology, 36,* 1202–1212.

Taylor, S. E., & Crocker, J. (1981). Schematic bases of social information processing. In E. T. Higgins, C. P. Herman, & M. P. Zanna (Eds.), *Social cognition: The Ontario Symposium in personality and social psychology.* Hillsdale, NJ: Erlbaum.

Tomkins, S. S. (1962). *Affect, imagery, and consciousness* (Vol. 1). New York: Springer.

———. (1963). *Affect, imagery, and consciousness.* (Vol. 2). New York: Springer.

———. (1979). Script theory: Differential magnification of affects. In H. E. Howe, Jr. & R. A. Dienstbier (Eds.), *Nebraska Symposium on Motivation, 1978* (Vol. 26). Lincoln: University of Nebraska Press.

Tversky, A., & Kahneman, D. (1974). Judgment under uncertainty: Heuristics and biases. *Science, 185,* 1124–1131.

Turk, D. C., & Salovey, P. (1985a). Cognitive structures, cognitive processes, and cognitive–behavior modification: I. Client issues. *Cognitive Therapy and Research, 9,* 1–17.

———. (1985b). Cognitive structures, cognitive processes, and cognitive–behavior modification: II. Judgments and inferences of the clinician. *Cognitive Therapy and Research, 9,* 19–33.

Turk, D. C., & Speers, M. A. (1983). Cognitive schemata and cognitive processes in cognitive–behavioral intervention: Going beyond the information given. In P. C. Kendall (Ed.), *Advances in cognitive–behavioral research and therapy* (Vol. 2). New York: Academic Press.

Wachtel, P. (1982). *Psychoanalysis and behavior therapy: Toward an integration.* New York: Basic Books.

Author Index

Subject Index